DBT Skills in Schools

The Guilford Practical Intervention in the Schools Series

Kenneth W. Merrell, *Founding Editor*
Sandra M. Chafouleas, *Series Editor*

www.guilford.com/practical

This series presents the most reader-friendly resources available in key areas of evidence-based practice in school settings. Practitioners will find trustworthy guides on effective behavioral, mental health, and academic interventions, and assessment and measurement approaches. Covering all aspects of planning, implementing, and evaluating high-quality services for students, books in the series are carefully crafted for everyday utility. Features include ready-to-use reproducibles, appealing visual elements, and an oversized format. Recent titles have Web pages where purchasers can download and print the reproducible materials.

Recent Volumes

Resilient Classrooms, Second Edition: Creating Healthy Environments for Learning
Beth Doll, Katherine Brehm, and Steven Zucker

The ABCs of Curriculum-Based Evaluation: A Practical Guide to Effective Decision Making
John L. Hosp, Michelle K. Hosp, Kenneth W. Howell, and Randy Allison

Curriculum-Based Assessment for Instructional Design:
Using Data to Individualize Instruction
Matthew K. Burns and David C. Parker

Dropout Prevention
C. Lee Goss and Kristina J. Andren

Stress Management for Teachers: A Proactive Guide
Keith C. Herman and Wendy M. Reinke

Interventions for Reading Problems, Second Edition:
Designing and Evaluating Effective Strategies
Edward J. Daly III, Sabina Neugebauer, Sandra Chafouleas, and Christopher H. Skinner

Classwide Positive Behavior Interventions and Supports:
A Guide to Proactive Classroom Management
Brandi Simonsen and Diane Myers

Promoting Academic Success with English Language Learners: Best Practices for RTI
Craig A. Albers and Rebecca S. Martinez

The ABCs of CBM, Second Edition: A Practical Guide to Curriculum-Based Measurement
Michelle K. Hosp, John L. Hosp, and Kenneth W. Howell

Integrated Multi-Tiered Systems of Support: Blending RTI and PBIS
Kent McIntosh and Steve Goodman

DBT Skills in Schools: Skills Training for Emotional Problem Solving
for Adolescents (DBT STEPS-A)
*James J. Mazza, Elizabeth T. Dexter-Mazza, Alec L. Miller, Jill H. Rathus,
and Heather E. Murphy*

Interventions for Disruptive Behaviors: Reducing Problems and Building Skills
Gregory A. Fabiano

Promoting Student Happiness: Positive Psychology Interventions in Schools
Shannon M. Suldo

DBT Skills in Schools

Skills Training for Emotional Problem Solving
for Adolescents
(DBT STEPS-A)

JAMES J. MAZZA
ELIZABETH T. DEXTER-MAZZA
ALEC L. MILLER
JILL H. RATHUS
HEATHER E. MURPHY

Foreword by Marsha M. Linehan

THE GUILFORD PRESS
New York   London

Copyright © 2016 The Guilford Press
A Division of Guilford Publications, Inc.
370 Seventh Avenue, Suite 1200, New York, NY 10001
www.guilford.com

Printed in the United States of America

This book is printed on acid-free paper.

Last digit is print number: 9   8

The authors have checked with sources believed to be reliable in their efforts to provide
information that is complete and generally in accord with the standards of practice that are
accepted at the time of publication. However, in view of the possibility of human error or changes
in behavioral, mental health, or medical sciences, neither the authors, nor the editors and publisher,
nor any other party who has been involved in the preparation or publication of this work warrants
that the information contained herein is in every respect accurate or complete, and they are not
responsible for any errors or omissions or the results obtained from the use of such information.
Readers are encouraged to confirm the information contained in this book with other sources.

Library of Congress Cataloging-in-Publication Data
Names: Mazza, James J., author.
Title: DBT skills in schools : skills training for emotional problem solving
    for adolescents (DBT STEPS-A) / by James J. Mazza [and four others].
Description: New York : The Guilford Press, [2016] | Series: The Guilford
    practical intervention in the schools series | Includes bibliographical
    references and index.
Identifiers: LCCN 2015044893 | ISBN 9781462525591 (paperback)
Subjects: LCSH: Dialectical behavior therapy. | Adolescent psychotherapy. |
    BISAC: PSYCHOLOGY / Psychotherapy / Child & Adolescent. | MEDICAL /
    Psychiatry / Child & Adolescent. | SOCIAL SCIENCE / Social Work. |
    EDUCATION / Counseling / General.
Classification: LCC RC489.B4 M39 2016 | DDC 616.89/142—dc23
LC record available at *http://lccn.loc.gov/2015044893*

This book is dedicated to the memory of two special people, Ray F. Dexter III and Mike Hackman. Lizz Dexter-Mazza never met her brother, Ray, who died by suicide at the young age of 15 in 1968 before Lizz was born. Jim Mazza supported his high school friend and teammate, Mike, as he battled mental health problems for over 30 years before he died by suicide in 2010. The legacy and memories of our loved ones, Ray and Mike, and countless others who confront similar challenges today, fuel our passion for helping adolescents develop effective emotion regulation skills and decision-making strategies. Our hope is that the DBT STEPS-A curriculum will make a difference in the lives of all adolescents.

About the Authors

James J. Mazza, PhD, is Professor in the College of Education at the University of Washington, where he teaches and conducts research in the field of adolescent mental health. Dr. Mazza's research focuses particularly on adolescent internalizing disorders, such as depression, anxiety, posttraumatic stress disorder, exposure to violence, and, especially, suicidal behavior. His work also examines the complex relationships among adolescent mental health issues, social–emotional abilities, and academic skills through multi-tiered systems of support. Dr. Mazza has written extensively on how to identify youth who are at risk for suicidal behavior, as well as on how to develop social–emotional learning (SEL) curricula to help all students learn emotion regulation skills. He has worked with over 30 school districts and thousands of school personnel in developing and implementing comprehensive school-based suicide identification and prevention strategies for adolescents. Dr. Mazza also provides consultation and training to school personnel internationally on implementing DBT STEPS-A in schools, on developing mental health intervention services within multi-tiered systems of support, and on integrating SEL curricula as a part of a school system's role in educating the whole child. He is the co-owner of Mazza Consulting and Psychological Services in Seattle, Washington.

Elizabeth T. Dexter-Mazza, PsyD, is the co-owner of Mazza Consulting and Psychological Services, where she conducts comprehensive dialectical behavior therapy (DBT) and skills-based coaching for adolescents and adults and provides parent coaching and support to family members and friends of individuals with emotion dysregulation. Dr. Dexter-Mazza provides training and consultation to schools, mental health agencies, and individuals in implementing DBT skills and therapy. She is also a trainer for Behavioral Tech, a company that offers DBT trainings to mental health professionals around the world. Dr. Dexter-Mazza completed her postdoctoral fellowship under the direction of Marsha M. Linehan at the Behavioral Research and Therapy Clinics (BRTC) at the University of Washington. She served as Clinical Director and a research therapist at the BRTC for Dr. Linehan's research studies, which provided both individual DBT and DBT group skills training. Dr. Dexter-Mazza has published several book chapters and peer-reviewed articles on DBT, borderline personality disorder, and graduate school training in managing suicidal clients.

Alec L. Miller, PsyD, is Clinical Professor of Psychiatry and Behavioral Sciences at Montefiore Medical Center of the Albert Einstein College of Medicine, Bronx, New York. He is also Co-Founder and Clinical Director of Cognitive and Behavioral Consultants, a training and consultation center in White Plains and Manhattan. For over 20 years, Dr. Miller has adapted and applied DBT to youth in outpatient, inpatient, and school settings, as well as to youth who have chronic medical illnesses. His publications include over 80 peer-reviewed articles and book chapters, as well as four books, including *Dialectical Behavior Therapy with Suicidal Adolescents* (coauthored with Jill H. Rathus and Marsha M. Linehan) and *DBT Skills Manual for Adolescents* (coauthored with Jill H. Rathus). Dr. Miller has trained thousands of clinicians and school personnel in DBT internationally.

Jill H. Rathus, PhD, is Professor of Psychology at Long Island University—C. W. Post Campus, in Brookville, New York, where she directs DBT scientist-practitioner training within the clinical psychology doctoral program. She is also Co-Director and Co-Founder of Cognitive Behavioral Associates, a group practice in Great Neck, New York, specializing in DBT and cognitive-behavioral therapy (CBT). Dr. Rathus codeveloped the adolescent adaptation of DBT with Alec L. Miller, and her current research includes psychometric evaluation of the Life Problems Inventory, of the Acceptability of Walking the Middle Path Skills Module, and of factors in training and implementing adolescent DBT. Her interests include DBT, CBT, adolescent suicidality, relationship distress, and assessment, and she publishes widely in these areas. Dr. Rathus is also a trainer with Behavioral Tech and a lecturer internationally on DBT with adolescents. She is a coauthor of six books, including *Dialectical Behavior Therapy with Suicidal Adolescents* and *DBT Skills Manual for Adolescents.*

Heather E. Murphy, PhD, NCSP, has a private practice in Seattle, Washington, where she works with self-harming and suicidal adolescents. She is adjunct faculty in educational psychology at the University of Washington. Dr. Murphy previously worked as a school psychologist in elementary, middle, and high schools for 7 years. During that time, she developed districtwide procedures for intervening with suicidal youth and standard practices for responding to a suicide. Dr. Murphy's research, publications, and clinical work focus on adolescent mental health, LGBT youth, and suicide intervention with adolescents.

Foreword

The DBT skills were first presented in published book format in 1993. They were originally developed for high-risk suicidal individuals with complex disorders who had trouble functioning and regulating their emotions effectively. For many years, the skills were used routinely with adults, and some time later they became widely used with adolescents who were having the same sorts of difficulties. The idea that DBT skills could be useful for everyone took a long time to emerge. When my research and graduate training clinic started conducting DBT skills training for friends and families of people who had difficulties with emotion regulation and general functioning, and then with parents of children with such difficulties, we began to realize that the skills were widely applicable. Next we heard that corporations were interested in the skills, then we found that football players were interested, and then we heard from parents that they wanted DBT skills taught in their school systems. In short, although it took a long time, the value of DBT skills training for the general public eventually became evident. Once it was evident, however, another major problem arose: How could we get the skills training out to members of the public? It was not so hard to get it to adults; all we had to do was make it available, and in they came. It wasn't too hard to get it to adolescents with psychological difficulties, either; we let them know we had a program, and they came as well.

Parents and even some schoolchildren, however, said, "We want these skills in schools!" But how were we to get DBT skills delivered to a broad range of children both with and without emotional difficulties? This did not seem easy. It is this problem that James J. Mazza, Elizabeth T. Dexter-Mazza, and their coauthors have solved. Jim, as an expert in school-based intervention, and Lizz, as an expert in DBT, put their respective skills together and came up with a solution that is clearly outlined in this book. The curriculum they have put together is a unique social–emotional learning (SEL) curriculum that focuses on helping adolescents develop and practice emotion management skills, interpersonal effectiveness strategies, and decision-making skills—the very same DBT skills that have been shown to be effective in working with high-risk adolescents (Mehlum et al., 2014; Miller, Rathus, & Linehan, 2007) and adults (Linehan, 1993, 2015a). Consistent with DBT and dialectics, the authors have found an ingenious way of expanding the reach and implementation of DBT skills to the universal population of adolescents in educational settings. The DBT STEPS-A curriculum offers a fabulous upstream approach for all adolescents to develop DBT skills and reduce the likelihood of emotionally dysregulated behaviors.

This SEL curriculum is designed to be taught by general education teachers or school personnel who have a vested interest in helping adolescents learn to help themselves. The 30 standardized lesson plans are structured to allow for peer-to-peer support and coaching, as well as teacher instruction and modeling. The lessons are based on the four standard modules of DBT: Mindfulness, Distress Tolerance, Emotion Regulation, and Interpersonal Effectiveness. Each of the DBT STEPS-A lessons is intended to be taught in a 50-minute period, so that the lessons can be easily integrated into a general education curriculum schedule. In addition, the authors have provided supplemental strategies that build upon the universal application of DBT STEPS-A for students who may be at greater risk within a multi-tiered system of support. Thus the DBT STEPS-A curriculum provides explicit DBT skills building to students along a continuum of emotional needs that also promotes both academic learning and SEL within the school structure.

The authors of this book represent a unique combination of experts from the fields of school and clinical psychology. James J. Mazza, a school psychologist by training, has worked with adolescents' social–emotional needs within school-based settings for over 20 years and has implemented other SEL programs, such as Reconnecting Youth. Elizabeth T. Dexter-Mazza, a clinical psychologist and a previous postdoctoral fellow of mine, is an expert in both training other mental health professionals and delivering DBT to high-risk adolescent and adults. They have been developing and revising this curriculum together for over 10 years. Jill H. Rathus and Alec L. Miller, who published the *DBT Skills Manual for Adolescents* in 2015, provided their expertise in working with high-risk adolescents and graciously offered handouts from their book to adapt and integrate into the DBT STEPS-A curriculum—creating a seamless continuum of DBT skill development and practice for all students, with the same language and strategies. The book also includes handouts and worksheets adapted from the second edition of my *DBT Skills Training Handouts and Worksheets* (Linehan, 2015b), all of which have been used effectively in our adolescent clinical trials and are also used in ongoing clinical programs with highly suicidal adolescents. Finally, Heather E. Murphy is a school psychologist who helped put together the first version of this curriculum and was the first instructor to pilot-test it. Together, this team of writers has tapped their years of experience and knowledge regarding school-based settings and the delivery of DBT skills to adolescents to produce an outstanding product for schools to use.

This book offers the next step in expanding DBT skills to a greater audience: adolescents in educational settings. DBT STEPS-A offers a novel approach in targeting school-based systems rather than individuals, and provides an opportunity for all adolescents to develop and practice DBT skills. With the numerous pressures and stressors that many adolescents experience, the skills highlighted in this curriculum will probably help adolescents to make better decisions when emotionally distressed and will equip schools with an SEL curriculum that has a positive impact on academic and social–emotional needs alike.

A mother just recently said to me, almost in tears, "I can't wait for you to get these skills into my child's school. I need them now!" Your ability to take this book and use it to teach schoolchildren a wealth of effective life and emotion regulation skills has the possibility of helping more than you can imagine. I wish you skillful means. The authors of this book have provided such means for you.

MARSHA M. LINEHAN, PhD, ABPP
University of Washington

Preface

The development of the DBT Skills Training for Emotional Problem Solving for Adolescents (DBT STEPS-A) curriculum has been an ongoing project for more than a decade. Our purpose in creating DBT STEPS-A was to provide a meaningful set of skills for emotion management, relationship building, and decision making that adolescents could acquire and apply to navigating the emotionally difficult situations and stressors that accompany adolescence. Most adolescents experience at least some such situations at home, at school, or with peers (including romantic partners). The curriculum was designed for students in middle and high schools.

THE DEVELOPMENT OF DBT STEPS-A

DBT STEPS-A is an adaptation for students in middle and high schools of the skills training components of dialectical behavior therapy (DBT). In developing the DBT STEPS-A curriculum, we consulted and exchanged information with Marsha M. Linehan (the creator and primary developer of DBT), and with Alec L. Miller and Jill H. Rathus (adapters of DBT for outpatient adolescents). Throughout our conversations, each expert emphasized that DBT skills help clients learn to manage emotions, improve relationships, and enhance their decision-making abilities. Adolescence in general can be an emotionally difficult time for many youth, and the onset of most mental health disorders occurs during this time (American Psychiatric Association, 2013). Given these two important issues, we believe that a curriculum focusing on the acquisition and practice of skills for emotion management and decision making will be beneficial for all adolescents. Unfortunately, most schools do not offer courses on coping with stress or decision making, and yet the need for such skills and abilities is continuing to grow among this young adult population (Rathus & Miller, 2015). The DBT STEPS-A curriculum was designed and developed to meet this need.

The rationale for developing DBT STEPS-A for educational settings was twofold. First, educational settings have been transforming their service delivery model to meet students' academic and/or social–emotional needs along a continuum from the day they start school. For example, the use of the response-to-intervention framework of assessment, intervention, and monitoring of the intervention occurs at the individual level. Current research has shown this model to be successful in delivering educational services to students (Cook, Burns, Browning-Wright, & Gresham, 2010). Unfortunately, more traditional models of mental health follow what is sometimes called a "waiting to fail" approach—in other words, waiting until symptoms become unmanageable and are interfering with school, social relationships, and/ or emotional control. Adolescents who are seen in outpatient settings have typically already experienced problematic behaviors and/or failures that are symptomatic of mental health issues (Rathus & Miller, 2002).

The educational setting (most often, schools) is also the most likely place for students to receive services, whether psychologically or academically focused. According to researchers and school practitioners (Burns et al., 1995; Cook et al., 2010; Hoagwood & Erwin, 1997), schools represent the de facto setting (Cook et al., 2015) for the delivery of mental health services. A review of three national surveys examining mental health services to students between the ages of 6 and 17 years found that approximately 80% of students identified as being in need of mental health services had not received them in the preceding 12 months (Kataoka, Zhang, & Wells, 2002), and that the small proportion of students who did receive them overwhelmingly received those services at their schools. Furthermore, Catron and Weiss (1994) found that 98% of students referred for mental health treatment in their schools received services, compared to less than 20% of students referred to outside agencies who actually received services. These data indicate that the implementation of DBT STEPS-A in an educational setting has several important advantages:

1. The educational setting has a "captive audience," so to speak. In other words, students are already coming to this setting to learn academically, and thus adding skill acquisition and training should be a natural fit. In fact, having DBT STEPS-A as a class within the curriculum that students are required to take would be ideal. Detailed discussions of what this would look like, and of issues that may arise in such a class, are provided in Chapter 2.

2. Schools are places where adolescents experience some significant stressors; however, schools can also offer positive support and assistance to students who are struggling.

3. The educational setting offers numerous opportunities for students in DBT STEPS-A to practice some of their acquired skills. School-related factors such as bullying, punitive discipline, and peer rejection exacerbate mental health problems (Cook et al., 2010). It is therefore beneficial to learn and practice skills in that same setting.

4. The educational setting is not parent dependent, meaning that adolescents do not need to rely on their parents to take them to a mental health agency in the community. Although parents are an important part of a therapeutic process, their inconsistencies can often lead to a lack of adolescent involvement. Wagner (1997) reported that parents' own life stressors can often be obstacles to helping their children get the mental health services they need.

5. Finally, social–emotional programs such as DBT STEPS-A require resources of time and money, both of which are scarce commodities in school districts. However, if the implementation of DBT STEPS-A is able to reduce (even by one) the number of students needing specialized placements, such as residential treatment, then the curriculum should be viewed as cost-effective and as saving school districts money in the long run.

LIFE ENHANCEMENT STRATEGIES

One of our major aims in developing DBT STEPS-A has been to help adolescents develop their own toolboxes of effective behavioral strategies, or what we call "life enhancement" strategies. We use the term "life enhancement" because the timely and appropriate use of these skills can have a significant impact on individual students beyond simply enabling them to solve current problems. They can use these skills to solve problems well into their futures, such as remaining in school and going on to college, maintaining important romantic relationships, or keeping important jobs. DBT STEPS-A helps adolescents acquire and practice these skills before making life choices that may have detrimental consequences. Thus we are hoping that DBT STEPS-A will provide the tools and the strategies for helping adolescents to manage difficult and emotional situations and to make better decisions when they are experiencing emotional distress.

Acknowledgments

All five authors:

This book could not have been written without the support, guidance, and input of many people.

First and foremost, we would like to thank Marsha M. Linehan for her unique brilliance in developing such a comprehensive treatment as DBT, which has helped clients throughout the world build lives worth living. We often refer to the DBT skills as "skills we all need—some of us learned them along the way, and some of us didn't." This project grew from the desire to ensure that everyone learns DBT skills in a proactive way to assist in the challenges of adolescence and adulthood. When Jim and Lizz first started thinking about teaching the skills to middle and high school students in 2006 and presented the idea to Marsha, she was on board immediately; in fact, she regularly encouraged us to move faster than we physically could. Marsha also mentored each of us, and she provided constructive guidance in making sure the skills being taught adhered to her conceptualizations of DBT skills. In addition, Marsha allowed us to adapt some of her new handouts and worksheets for use in the DBT STEPS-A curriculum. We are grateful for her trusting us to translate her DBT skills into a curriculum for all students.

We are incredibly grateful to Natalie Graham, Editor at The Guilford Press, for all of the support and guidance she has given us over the last 5 years in helping us to meet deadlines and manage the many details of putting a work like this into writing. Barbara Watkins, our developmental editor at Guilford, also provided us with instrumental feedback and editing that have improved the quality of this book immensely and helped us navigate DBT from a clinical treatment setting to a universal school-based curriculum. Finally, we thank Marie Sprayberry, copyeditor, and Louise Farkas, senior production editor, and all of the staff at Guilford who have worked on making this book a reality.

James J. Mazza and Elizabeth T. Dexter-Mazza:

This book has been a part of our lives for more than a decade, from conception to publication. The scope of and effort involved in such a project required a great deal of dedication from multiple people, and fortunately we had a great team of authors for this book. The contributions of Jill H. Rathus and Alec L. Miller have been nothing short of extraordinary, from providing content about adolescent DBT to furnishing emotional support during challenging times. Alec and Jill also assisted us in creating a manageable path toward completing our book, and generously offered the use of many handouts for adaptation from their own book, *DBT Skills Manual for Adolescents*. Their contributions have allowed us to create continuity of care in services; the same DBT skills and language are used throughout, regardless of setting. In particular, this collaboration helps fill a major gap in helping students make the transition from clinical/residential treatment settings back to school or vice versa. Finally, we sincerely thank Heather E. Murphy for assisting in the initial drafts of the lessons and for helping us to get this project off the ground. To Marsha Linehan and our wonderful writing team, we are forever indebted to all your insight, knowledge, materials, support, and (most of all) friendship.

We have been fortunate to work with several school districts and programs that have implemented earlier versions of the DBT STEPS-A curriculum and generously provided us with feedback on each of the lessons. In particular, we want to thank the staff of Project GRAD LA in Los Angeles, who embraced the curriculum as a missing link and trained each of its College Success Advisors to teach the skills to their high school students. Their dedication to implementing the lessons as designed has been unparalleled. Patty Geiselman has been our constant cheerleader and support in this program, and we are grateful for all she has done for DBT STEPS-A and Project GRAD LA.

We are both enormously grateful to our friends and family, especially our parents and siblings, for their constant encouragement and their understanding of why we were so busy and missing out on life events because of "the book." Their unending support in all of our endeavors is part of the true meaning of "family." Finally, we thank our incredible children, Jackson, Ashton, and Grace, who every day make us laugh and keep us on our toes. Because of them, we never lost our motivation and mission to ensure that all kids learn these skills so they can create meaningful and fulfilling lives. We are forever grateful to them and in awe of their patience and understanding of why Mom and Dad had to write. This project started just before our oldest child was born, so our kids have no experience of life without our writing this book.

James J. Mazza:
There is an extensive list of people I would like to acknowledge throughout the development of the idea and product of this book. First, I thank William (Bill) Reynolds, who was my academic advisor and helped cultivate my interests in the field of adolescent mental health in general, and suicidal behavior in particular, while I was a graduate student at the University of Wisconsin–Madison. I have had several mentors in the field of suicidology—Mort Silverman, Alan Berman, David Jobes, Cheryl King, Peter Gutierrez, David Rudd, David Miller, and John Kalafat—who continued to support and challenge me to make a difference for school-based students. Thank you to the University of Washington School Psychology Program, which I have called home for 20 years, in supporting my pursuit of this curriculum. In particular, Janine Jones has been unconditionally supportive throughout this 10-year journey and has always stepped up at a moment's notice to help out; one could not have a better colleague. Thanks also to Clayton Cook for his ability to provide a global perspective on the continuum of mental health services that students need. I am grateful to the many graduate students I have had the honor of working with over the years for asking critical questions and

pushing me to articulate my own ideas so clearly. In particular, I thank two former students who have become both colleagues and friends, Ronald Cunningham and Heather E. Murphy, for their unending emotional support through this process.

My final acknowledgment goes to Lizz Dexter-Mazza for all of her incredible patience, skillful words, encouragement, flexibility, and perseverance throughout 10 busy years of our lives. As the second author of the book, Lizz provided expert content knowledge of DBT that was invaluable. Her relentless encouragement and support never wavered. She is the best wife, mom, friend, and second author one could ever have.

Elizabeth T. Dexter-Mazza:

I am overwhelmed about where to start and whom to thank, because so many people have supported me over the years. We have been working on moving DBT skills into the schools for 10 years, but my journey through the DBT world started years before in graduate school, when Soonie Kim offered me an opportunity to volunteer in her clinic, Portland DBT. That experience began my journey into DBT and set my future career path. I am so thankful to Soonie for taking me in and offering all she had in order to make me a DBT therapist. After Soonie, I was fortunate to work with Alec Miller. Alec has been my mentor, colleague, and dear friend. He taught me everything I know about working with adolescents and families, and his endless support in this project has been invaluable.

I also owe many thanks to the numerous DBT experts, trainers, and therapists I have been blessed to work with through Marsha Linehan's research lab, the BRTC, at the University of Washington; to the staff of Behavioral Tech; and to my Seattle-based consultation team. I have learned so much from all of you. Jill Rathus, in particular, has become an incredible friend and colleague, who never wavers in her brilliance and support. I am very grateful to her for everything she has done for this book and for me. In addition, I am appreciative of the unending support, wisdom, and friendships of Melanie Harned, Katie Korslund, Elaine Franks, Jennifer Sayrs, Adam Payne, Laurence Katz, Kate Comtois, Tony Dubose, Andre Ivanoff, Helen Best, Bob Goettle, Annie McCall, and Rebecca Schneir. I will be forever grateful to these amazing people for helping us in making the mission of getting DBT skills to the masses a reality!

Over the past 15 years, I have repeatedly heard both clients and their families say that they wish they had learned these skills in school. I am grateful to all the clients I have worked with, who have taught me invaluable lessons, made me a better DBT therapist, and constantly encouraged me to write this book.

Finally, words cannot begin to describe the incredible amount of love, wisdom, and encouragement I have received from Jim Mazza. He constantly balanced being a task-focused first author, pushing me for deadlines, with being the first to step up as a supportive husband and father so I could meet those deadlines. Even in moments when I wanted to give up, he encouraged me and kept me going. He truly exemplifies the definition of a "whole partner."

Alec L. Miller:

I want to acknowledge the many people who have contributed to my thinking about and applying DBT to schools. First, I would like to thank Jim and Lizz for their invitation to join them on this book. Their fund of knowledge about schools and DBT, as well as their creativity, passion, leadership, and friendship, made this collaborative effort seamless and fun. Second,

I thank the many school districts in New York State that have allowed our group from Cognitive and Behavioral Consultants to train their elementary, middle, and high school staffs in DBT. These districts include Ardsley, Pleasantville, Mamaroneck, New Rochelle, Briarcliff Manor, Irvington, Hastings, Rockland BOCES, the village of Florida, and many others. One school psychologist in particular, Dawn Catucci, deserves special thanks. Not only was she single-handedly responsible for convincing the Ardsley Union Free School District in 2007 to implement DBT in all of its schools, she has also been an ambassador of DBT for the entire New York school system. In fact, she and her colleagues have collected data, spoken at conferences, and inspired many other districts in New York to consider adding DBT to their schools as well. Third, during my 10 years as the director of clinical services at P.S. 8, an elementary school in the Bronx, New York, I collaborated with Erica Lander, Amanda Edwards, and many other colleagues in adapting DBT for use with elementary school-age children. Their clinical prowess and creativity helped further expand my knowledge of DBT for elementary school kids.

Finally, I thank the children and parents in these various schools who allowed us to pilot-test various versions of DBT in schools and provided us with feedback that has allowed us to improve our programs. It has always made intuitive sense to bring these DBT life skills that we were teaching to youth in clinical settings to children in schools. We have finally been able to do it.

Jill H. Rathus:

First, I thank my wonderful coauthors. It has been a delightful experience and an honor to be a part of this writing team. Jim and Lizz are incredible thinkers, colleagues, and now friends, and I could not be happier to have worked with them.

I am very grateful to my many colleagues and friends in the DBT community, who have been so supportive at Behavioral Tech and elsewhere. This list includes, but is not limited to, Tony DuBose, Laurence Katz, Melanie Harned, Lorie Ritchel, Adam Payne, Jennifer Byrnes, and Aaron Drucker. In addition, I thank my colleagues and friends at Long Island University—C. W. Post Campus (LIU–Post) for being a long-standing source of support, both personally and professionally: Bob Keisner, Eva Feindler, Pam Gustafson, David Roll, Camilo Ortiz, Danielle Knafo, Hilary Vidair, Geoff Goodman, Marc Deiner, Cathy Kudlak, and Katherine Hill Miller. I also want to acknowledge my intelligent, funny, and dedicated graduate students at LIU–Post, and, in particular, my DBT clinical research lab students.

I extend my appreciation to my dear friend, partner, and cofounder at Cognitive Behavioral Associates, Ruth DeRosa. I also thank my other talented and supportive DBT team members: Michelle Chung, Nira Nafisi, Shamshy Schlager, Gus Cutz, Hilary Vidair, Lisa Shull Gettings, Avigail Margolis, Steve Mazza, Shimon Littman, and Shannon York. My influential mentors, Dan O'Leary, Bill Sanderson, Marvin Goldfried, Dina Vivian, Dan Klein, Everett Waters, and the late Ted Carr, deserve many thanks as well.

I also thank the members of my family for their endless support, and especially my teenage children for their wisdom, love, and wit, and for bringing me so much joy. Conveniently, my children also supply me with lots of skills-teaching material and examples.

Finally, I thank my clients and their family members, who continue to inspire and touch me with their courage, motivation, and perseverance as they learn and practice more skillful means.

Heather E. Murphy:

First and foremost, I thank Marsha Linehan for the creation of DBT. DBT has reached and helped so many people, and I am very grateful to have worked with and learned from her in order to contribute what I can in helping others. I thank James Mazza for his immense support throughout my graduate training and also for bringing me on board with this project at its inception. Over the years, I have worked with many skilled DBT therapists who have challenged me and helped me grow; I especially acknowledge Linda Dimeff, Peggilee Wupperman, Barbara Kleine, Andre Ivanoff, and Benny Martin. I also acknowledge my coauthors, Elizabeth Dexter-Mazza, Jill Rathus, and Alec Miller, for their contributions.

DBT changed my life personally as well as professionally, because it was through my training that I met an incredibly kind and intelligent person who would later become my husband; I thank Cory Secrist for his enduring love, humor, and support. During this time, I also met someone who would become a dear friend and colleague, Sheila Crowell, whom I also acknowledge. I thank my sister, Bridget Murphy, for being a constant source of encouragement. Finally, I want to thank my parents, Tom and Denise Murphy, without whom I would not have been able to achieve all that I have; to them, I am perpetually grateful.

Contents

PART I

OVERVIEW OF DBT STEPS-A

CHAPTER 1

What Is DBT Skills Training for Emotional Problem Solving for Adolescents (DBT STEPS-A)?

WELCOME TO DBT STEPS-A

DBT Skills Training for Emotional Problem Solving for Adolescents (DBT STEPS-A) is a program for developing emotion management, interpersonal, and decision-making skills in middle school and high school students. Adolescents may face numerous social, developmental, and academic pressures, such as peer rejection, low self-confidence, confusion about self, impulsive behavior, involvement in drugs and alcohol, and issues related to intimacy and sexual relationships. Although schools often do not offer courses on coping with stress and decision making, adolescents' needs for such skills are continuing to grow (Rathus & Miller, 2015). As described in the preface, the DBT STEPS-A curriculum was developed to meet this need. It teaches practical skills for regulating emotions, reducing impulsive behaviors, solving problems, and building and repairing interpersonal relationships.

The DBT STEPS-A curriculum is designed to be taught by general education teachers or by school personnel with some background in adolescent mental health issues, such as health teachers, school counselors, or school psychologists. The curriculum consists of four primary skill areas or "modules" (Mindfulness, Distress Tolerance, Emotion Regulation, and Interpersonal Effectiveness); it is designed for approximately 30 weeks of lessons (1 class per week over two semesters, or twice a week over one semester) taught in standard 50-minute blocks. However, the curriculum is also flexible, so if the situation or circumstances only allow for 20 weeks or perhaps 40 weeks, the curriculum can be modified to fit the time schedule.

DBT STEPS-A is based on the skills training component of Dialectical Behavior Therapy (DBT), an empirically supported psychological treatment for adults and adolescents with problems caused by pervasive emotion dysregulation. Originally developed for adults by Linehan (1993, 2015a, 2015b) and adapted for suicidal adolescents by Miller and Rathus (Miller, Rathus, Leigh, Landsman, & Linehan, 1997; Rathus & Miller, 2002; Miller, Rathus, & Linehan, 2007; Rathus & Miller, 2015), DBT with adolescents is a comprehensive intervention that consists of weekly individual therapy, a weekly multifamily skills training group, between-session telephone coaching for skills generalization, and a therapist consultation team. This comprehensive model was used by Mehlum and colleagues (2014) in their recently published randomized controlled study, which demonstrated the effectiveness of DBT for adolescents with multiple problems. Those receiving DBT, as compared to those receiving enhanced usual care, had significant reductions in self-harm, depression, hopelessness, and borderline personality symptoms after 16 weeks of treatment (Mehlum et al., 2014). The skills taught in DBT have been found to be useful with a wide range of clinical and nonclinical populations (Mazza & Hanson, 2014a, 2014b; McMain, 2013; Hashim, Vadnais, & Miller, 2013). DBT skills can be considered basic social and emotional life skills.

DBT STEPS-A is not a therapy program. Rather, it is the skills training component of DBT modified for students of middle and high school age, to be delivered as a universal social–emotional learning curriculum. We believe that all adolescents, not just those who have difficulties regulating their emotions and behaviors, can benefit from the DBT STEPS-A curriculum. The goal of DBT STEPS-A is to help youth develop their own toolboxes of effective strategies to regulate emotions, solve problems, improve relationships, and enhance their lives.

HOW THIS BOOK IS ORGANIZED

This book is divided into three sections. In Part I, we present the rationale for DBT STEPS-A; the research background for its use with adolescents; an overview of its various components, including the lessons and the student handouts; and guidelines for its implementation, both in general classrooms and with more challenging students. In the present chapter, we briefly describe existing social–emotional learning curricula, their limitations for use with adolescents, how DBT STEPS-A addresses those limitations, and the research background for its use with adolescents. We then present a detailed overview of the curriculum, the four skills modules (Mindfulness, Emotional Regulation, Interpersonal Effectiveness, and Distress Tolerance), and the specific skills taught in each module. Chapter 2 examines the practical issues of implementing DBT STEPS-A into a school's overall curriculum, providing assignments and student grading, handling confidentiality issues, and making/enforcing rules of attendance; it also describes the use of the student handouts. Chapter 3 provides a brief overview of how to work with students who may need more intensive services (i.e., those in Tiers 2 and 3, where DBT STEPS-A is the foundational curriculum but other supportive services are recommended to address the students' current needs).

Parts II and III comprise the curriculum content itself. Part II consists of 30 detailed lesson plans for the DBT STEPS-A instructor to follow, as well as all the tests and answer keys. Part III contains all the student handouts (both informational/activity handouts and homework sheets) needed for teaching the class.

THE NEED FOR SOCIAL–EMOTIONAL LEARNING CURRICULA FOR ADOLESCENTS

Social–emotional learning (SEL) curricula are focused on helping students of all ages acquire and practice the skills they need for successfully navigating stressful life events; coping with emotional dysregulation; and developing/ maintaining important family, peer, school, and intimate relationships. The Collaborative for Academic, Social, and Emotional Learning (CASEL) highlights SEL as the "processes through which children and adults acquire and effectively apply the knowledge, attitudes, and skills necessary to understand and manage emotions" (CASEL, 2013, p. 4). For adolescents, SEL is particularly important because of the many social stressors and developmental factors that are typical for this age group, such as peer rejection, alcohol and drug use, dating and intimacy issues, bullying, social relationships, concerns about physical attractiveness, academic transitions from middle to high school, and becoming more independent of parents.

The stressors adolescents experience can range from mild to severe, and it is rare that an adolescent escapes this developmental stage without any stressful life events or emotional struggles. Problems that typically have a mild impact on academic and social functioning include feeling anxious about asking someone out on a date, skipping a class, managing a workload, or breaking curfew for the first time. Severe problems (which happen less frequently) may include self-harming, suicidal behavior, substance abuse, family conflict/aggression, or being arrested. These are typically either causes or results of intense emotional pain and dysregulation, and they are likely to have a significant impact on an adolescent's social and academic functioning.

The prevalence of mental health issues among adolescents is higher than many people realize. Cook et al. (2015) state that 20% of young adults experience mental problems each year (e.g., depression, anxiety, antisocial behavior)—and this percentage is unfortunately an underestimate, given that problems with academics, dating, intimacy, and other social issues (e.g., peer rejection, bullying) are not included in this number. Furthermore, Johnston, O'Malley, Bachman, and Schulenberg (2007) reported data from a national survey indicating that over 50% of high school seniors and nearly 20% of eighth graders reported using illicit drugs in their lifetimes. Thus it appears that the vast majority of youth could use good emotion management, problem-solving, and decision-making skills to navigate the emotional rollercoaster of adolescence.

Unfortunately, the current educational system in the United States is focused on academics, while ignoring the relationship between mental health issues and academic performance (Cook et al., 2010). When it comes to mental health and emotion regulation issues, most schools use a "waiting to fail" approach; as noted in the preface, this means that students must first engage in a problematic behavior before coming to the attention of appropriate school personnel. If the problematic behavior involves alcohol, drugs, or skipping school, punitive measures such as detention or suspension are commonly used—although these have not been shown to be effective (Monahan, VanDerhei, Bechtold, & Cauffman, 2014) and often lead to more problematic behavior.

Instead of using this reactionary approach, schools have begun to recognize that SEL curricula provide a proactive approach since these curricula are designed to help students develop appropriate skills in decision making and emotion management *before* they engage in problematic behavior. SEL curricula in elementary and middle school grades have been shown to reduce the number of disciplinary referrals and suspensions, while also increasing academic performance (Cook, Gresham, Kern, Barreras, & Crews, 2008). The use of SEL curricula therefore offers a "win–win" scenario: Students are not getting suspended or disciplined as much, and therefore are remaining in the classroom more frequently, which leads to more instructional time and learning for the students.

EXISTING SEL CURRICULA

Over the past 10 years, the number of SEL curricula has grown dramatically, as has support for using them (Kilgus, Reinke, & Jimerson, 2015). Several states (e.g., Pennsylvania, Illinois, and Kansas) have developed SEL standards and are working on aligning them with state education standards. Current SEL curricula are categorized by the age level of the intended audience, with substantially more such curricula focused on children in preschool and elementary school than on adolescents in middle and/or high school (CASEL, 2013, 2015). In fact, the *2013 CASEL Guide* (for preschool and elementary school ages) lists 19 SEL programs for elementary school, whereas the *2015 CASEL Guide* (for middle and high school ages) lists only 6 SEL programs for middle school and only 5 programs designed for high school. Table 1.1 lists and describes selected SEL curricula from the *2015 CASEL Guide*. The curricula chosen for this table are designed specifically for middle school (grades 6–8) and/or high school (grades 9–12); have assessment tools for monitoring implementation and measuring student behavior; are taught to all students (Tier 1 or universal level); and have empirical support in the form of specific student outcomes. There are other SEL curricula designed for middle and high school populations; however, CASEL has been recognized as a national leader in establishing competencies for inclusion in SEL programs and has developed a rigorous set of standards to evaluate these curricula (Durlak, Weissberg, Dymnicki, Taylor, & Schellinger, 2011). The table provides the name of each curriculum, the structure of the curriculum, the intended grade level, targeted behaviors, and student outcomes.

The research investigating SEL curricula designed specifically for adolescents has been limited (Durlak et al., 2011). As we reviewed the *2015 CASEL Guide*, it was striking to note that none of the research studies supporting the middle or high school programs has demonstrated significant student outcomes in the area of reduced emotional distress. At the high school level, only the Student Success Skills curriculum provides free-standing SEL lessons (of which there are eight). The review also highlighted that students in all five high school SEL programs showed significantly improved academic performance; yet only students taking Facing History and Ourselves showed improved SEL skills and attitudes, while only students in the Reading Apprenticeship program showed a reduction in problem behaviors. Similar findings were reported among the four selected middle school SEL programs: Only two of the four programs reported improved SEL skills and attitudes (Student Success Skills; Facing History and Ourselves), and only two of the four showed reductions in problem behaviors (Second Step: Student Success through Prevention for Middle School; Facing History and Ourselves). Finally, only Facing History and Ourselves reported improved positive social behaviors at the middle school level. Thus our examination of the *2015 CASEL Guide*, along with the meta-analysis conducted by Durlak and colleagues (2011), suggests (1) that there are significantly fewer SEL programs designed for middle and high school students than for younger students and (2) that among the existing programs for older students, effectiveness in reducing emotional distress remains largely undocumented.

In two other relevant studies, the utility of implementing SEL curricula among adolescent students is supported (Cook et al., 2008; McMain, 2013). In a review of the meta-analytic literature on social skills training programs for students with emotional and/or behavioral disorders (EBD), Cook and colleagues (2008) reported that two-thirds of such students receiving social skills training programs improved their social competence, com-

TABLE 1.1. Selected SEL Curricula

Curriculum name	Structure	Intended grade level	Targeted behaviors	Outcomes
Middle school SEL programs				
Expeditionary Learning	Organizational approach; uses teaching practices infused in academic curricula (English language arts)	6–12	Relational character (kindness, honesty, integrity) and performance character (organization, perseverance, craftsmanship)	Grades 6–8: ↑ **academic performance**
Facing History and Ourselves	Teaching practices that are infused in the academic curriculum (history, social studies, or language arts)	6–12	Positive youth development in the form of social and ethical reflection and civic learning	Grades 7, 8: ↑ **positive social behavior,** ↓ **problem behaviors,** ↑ **SEL skills and attitudes**
Second Step: Student Success Through Prevention for Middle School	Free-standing lessons (40 lessons)	6–8	Empathy, communication, problem solving, bullying prevention, substance abuse prevention	Grade 6: ↓ **problem behaviors**
Student Success Skills	Teaching practices and free-standing lessons (8 lessons)	6–12	Goal setting (along with progress monitoring); providing a supportive environment; memory and cognitive skills; emotion management; developing healthy optimism	Grade 7: ↑ **academic performance,** ↑ **SEL skills and attitudes**
High school SEL programs				
Consistency Management and Cooperative Discipline	Teacher training program—uses teaching practices	6–12	Teacher–student interactions, classroom environment, classroom management	Grade 9: ↑ **academic performance**
Facing History and Ourselves	Teaching practices that are infused in the academic curriculum (history, social studies, or language arts)	6–12	Positive youth development in the form of social and ethical reflection and civic learning	Grades 9, 10: ↑ **academic performance,** ↑ **SEL skills and attitudes,** ↑ **teaching practices**
Project Based Learning by Buck Institute for Education	Instructional approach; uses teaching practices focused on designing projects that engage students	6–12	Goal setting, problem solving, self-management	Grade 12: ↑ **academic performance**

(continued)

TABLE 1.1. *(continued)*

Curriculum name	Structure	Intended grade level	Targeted behaviors	Outcomes
Reading Apprenticeship	Teaching practices infused in the academic curriculum (reading, social studies, and science)	6–12	Building community and developing a safe environment; developing identity and self-awareness as a reader; cognitive skills; problem solving	Grades 9, 11: ↑ **academic performance**, ↓ **problem behaviors**, ↑ **teaching practices**
Student Success Skills	Teaching practices and free-standing lessons (8 lessons)	6–12	Goal setting (along with progress monitoring); providing a supportive environment; memory and cognitive skills; emotion management; developing healthy optimism	Grades 9, 10: ↑ **academic performance**

Note. Data from CASEL (2015).

pared to one-third in the control groups. In a related study of a social competence and emotion management skills program, McMain (2013) examined the effectiveness of a DBT-skills-only group versus a wait-list control group over a 20-week period for a clinical population of adults diagnosed with borderline personality disorder. The skills-only group was taught skills from the four DBT modules (Mindfulness, Distress Tolerance, Emotion Regulation, and Interpersonal Effectiveness) plus dialectics. This group showed a greater reduction in anger expression, less impulsive behavior, better distress tolerance, and better emotion management skills than their wait-list peers. The results from the McMain (2013) and Cook et al. (2008) studies suggest that skills training focused on interpersonal and emotion management issues can be an effective strategy for school-based adolescents, especially in the area of reducing emotional distress.

In addition to the lack of outcome research, the existing SEL curricula designed specifically for students of middle and high school ages have some notable limitations. First, they often involve broader systems that go beyond the individual level, such as family and community involvement, the creation of supportive learning environments, and the development of a positive school climate. Although these are important components for improving environments in which individual students may experience social or emotional distress, there are many situational factors in these environments that are outside the students' control. Second, the level of skill specificity being taught is unclear. For example, most of the curricula teach self-awareness and management skills; yet it is difficult to identify what specific skills the students have learned when the lessons are completed. Finally, the curriculum components often adhere to the five core components of CASEL (self-management, self-awareness, social awareness, relationship skills, and responsible decision making), which fundamentally represent SEL but do not have an underlying theoretical foundation for their inclusion. Thus our present understanding of how these components interact and how they are related to specific cognitive and/or emotional behaviors remains vague.

WHY DBT STEPS-A?

DBT STEPS-A offers an alternative SEL curriculum that addresses the limitations of the existing SEL approach. First, DBT STEPS-A is a universal curriculum that teaches emotion management strategies, decision-making skills, and interpersonal skills at the individual level. Thus the program does not require the involvement of broader systems, such as family or community.

Second, students are taught skills with a high degree of specificity and with explicit definitions, which are geared toward issues and stressors that adolescents often face. Many of the skills are identified by mnemonics representing the specific skills that are to be used; these mnemonics enhance students' ability to recall the skills and practice them when appropriate.

Third, the skills taught in DBT STEPS-A are drawn from DBT, which is based on Linehan's (1993, 2015a) biosocial theory of pervasive emotional dysregulation. According to this theory, a vulnerable biology coupled with an "invalidating environment" (i.e., lack of support or outright hindrance or mistreatment by family, peers, and/or teachers/coaches) can result in problems in four key areas: difficulty regulating emotions, which leads to confusion about the self, impulsive behaviors, and interpersonal problems. The four DBT skills modules are specifically designed to address deficits in each of these areas

1. The Emotion Regulation module teaches skills for decreasing unpleasant, distressing emotions and increasing positive emotions.
2. The Mindfulness module teaches skills for increasing self-awareness, becoming less judgmental, and gaining control of one's attention.
3. The Distress Tolerance module teaches skills for making distress endurable, so that an upsetting situation is not made worse by impulsive action.
4. The Interpersonal Effectiveness module teaches skills for asking for something or saying no to another person, while maintaining a good relationship and one's self-respect.

Although the DBT skills were originally developed to remediate severe problems in persons with serious mental disorders, the skills themselves are basic social and emotional life skills that are useful for everyone. Many people learn these skills on their own, but many do not, and others learn some but not all of them. The skills are particularly useful for adolescents, since confusion about the self, difficulty managing emotions, impulsiveness, and interpersonal difficulties can all be aspects of the developmental stage of adolescence.

Finally, preliminary outcome research now empirically supports the effectiveness of implementing the DBT STEPS-A curriculum across multiple middle and high school settings (Haskell et al., 2014; Mazza & Hanson, 2014a, 2014b; Miller, Mazza, Dexter-Mazza, Steinberg, & Courtney-Seidler, 2014). The results of these studies are discussed next. Studies examining the efficacy of the DBT STEPS-A curriculum in school-based populations are ongoing.

Preliminary Research on the DBT STEPS-A Curriculum in School-Based Settings

As a comprehensive treatment for pervasive emotional difficulties, DBT has gained empirical support for its effectiveness from research with adults (Dimeff, Woodcock, Harned, & Beadnell, 2011; Harned, Rizvi, & Linehan, 2010; Neacsiu, Rizvi, Vitaliano, Lynch, & Linehan, 2010) and more recently with adolescents (Mehlum et al., 2014). The skills component of DBT as a stand-alone treatment has been recently studied through the use of the DBT STEPS-A curriculum with school-based adolescents, and the findings have been encouraging (Haskell et al., 2014; Mazza & Hanson, 2014a; Miller et al., 2014).

One of the first schools to implement the DBT STEPS-A curriculum was a group of selected inner-city middle and high schools in Philadelphia, Pennsylvania, through Mastery Charter Schools. After the first year, the preliminary results comparing pretest versus post-test emotional distress scores looked promising; in particular, ninth graders who received DBT STEPS-A showed a significant reduction in their overall emotional distress scores, compared to those of peer controls (Haskell et al., 2014). In a second preliminary study, Mazza and Hanson (2014b) looked at eighth graders who were attending an alternative school in Battle Ground, Washington, and receiving the first two modules of the DBT STEPS-A curriculum (Mindfulness and Distress Tolerance). Of these students, 80% reported that they would use the skills themselves, and approximately 90% thought that the skills would be useful to others.

Potential Benefits to Schools in Using DBT STEPS-A

Schools that choose to implement DBT STEPS-A receive two related benefits. First, school administrators usually spend a significant amount of time dealing with students who present emotional and/or behavioral problems. Such students often receive disciplinary actions, such as detentions, suspensions, and even expulsions, because of behaviors that violate school rules; they may have made impulsive or poor decisions, perhaps acting out in distress, anger, or other intense emotions. Some of this administrative time is spent meeting with parents, while some of it is spent in teams developing appropriate individualized education plans (IEPs) and intervention strategies. These are "lose–lose" situations for schools because suspended or expelled students are no longer in the classrooms to learn, and because the amount of time school personnel spend on documenting disciplinary actions and reintegration plans is often significant. SEL programs, such as DBT STEPS-A, have been shown to reduce office referrals and disciplinary actions, thus saving valuable school resources (Cook et al., 2008).

The second benefit for schools is the reduction in the likelihood of students' needing specialized placement, such as residential treatment, which can cost districts anywhere from $50,000 to $125,000 per year per student. Because DBT STEPS-A teaches effective skills for emotion management, problem solving, interpersonal effectiveness, and decision making, students who acquire these skills are less likely to need specialized placements due to EBD issues. Again, this can save school districts money while keeping students in schools.

OVERVIEW OF THE DBT STEPS-A CURRICULUM: SKILL MODULES AND SPECIFIC SKILLS

The overall goals of the DBT STEPS-A curriculum are for students to learn skills for managing their emotions, behaviors, and relationships, and to be able to apply (or "generalize") these skills to their lives outside the classroom. Thus the main foci of the DBT STEPS-A curriculum and class are skill acquisition and generalization.

When youth have better control of their emotions, are less impulsive, and have better relationships, they are better able to learn, and the impact of adverse outside-of-school factors on learning is reduced. The life skills learned through DBT STEPS-A can increase students' chances of success in the present and beyond graduation.

Curriculum Sequence

The recommended sequence of skill modules and lessons is shown in Figure 1.1. The first two lessons of the program are introductory lessons that focus on the DBT STEPS-A curriculum structure, four areas where teens typically have problems, the classroom guidelines, and the definition of dialectics. Of the four modules shown in Figure 1.1, the Mindfulness module should be taught first. Because mindfulness skills are the "core" skills—the foundation for all subsequent skills and modules—it is important that students gain a basic understanding of these skills before moving on. Furthermore, the Mindfulness module is taught again before each of the subsequent modules. We recommend teaching Distress Tolerance as the second module, although the order is not set in stone, and some instructors may choose to alter the sequence to fit their particular situations and/or current events.

Table 1.2 provides a list of each DBT STEPS-A lesson by its number, the corresponding skill(s), and the module in which the lesson is being taught. The specific lessons and skills are described in detail below, starting with the two introductory lessons.

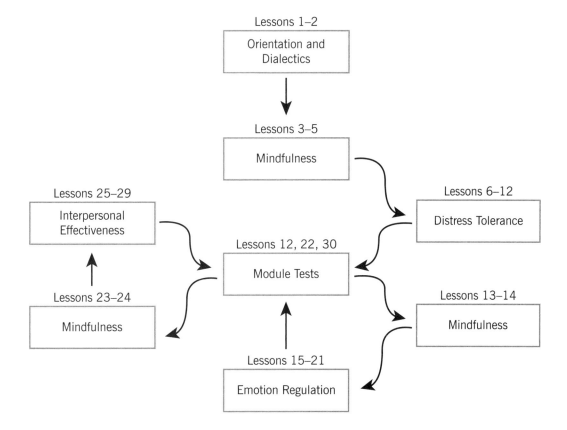

FIGURE 1.1. DBT STEPS-A curriculum: Recommended sequence of the curriculum modules.

TABLE 1.2. List of the Skills and Lesson Numbers

Module	Skill(s)	Lesson no.
Orientation	Classroom guidelines	Lesson 1
Dialectics	Principles of Dialectics	Lesson 2
Mindfulness	Wise mind	Lesson 3
	"What" skills	Lesson 4
	"How" skills	Lesson 5
Distress Tolerance	Intro. to crisis survival, and ACCEPTS	Lesson 6
	Self-soothe and IMPROVE	Lesson 7
	TIP Skills	Lesson 8
	Pros and cons	Lesson 9
	Intro. to reality acceptance and radical acceptance	Lesson 10
	Turning the mind and willingness	Lesson 11
	Mindfulness of current thoughts; Distress Tolerance Test, if given	Lesson 12
Mindfulness	Wise mind	Lesson 13
	"What" and "how" skills	Lesson 14
Emotion Regulation	Goals of emotion regulation; functions of emotions	Lesson 15
	Describing emotions	Lesson 16
	Checking the facts and opposite action	Lesson 17
	Problem solving	Lesson 18
	A of ABC PLEASE	Lesson 19
	BC PLEASE of ABC PLEASE	Lesson 20
	Wave skill—mindfulness of current emotions	Lesson 21
	Emotion Regulation Test	Lesson 22
Mindfulness	Wise mind	Lesson 23
	"What" and "how" skills	Lesson 24
Interpersonal Effectiveness	Goal setting	Lesson 25
	DEAR MAN	Lesson 26
	GIVE	Lesson 27
	FAST	Lesson 28
	Evaluating options	Lesson 29
	Interpersonal Effectiveness Test	Lesson 30

Orientation (Lesson 1)

In Lesson 1, students are introduced to the class, given classroom rules and guidelines, and oriented to the class schedule. They are also oriented to the four main areas in which teens typically have problems (difficulty managing emotions, confusion about self/distraction, impulsive behaviors, and interpersonal problems)—and the four DBT skills modules that can address the problems (Emotion Regulation, Mindfulness, Distress Tolerance, and Interpersonal Effectiveness, respectively).

1. *Difficulty managing emotions.* Adolescents often experience intense, quickly changing emotions, and these can lead to impulsive, emotion-based behaviors. Sometimes teens don't even recognize their emotions or the physical sensations that go along with the emotions. The skills in the Emotion Regulation module teach first how to recognize and name emotions, and then how to decrease unpleasant emotions and increase positive emotions.

2. *Confusion about self/distraction.* Adolescence is a time when students are developing who they are, what they like, their values, and their goals. Peer pressure, social media, and other environmental pressures can make it difficult for teenagers to understand themselves. It is also a time when distraction and loss of focus are problems. Confusion about the self and distraction can be improved by using the skills taught in the Mindfulness module (again, often referred to as "core" mindfulness skills to emphasize their importance). These skills increase self-awareness and control of attention. These skills are necessary for making centered, grounded decisions about the self, as well as focusing the mind (on classwork or other activities).

3. *Impulsiveness.* Teens can engage in a variety of problematic impulsive behaviors—ranging from skipping class, using drugs, and consuming alcohol to risky unprotected sexual behaviors, self-injurious behaviors (e.g., cutting, burning, or hitting oneself), and suicidal behaviors. Sometimes impulsive behaviors function as an escape from painful emotions. The skills taught in the Distress Tolerance module help make distress more endurable so that students do not act impulsively and make the situation worse.

4. *Interpersonal problems.* Many people struggle with how to ask others for things they want, say no to things they don't want, build and maintain long-term relationships, and maintain self-respect during interpersonal interactions. The three primary sets of skills in the Interpersonal Effectiveness module are strategies for increasing success in each of these difficult areas.

Students are then asked to identify specific behaviors that they want to work on increasing and decreasing over the course of the class. Behaviors to be decreased can include missing curfew, skipping class, not doing schoolwork, relationship and family problems, physical or verbal abuse toward others, gambling, drug or alcohol use, and chronic lateness to work or school. Some of these behaviors may seem fine to bring up in class, and others may not. In order to maintain confidentiality and to keep everyone focused, we encourage that the term "target behavior" be used in class discussions, so that students are not tempted to think, "Since this behavior isn't *my* problem, I do not have to pay attention."

Dialectics (Lesson 2)

The underlying philosophy of DBT and of DBT skills is "dialectics." Dialectics is a worldview in which reality as a whole consists of opposing forces—a "thesis" in tension with an "antithesis." A "synthesis" emerges from this tension. From a dialectical perspective, change is constant: A synthesis becomes a new thesis with a new antithesis. Opposites can both be true as parts of the larger whole, and contradictions may not cancel each other out. A premise of dialectics is that no one person can know all of reality, and so one person's truth can only be a partial truth. There is always more to know.

A dialectical perspective can help individuals think, feel, and behave in a balanced way. The fundamental dialectic in DBT is that of acceptance *and* change. We must accept things as they are, including ourselves, *and* at the same time recognize the need to change things, including ourselves. There are change-oriented skills in DBT STEPS-A, such as emotion regulation and interpersonal effectiveness skills; there are also acceptance-oriented skills, such as mindfulness and distress tolerance skills. The goal of dialectical thinking in DBT STEPS-A is to help students reduce "black-or-white," "all-or-nothing" thinking and increase their ability to recognize that there can be multiple perspectives to any situation. We want students to move away from "either–or" thinking and move toward "both–and" thinking. For example, it is useful for students to remind themselves of this common dialectical statement when the going gets tough: "I'm doing the best I can in this moment, *and* I need to do better."

Recognizing different perspectives does not necessarily mean approving or agreeing with other perspectives; it simply allows us to consider both sides of a situation. Once both sides of a dilemma or conflict can be understood, a search for synthesis can begin. A dialectical synthesis is not simply a compromise. Rather, it is a solution that honors the truth in both sides. For example, when we are stuck in a black-or-white dilemma, the synthesis will *not* be gray, but will be like black-and-white polka dots or like a checkerboard.

Mindfulness (Lessons 3–5, 13–14, and 23–24)

As we've noted, mindfulness skills are the foundation of the DBT STEPS-A curriculum, and the skills in the other three modules build on them. As shown in Figure 1.1, the Mindfulness module is repeated after each subsequent module.

Why Teach Mindfulness Skills?

Mindfulness skills teach youth how to focus their attention, pay attention to one thing at a time, and increase their awareness of the present rather than being distracted by thoughts about the past and future. These are critical skills—not only for regulating emotions, but for studying and for focusing in school. Mindfulness skills also help students notice and label their emotions, thoughts, and urges; doing this increases their self-awareness while reducing potential impulse control problems. Furthermore, these skills help students notice when they are making overly emotional decisions or overly logical ones, and assist them in finding a balance. With greater awareness, student will have more choices and can make more effective decisions. Mindfulness skills can help students enhance their identity, develop future goals, and identify their values.

The DBT core mindfulness skills developed by Linehan (1993, 2015a) are secular. Although Linehan drew from Buddhist practices, the mindfulness skills are not meant to teach Buddhism, spirituality, or any type of religion. The skills help individuals become more aware of living in the present moment and to be more mindful in our current lives. According to Jon Kabat-Zinn, the treatment developer of Mindfulness-Based Stress Reduction, mindfulness is "paying attention in a particular way, on purpose, in the present moment nonjudgmentally" (Kabat-Zinn, 1994, p. 4). In contrast, mindlessness is like being on automatic pilot—not being aware of what we are doing or what is going on around us in this one moment. Thus mindfulness skills focus on increasing awareness and control of attention.

According to Linehan (2015a), there are three main goals of mindfulness: (1) Reduce suffering and increase happiness, (2) increase control of our minds, and (3) experience reality as it is.

1. *Reduce suffering and increase happiness.* Research has found that regularly practicing mindfulness has been associated with increased emotional stability (e.g., decreased depression, anxiety, anger) and increased sense of well-being (e.g., improved body image, reduction of physical problems) in both clinical and nonclinical populations (Kabat-Zinn et al., 1992; Vøllestad, Nielsen, & Høstmark, 2012; Kaviani, Javaheri, & Hatami, 2011). This does not mean that mindfulness will take away all pain and troubles; it means that mindfulness can help reduce misery and increase overall joy in day-to-day life.

2. *Increase control of our minds.* Being in control of our minds is learning to be in control of our attention. It is being in control of what we pay attention to and for how long. It is the difference between walking or driving home and wondering how we got there and really noticing the route and the experience of driving. The first way is mindlessness. Mindfulness is taking control of what we pay attention to and being aware of it in the present, rather than getting lost in thought.

3. *Experience reality as it is.* Experiencing reality as it is means being present to life as it is, rather than as we think life should be. It is the opposite of avoiding life or escaping problems. Escape often causes even more problems, and suppressing thoughts and emotions can increase their frequency.

Specific Mindfulness Skills

The Mindfulness module teaches seven core skills aimed at increasing students' ability to be more mindful during their everyday interactions: wise mind; the three "what" skills (observing, describing, and participating); and the three "how" skills (nonjudgmentally, one-mindfully, and effectively).

WISE MIND

The first mindfulness skill taught is called "wise mind." Students are first oriented to the three states of mind: "reasonable mind," "emotion mind," and "wise mind." Reasonable mind is acting out of reason and logic in the absence of emotion. Being in reasonable mind may be helpful when one is working on a chemistry experiment in the lab and must add the chemicals very carefully and strategically so that the substances do not explode. Emotion mind is thinking and acting from intense emotion, disregarding all reason and logic. For example, a student named Katy finds out that she received a D on her chemistry final, just as she is about to take her English final. She is so upset that she cannot concentrate on her English final and starts to believe she is going to fail this second exam (and perhaps the whole semester). Wise mind is the synthesis of reasonable mind and emotion mind. It is the place from which we can make wise decisions that acknowledge both our logic and our emotions. It is not a place of compromise; rather, it is a place that allows us to see reality for what it is and experience our emotions about it without becoming overwhelmed. Wise mind is the state of mind in which

Katy can validate her emotions of sadness and fear about the chemistry exam, while also holding the logic that if she skips the English final, she will fall even further behind and most certainly fail. Right now, she only thinks she will fail and does not know it for sure. Once she is able to reach wise mind, she will be able to determine what other skills she can use to help decrease her emotions.

THE "WHAT" SKILLS

The remaining six mindfulness skills—the "what" skills and the "how" skills—focus on how we can practice mindfulness and access our wise mind. The "what" skills are practiced one at a time, not together. We observe or describe or participate.

- *Observing.* To observe mindfully is simply to notice or observe things either inside or outside of ourselves, without putting words on our observations. We observe the world outside ourselves through our five senses. We observe our own thoughts and emotions through our internal sensations. However, we cannot observe the thoughts, emotions, or intentions of other people. We can only observe other people's behaviors and facial expressions.

- *Describing.* To describe is to put an observation into words. We cannot mindfully describe something we have not observed. To describe it mindfully is to stick to the observable facts without judgments, interpretations, or opinions.

- *Participating.* To participate mindfully is to completely engage in an activity completely, throwing oneself into it 100%. To participate means going to a school dance and throwing oneself into the dancing without self-consciousness, without constantly watching to see whether people are looking and wondering what they think.

THE "HOW" SKILLS

As the names of these skill groups indicate, the "what" skills are *what* we do; the "how" skills are *how* we observe, describe, or participate. Unlike the "what" skills, the "how" skills— nonjudgmentally, one-mindfully, and effectively—are to be practiced together.

- *Nonjudgmentally.* To observe, describe, or participate nonjudgmentally means just that: not to judge. To describe, for example, is to verbalize only what one sees, without evaluating it as good or bad. Judgments tend to fuel the intensity of emotions; therefore, the more judgmental thinking and communicating are, the more intense the emotions are likely to be.

- *One-mindfully.* One-mindfully means doing only one thing at a time in the moment; it is the opposite of multitasking. It is focusing attention on this moment, rather than on what might happen in the future or what has happened in the past.

- *Effectively.* Last, acting effectively means doing what works—that is, choosing actions that move one toward his or her long-term goals. It is the opposite of cutting off one's nose to spite one's face, similar to doing something based on principle, even though it moves one further away from his or her goals.

Distress Tolerance (Lessons 6–12)

The next module is Distress Tolerance. The skills in this module help students cope with emotional distress so that they do not act impulsively and make matters worse. Students must have some ability to tolerate distress in order to consider using other effective skills, such as those from the Emotion Regulation module.

Why Teach Distress Tolerance Skills?

The goal of the distress tolerance skills in DBT STEPS-A is to reduce impulsiveness across different environments. Ultimately, this means fewer outbursts, conflicts, skipped classes, and aggressive incidents in school. Thus the reduction of impulsiveness through distress tolerance strategies has significant benefits in reducing disciplinary issues and concerns, while also enhancing academic progress.

The distress tolerance skills are divided into two categories: the crisis survival skills and the reality acceptance skills. A person can use crisis survival skills when dealing with a major problem or crisis that cannot be solved right away. If the crisis is causing the individual to experience a significant amount of distress (about 65 or higher on a scale of 0–100), and the person is in danger of acting from emotion mind in an ineffective way, then crisis survival skills should be employed.

Crisis Survival Skills (Lessons 6–9)

Several sets of crisis survival skills are taught in the DBT STEPS-A curriculum: distracting with wise mind ACCEPTS; IMPROVE the moment; self-soothing with the five senses, plus movement; TIP skills; and pros and cons. Several of these skill names are mnemonics standing for a variety of distraction methods. Crisis survival skills are not intended to eliminate distress, nor do they solve the problem causing the distress. These skills only make distress more tolerable in the short term and reduce the likelihood of making the situation worse. They are not to be used to escape or avoid problems over the long term.

DISTRACTING WITH WISE MIND ACCEPTS (LESSON 6)

The ACCEPTS skills are methods for distracting from a painful situation by mindfully participating: Activities, Contributing, Comparisons, Emotions, Pushing away, Thoughts, and Sensations. The key here, and with all other skills in DBT STEPS-A, is for students to engage in the skills *mindfully*. Through participating one-mindfully in other behaviors, students will be able to distract themselves from their current problems and emotions (As we all know, it is not effective to practice distraction all the time. The Emotion Regulation module teaches effective skills to help students tolerate and experience emotions as well.).

IMPROVE THE MOMENT (LESSON 7)

The IMPROVE skills focus on how to get through the current moment: Imagery, Meaning, Prayer, Relaxation, doing only One thing in the moment, taking a brief Vacation, and Encouragement.

SELF-SOOTHING WITH THE FIVE SENSES AND MOVEMENT (LESSON 7)

The premise of self-soothing is to make distress more tolerable by engaging in sensual comforts, such as looking at something beautiful (vision), listening to favorite music (hearing), lighting a scented candle (smell), eating a favorite food (taste), or having a warm bath (touch). Movement (walking, yoga, tai chi, etc.) is also used as a form of self-soothing.

TIP SKILLS (LESSON 8)

The TIP skills are ways to reduce intense emotions quickly for a brief amount of time. They work by activating the parasympathetic nervous system (PNS). The PNS is the body's physiological emotion regulation system that calls the body into rest (i.e., heart rate slows down, blood pressure decreases, saliva production decreases, pupils constrict, and digestion increases). Activation of the PNS counters the effect of the sympathetic nervous system (SNS), which is the "fight-or-flight" system that calls the body into action.

TIP stands for three ways that one can activate the PNS—by changing body Temperature, using Intense exercise, and engaging in Paced breathing.

- *Temperature.* Putting the face in a bowl of cold water can activate the PNS.

- *Intense exercise.* Intense exercise (e.g., running, power walking, jumping jacks, air boxing, sit-ups, push-ups) can quickly decrease intense emotions. It's best to exercise for 20 minutes mindfully; the PNS will be activated once the exercise stops and the body slows down.

- *Paced breathing.* Paced breathing entails slowing down the breath and engaging in deep breathing where the exhale is longer than the inhale. Typically, the goal is 4 seconds for the inhale and 6–8 seconds for the exhale. This will decrease the total number of breath cycles per minute to between 5 and 7 breaths per minute. The average pace of breathing for a teenager is about 12–16 breaths per minute.

PROS AND CONS (LESSON 9)

The skill of pros and cons is a decision-making strategy that is useful for a wide variety of issues. Within the Distress Tolerance module, students use it to determine the short- and long-term advantages and disadvantages of engaging in problematic impulsive behaviors (i.e., the students' target behaviors). This model of pros and cons is different from the typical model, in that the pros and cons of engaging in a target behavior and the pros and cons of not engaging in it must both be identified. This results in a four-cell list rather than a two-column list. By comparing the pros and cons of acting on urges with the pros and cons of tolerating the urges, students are able to identify effective reasons for tolerating their urges and acting skillfully. The long-term pros of tolerating the urge usually outweigh the short-term pros of acting impulsively. Pros and cons are best completed when a student is not distressed and in advance of emotional situations. The list should then be kept handy so it can be referred to when impulsive urges arise. Once students decide that they are going to tolerate their urges and not act on their emotions, then they can use one of the other crisis survival skills to help them tolerate the urges (e.g., distracting with wise mind ACCEPTS, IMPROVE the moment, or self-soothing).

Reality Acceptance Skills (Lessons 10–12)

The second half of the Distress Tolerance module focuses on skills for accepting reality. Whereas the crisis survival skills focus on tolerating distress in the short term, the reality acceptance skills focus on tolerating distress for problems that cannot be solved in the longer term—either because the past cannot be changed, because present circumstances are outside our control, or because solutions are only possible in the future. Before we can change reality, we must first see and accept reality as it is. Reality acceptance skills are tools for how to make the best of a bad situation. These skills are radical acceptance, turning the mind, willingness, and mindfulness of current thoughts.

RADICAL ACCEPTANCE (LESSON 10)

Radical acceptance is acknowledging and accepting reality as it is, rather than how we think it should be or want it to be. "Radical" refers to accepting something "all the way," completely, 100%. We must be able to see the facts without judgment in order to begin acceptance. The key concept behind radical acceptance is that pain in life is inevitable, but suffering is optional. Fighting a difficult reality (non-acceptance) adds suffering and misery to pain.

For example, a student named Tom is expelled from school for cheating when he did not cheat. As a result, he has missed 6 months of school, has had to repeat the school year, has not been able to attend school functions, and has lost contact with many of his friends. This is a painful situation. But when Tom fights the reality by insisting that "It shouldn't have happened," or asking "Why me?", he adds suffering to his pain. Fighting reality does not change reality. Acceptance of reality does not mean approval or passivity. Accepting what has happened does not mean that Tom agrees with the expulsion or gives up. Although acceptance may bring up much anger, sadness, and grief about the loss, it can also move Tom toward completing schoolwork in order to catch up, get back on track, repair old relationships, or build new ones.

Acceptance is about letting go of all the "shoulds" in our lives, such as "Things should be easier," "It shouldn't have happened this way," or "I should be able to do the things I want to do." Acceptance means acknowledging the reality of our lives, such as "My parents do have the right to place restrictions on me," "Everything is caused, so this could not have happened any other way unless I [or someone else] did something different earlier," or "I may not have caused all the problems in my life, *and* I still have to solve them."

TURNING THE MIND (LESSON 11)

Radical acceptance is not a one-time skill. Once something is radically accepted, it is probably not accepted forever. Acceptance can come and go, and when we find ourselves in a place of nonacceptance, we must turn our minds back to acceptance. Turning the mind is choosing to turn toward accepting reality, like coming to a fork in the road and turning toward the road of acceptance. Signs that we have gone back to nonacceptance and are rejecting reality include anger or willfulness.

For example, on Monday a student named Erica may be able to radically accept that she did not get the lead in the class play; then on Thursday she sees the student who has the lead make mistakes, and she gets angry again that she wasn't picked. Erica will have to use the skill of turning the mind to turn herself back toward acceptance. She may have to do this over and over again to let go of the suffering. Turning the mind may need to occur once a year, once a month, once a week, once an hour, or 30 times a minute. Students must practice being mindful to notice when nonacceptance of reality reappears.

WILLINGNESS (LESSON 11)

Willingness is the skill of doing what is needed in any given situation. It is similar to the skill of acting effectively from the mindfulness "how" skills. Willingness is often easier to teach by contrasting it with willfulness. Willfulness is refusing to tolerate the moment, to act as if it is not occurring. Willfulness can take the form of sitting on our hands, being passive at a time when action is called for. Willfulness can also take the form of trying to control things that are out of our control. For example, a student named Nia might try to get her friends to see the movie she wants to see, when everyone else wants to see a different movie. When Nia doesn't succeed, she may go with everyone else but complain, making them unhappy. Willfulness is the inability to move from our own stance. It is doing something grudgingly. Willingness is doing what is needed nonjudgmentally and without reservation. It is doing and acting completely from wise mind.

MINDFULNESS OF CURRENT THOUGHTS (LESSON 12)

Mindfulness of current thoughts is the final skill taught in the Distress Tolerance module. We have all had painful thoughts, and dwelling on those thoughts tends to increase our distress and pain. It's understandable to want to push painful thoughts out of our minds, to suppress them. This can help temporarily, but research (Wegner, 1989) has found that thought suppression tends to increase the frequency of the suppressed thought. Mindfulness of current thoughts is the opposite of trying to change or suppress thoughts; it is about allowing thoughts to come and go out without holding on to them or trying to push them away. All thoughts are mental events, neural firings of the brain. In this sense, all thoughts are essentially the same. Mindfulness of current thoughts is mindful observing and describing of a thought as just a thought. Through observing thoughts, we gain distance from them and can watch them come and go without holding on to them or believing that "Since I thought it, it must be true." We can let go of analyzing the thoughts.

Emotion Regulation (Lessons 15–21)

After the Mindfulness module is revisited briefly, the Emotion Regulation module is taught. It is designed to help students acquire a better understanding of emotions and develop a greater capacity to regulate their emotions. This module includes skills to reduce unpleasant emotions (vulnerability to emotion mind) and skills to increase positive emotions.

Why Teach Emotion Regulation Skills?

Emotion regulation skills are crucial for adolescents, especially those who may be emotionally sensitive and reactive, and for whom calming down from emotional arousal does not come easily. Developing the ability to make decisions that are not made under emotional duress provides these students with a greater likelihood of making effective decisions. Whereas the mindfulness skills and the distress tolerance skills are both acceptance-based sets of skills, the skills taught in this module and the Interpersonal Effectiveness module are considered change-based skills.

There are four categories of emotion regulation skills: (1) understanding and naming emotions, (2) changing emotional responses, (3) reducing vulnerability to emotion mind, and (4) letting go of emotional suffering.

Understanding and Naming Emotions

GOALS OF EMOTION REGULATION AND FUNCTIONS OF EMOTIONS (LESSON 15)

The Emotion Regulation module begins by teaching students that basic emotions are biologically hard-wired and serve important functions. They motivate and prepare us for action; for instance, fear involves physiological arousal that urges us to move away from what is feared. Emotions communicate to and influence others through our facial expressions and our verbal and nonverbal behaviors. Finally, emotions give us information about ourselves and our environment. The goal of the module is not to get rid of emotions, but rather to understand and manage them better.

DESCRIBING EMOTIONS (LESSON 16)

Students are then taught how to observe and describe the parts of the emotion system, as shown in the model of emotions (depicted in Handout 16.1). This model presents an emotion as a full-system response that includes vulnerability factors; a prompting event; thoughts or interpretations about the event; internal physiological responses and action urges; external responses such as facial expressions and behaviors; and consequences of actions. Being able to observe and describe the process helps students identify the specific emotion. Changing any one part of the emotion system can change the emotion or reduce its intensity.

Once students are able to understand and label their emotions, they must decide whether they want to change their emotion or continue to experience the emotion.

Changing Emotional Responses

CHECKING THE FACTS (LESSON 17)

Thoughts and interpretations of a prompting event can intensify or change an emotion; they can be also what prompts an emotion in the first place. Interpretations, however, can be wrong. We may think we see a snake in our path and jump away from it, heart pounding. On second look, it turns out to be a stick, and we start to calm down. The skill of checking the facts asks students to make sure that what they think happened actually did happen. Revising an initial interpretation to match the facts more closely can change the initial emotion.

OPPOSITE ACTION (LESSON 17)

The skill of opposite action focuses on changing an emotion by acting opposite to the emotion's action urge or behavior tendency. Every emotion naturally comes with an action urge.

For example, when we are angry, we often have the urge to attack; if we are scared, we have the urge to avoid; and when we are sad, we tend to want to withdraw. Changing behavior can change the emotion. This skill is based on empirically supported treatments for depression and anxiety disorders that call for getting active in the case of depression, and approaching rather than avoiding for phobias and other anxiety disorders. The key to opposite action is that students must engage in the opposite action 100%; maintaining thoughts of frustration and anger while smiling at someone will not reduce or change the emotion associated with the other person. Furthermore, the goal must be to change the emotion.

PROBLEM SOLVING (LESSON 18)

When painful emotions are caused by a situation or life problem, solving the problem is the best way to change the emotion. This skill includes a seven-step problem-solving process.

Reducing Vulnerability to Emotion Mind: ABC PLEASE

The third set of emotion regulation skills focuses on preventing painful emotions from starting by decreasing vulnerability to emotion mind. These skills are known by the mnemonic ABC PLEASE.

ACCUMULATING POSITIVES (LESSON 19)

Increasing positive experiences relieves stress and builds emotional resilience. Students are encouraged to accumulate positives in the short term by doing at least one thing every day that they find pleasant and enjoyable. They are also encouraged to plan for the long term by identifying their personal values, choosing long-term goals based on those values, and identifying specific steps they can take now to begin moving toward those goals.

BUILDING MASTERY (LESSON 20)

Building mastery is as important as accumulating positives. Building mastery is the skill of engaging in activities that are difficult but not impossible. By engaging in and completing difficult tasks on a regular basis, individuals will increase their overall sense of self-confidence, self-worth, and competence. These activities may include tasks that are not particularly enjoyable, but that confer a sense of accomplishment and pride once they are completed.

COPING AHEAD OF TIME WITH EMOTIONAL SITUATIONS (LESSON 20)

The next skill involves selecting and rehearsing coping skills in advance of a situation that is likely to trigger difficult emotions. Advance rehearsal increases the likelihood that a person will actually carry out that behavior during the emotional situation, and it reduces the likelihood that the person will become emotionally overwhelmed. There are two methods of rehearsing in advance: imaginal practice and *in vivo* practice. *In vivo* practice is practice as close to the actual situation as possible, such as role-playing the situation with another person. Imaginal practice is imagining the situation and engaging in the skills. Research (Atienza, Balaguer, & Garcia-Merita, 1998, Jeannerod & Frak, 1999; Kazdin & Mascitelli, 1982) has found that imaginal practice can be as effective as live practice for some behaviors. This is true for athletes practicing new skills, as well as individuals who know they are going to experience an emotionally difficult situation.

PLEASE SKILLS (LESSON 20)

The PLEASE skills decrease vulnerability to emotion mind by taking care of the body. PLEASE stands for the following: treat PhysicaL illness, balance Eating, Avoid mood-altering drugs, balance Sleep, and get Exercise. Although the PLEASE skills are essentially commonsense practices, teens and adults often overlook them or do not make the connection between these health-related behaviors and their moods. They are among the most important skill sets, and we stress their importance to our students.

Letting Go of Emotional Suffering

THE WAVE SKILL—MINDFULNESS OF CURRENT EMOTIONS (LESSON 21)

There are times when a student must experience a difficult emotion in order to respond effectively. In such situations, the student should use the "wave" skill, which is also referred to as "mindfulness of current emotions." In the Distress Tolerance module, the students learn how to distract from their emotions and emotion-based behavioral urges. At times, distraction is very effective; however, it is just as important for students to learn how to experience and tolerate their emotions as well. This skill will teach students how to be mindful of and experience the physical sensations that accompany emotions, without distracting themselves from or avoiding them.

Interpersonal Effectiveness (Lessons 25–29)

The last module of the DBT STEPS-A curriculum is Interpersonal Effectiveness. It is taught after the Mindfulness module lessons have once again been reviewed. The overall goal of the Interpersonal Effectiveness module is to help students develop and maintain better interpersonal relationships by improving assertiveness, reducing conflict, and increasing self-respect.

Why Teach Interpersonal Effectiveness Skills?

It is no surprise that one often hears that the event prompting an intense emotional or problem behavior was an interpersonal situation. These situations can include problems with boyfriends or girlfriends, teachers, family members, or friends. Thus the Interpersonal Effectiveness module is extremely important. The interpersonal effectiveness skills benefit all types of relationships: peer to peer, student to teacher and staff, and family. Strains from school problems such as peer exclusion, bullying, or not connecting with teachers can be reduced with good interpersonal effectiveness skills. In addition, improving overall interpersonal effectiveness among students creates the potential for an overall change in the culture of students' (and perhaps also staff members') interactions throughout the school. The interpersonal effectiveness skills help students learn how to ask effectively for things they want or say no to things they don't want, while maintaining or improving the relationship and maintaining self-respect.

Specific Interpersonal Effectiveness Skills

OVERVIEW AND GOAL SETTING/PRIORITIZING (LESSON 25)

The first lesson in this module teaches how to identify and prioritize three main goals in any given interpersonal situation: (1) "objectives effectiveness," or being able to ask for things students want or say no to things they do not want; (2) "relationship effectiveness," or maintaining and even improving the relationship when asking or saying no; and (3) "self-respect effectiveness," or maintaining and improving self-respect in the interaction. All three goals may be met in any interpersonal situation; however, each situation may differ in the degree to which the goals can be met. Students are taught to consider the three goals listed above and rank their importance for an interaction. When it is not possible to obtain all the goals, prioritizing them allows students to emphasize one set of skills over another to obtain the most important goal in a given situation. In the subsequent lessons, skills that correspond to each of these goals are then taught.

OBJECTIVES EFFECTIVENESS SKILLS: DEAR MAN (LESSON 26)

The objectives effectiveness skills are assertiveness skills that individuals can use to ask for things they want or say no to things they do not want. DEAR MAN is a mnemonic for this set of skills: Describe the situation, Express your emotion or opinion, Assert your request, Reinforce the other person ahead of time, stay Mindful of this moment, Appear confident, and Negotiate as needed.

RELATIONSHIP EFFECTIVENESS SKILLS: GIVE (LESSON 27)

The DEAR MAN skills can be thought of as what to say to obtain an objective. The GIVE skills can be thought of as how to say it to maintain or improve the relationship with the other person in both the short and long term. GIVE is a mnemonic for be Gentle, act Interested, Validate, and use an Easy manner. Students are taught to consider how they want the other person to feel about them after the interaction is over.

SELF-RESPECT EFFECTIVENESS SKILLS: FAST (LESSON 28)

The FAST skills can be thought of as how to ask or say no in order to maintain or improve self-respect in the interaction. FAST stands for be Fair, no Apologies, Stick to values, and be Truthful. As compared to the GIVE skills, students are taught to consider how they want to feel about themselves after the interaction is over. Students' values identified during the Emotion Regulation module (as they accumulate positives in the long term—part of the A of ABC PLEASE) are relevant here.

EVALUATING OPTIONS (LESSON 29)

Finally, being interpersonally effective also includes being able to determine the intensity with which to ask for things or say no to someone else. In some situations, it is imperative to ask firmly and not to take no for an answer; in other situations, it is more effective to ask softly and take no for the answer. The final set of skills in this module, evaluating options, describes the factors that should influence the intensity of asking or saying no and how to weigh them. These 10 factors are (1) your own or the other person's capability to give what is asked; (2) your priorities; (3) the effect of your actions on your self-respect; (4) your and the other person's moral and legal rights in the situation; (5) your authority over the other person or the other person's authority over you; (6) the type of relationship you have with the person; (7) the effect of your action on your long-term versus short-term goals; (8) the degree of reciprocity, or give and take, in the relationship; (9) whether you have (or the other person has) done adequate homework to prepare; and (10) the timing of your request or refusal. Students will weigh these factors to determine the intensity of asking for something or saying no after they have prioritized their goals for the interpersonal situation.

CONCLUSION

The 30 lessons (tests included) constitute the DBT STEPS-A curriculum. The recommended sequence of delivery has been provided: starting with Mindfulness, proceeding to Distress Tolerance and then Emotion Regulation, and finishing with Interpersonal Effectiveness. However, instructors can use a sequence of Mindfulness, Interpersonal Effectiveness, Emotion Regulation, and Distress Tolerance. The decision of which module to implement after Mindfulness is based on the teachers' familiarity with or knowledge of the students in the class. The specific lessons and student handouts are provided in Parts II and III, respectively.

CHAPTER 2

Practical Issues in Schools

The DBT STEPS-A curriculum and skills are designed for universal implementation. We believe that all adolescents can benefit from the DBT STEPS-A curriculum, but it is ultimately up to the personnel of each school district or educational setting to decide how they want to implement the curriculum, depending on their state requirements and educational standards. The DBT STEPS-A curriculum is designed to be taught within a class structure, and several options for class implementation are discussed below.

OPTIONS FOR IMPLEMENTATION

The first option is implementing DBT STEPS-A as an independent, mandatory course for all students. There are several advantages to this option. First, all students will receive the curriculum and thus will have the opportunity to develop the DBT skills. Second, as an independent course, its content will be viewed as just as important as the content of other courses (such as English language arts, math, and science), and as part of the basic education received by students. Some states (e.g., Kansas and Pennsylvania) are beginning to develop school-based SEL standards that are aligned with state academic standards; the DBT STEPS-A course could be used to meet those standards. The last advantage is that making DBT STEPS-A an independent, required course should have a positive impact on the entire school environment. With every student exposed to the curriculum, school administrators and personnel can use the skills in their interactions with adolescents. For example, when an adolescent appears distracted in class, the teacher can remind the student, "Use your mindfulness skills to help you refocus." Similarly, athletic coaches can remind team members to use their emotion regulation skills during the next match in order to perform better. The disadvantage of this option is that schools need to find a place in their educational schedule to include the DBT STEPS-A class.

The second option is for the DBT STEPS-A class to be taught in conjunction with a course that is already required, such as health. The advantage of this option is that a health course is already required in most states, and thus the educational schedule does not need to be altered to accommodate the DBT STEPS-A class. Also, this option (like the first option) has the advantages of exposing all students to the curriculum, addressing SEL standards, and having positive effects on the entire school environment. The disadvantage is that the DBT STEPS-A curriculum may need to compete for limited time resources with the requirements to cover specific health material. Although the content of many health courses overlaps with the skills taught in DBT STEPS-A (such as skills for assertive refusal, healthy decision making, and stress management), state standards for the health class may require class content to be tipped toward the health curriculum. Advocates for CASEL (Weissberg & Cascarino, 2013) have discussed the limitations of this option and the need to integrate SEL curricula into the standard core curricula being taught in schools.

A third option is to offer DBT STEPS-A as an elective course. If this option is chosen, then several mechanisms can be used to encourage enrollment. First, teachers can send lists of students they believe would benefit from the DBT STEPS-A class to the school principal or administrators. Second, students can self-select enrollment in the class, as they do for other elective courses. If there are too many students wanting to enroll in the DBT STEPS-A class, random assignment or other schoolwide procedures can be used to select the participants. Finally, students who come to the attention of school personnel because of difficulty in managing emotions or behaviors can be chosen for this class. However, this selection strategy may result in a class of students who need more support than a universal program can provide.

OPTIONS FOR SCHEDULING

In regard to scheduling, the DBT STEPS-A course should be treated like other courses in the curriculum. This means that if the course is designated as a health course, it should meet as frequently and for the same length of time as other health courses. The DBT STEPS-A curriculum is flexible for varying school schedules; we recommend providing it in a class taught either once a week over the course of a year or twice a week per semester. Each lesson is presented in Part II of this book as a 50-minute lesson plan; however, the content can be adjusted, depending on the length of the class or the requirements of block scheduling. Finally, the curriculum is not designed to be taught in a class that meets every day, because students need time and opportunities to practice their newly learned skills outside the DBT STEPS-A classroom, which helps with the generalization of the skills.

CURRICULUM GOALS

Skill Acquisition and Generalization

The ultimate goals of the DBT STEPS-A curriculum are for students to learn the skills (skill acquisition) and to be able to apply them to their lives outside the classroom (skill generalization). Thus the DBT STEPS-A curriculum focuses on helping students learn different skills, while also providing structured opportunities for students to practice those skills. Skill acquisition and generalization are the main foci of the DBT STEPS-A curriculum and class.

Skill acquisition in DBT STEPS-A is a two-part process: instruction and skill practice. The lessons are designed to teach students the underlying reasons for the skills, such as why our bodies and minds react the way they do under certain circumstances. Students are given information about emotions and their emotional reactions, and are taught that they can change those reactions or reduce the intensity of the reactions through specific coping strategies.

The majority of time during each lesson is spent on helping students understanding what the skill (or skills) being taught is, the rationale behind the skill, examples of the skill, and when to implement the skill. This part of the lesson uses examples and involves student participation in order to ensure that the skill is properly understood.

The homework is assigned after each lesson and promotes generalization by requiring practice of the taught skills in environments outside the DBT STEPS-A classroom. As with most other skills, such as riding a bike or learning to swim, students will need to practice these skills over and over again to gain proficiency and confidence in using them.

We expect that some skills will work better for some students than for others. Thus each module contains multiple skills that can be used for the same purpose. Students should be encouraged to try all the skills and choose those that work best for them. It is highly likely that students attending the same DBT STEPS-A class will choose to implement different skills for similar situations.

CLASS SIZE AND GENERAL FORMAT

The DBT STEPS-A curriculum has been designed for class periods that are 50 minutes in length, and the lessons are written to maximize peer-to-peer interactions and student participation. With a smaller class size of 8–10 students, there are greater opportunities for class participation, homework review, and skills practice. However, throughout all the lesson plans, the structured interactions and times can be easily modified for smaller or larger groups and different class lengths. We recognize that small group sizes may be unrealistic for most schools, given the demands of school districts and the needs of the students, and thus the lessons are easily adaptable to larger groups. However, research has shown that small groups are an efficient means for increased participation and increased performance and coordination of activities and facilitate peer interactions in assisting or helping others to develop their skills or expertise (Moreland, Levine, & Wingert, 1996); this reviewed research thus suggests that when a smaller group is possible, it is likely to be more efficient and effective.

The general format of the DBT STEPS-A class, open versus closed, also needs to be considered. Instructors implementing a DBT STEPS-A class must carefully consider the advantages and disadvantages of making the class closed versus open, as well as other details regarding the class structure.

There are several advantages of using a closed-group format, meaning that once the class starts (i.e., at the beginning of the school year, semester, or quarter), it is closed to additional students; even if a student drops out, he or she is not replaced. The first advantage of this format is that the group dynamics begin to form at the beginning of the class and are not disrupted by the addition of new students. Second, given that the DBT STEPS-A curriculum relies on students' providing some degree of self-disclosure, a closed-group format promotes a sense of stability and safety, so that classmates can begin to support and trust one another. Third, the closed format provides a sense of flow and continuity, which also enables the students to provide support, practice opportunities, and coaching for each other.

The main disadvantage of a closed-group format, of course, is that students cannot be added to the class once it starts. Therefore, a student who makes a poor decision 2 weeks into the school year and realizes that he or she could benefit from the class is not able to enroll in it if a closed format is adopted. Similarly, students who transfer from other schools during the middle of the academic year are also ineligible to take the class until the next time it is offered. Finally once the class has started, the closed format does not allow for additions to achieve a more balanced group, such as the number of male to female students.

In addition, we recognize that schools may not have the option of using a closed-group format, given district rules and policies. If a student joins an ongoing DBT STEPS-A class, the student should have a one-on-one meeting with the teacher first to go over the class orientation materials, especially the classroom rules. The decision of whether to adopt an open or closed format also may be determined by the intended population: universal, selective, or indicated (Tier 1, 2, or 3, respectively; see Chapter 3 for a more detailed discussion).

INSTRUCTOR CHARACTERISTICS AND TRAINING

DBT STEPS-A is designed to be a universal (Tier 1) SEL curriculum, meaning that it can be taught by any general or special education teacher who has a minimal amount of mental health awareness. Health instructors, who often have some mental health awareness training, make excellent instructors for DBT STEPS-A. For schools that choose to use DBT STEPS-A with students who have been already identified with mental health or behavioral problems (Tiers 2 and 3), we recommend health teachers with greater mental health experience, as well as school counselors or school psychologists. These classes will be composed of students who need more intensive services and thus instructors with more training. (Again, this type of class is discussed more fully in Chapter 3.)

An important characteristic to consider when choosing a DBT STEPS-A teacher is his or her willingness to practice and use the skills before teaching them. Doing so will enable the instructor not only to teach the skills more successfully in the classroom, but to provide opportunities for students to see the skills in action and their effectiveness. The instructor needs to act as a role model for the students, identifying out loud what skill he or she is using, while also modeling vulnerability and self-monitoring—two important characteristics students will need to develop if they are going to be successful in the DBT STEPS-A class.

In fact, a second important teacher characteristic is a willingness to use his or her own experiences with the skills as classroom examples. Again, teachers should be aware that effective self-disclosure models successful skill use and should be appropriate for the classroom environment. Although each lesson provides examples pertinent to each skill, the more tangible or "real" the examples are, the more likely students will be to learn and retain the skill. Examples of skill use in the context of a particular school's crisis events are often of personal value to the students.

The classroom environment is often a reflection of the instructor's management style and ability to facilitate group discussions in a nonjudgmental manner. Because self-disclosure and participation are strongly encouraged in the DBT STEPS-A curriculum, it is essential that instructors provide a nonjudgmental environment and one that promotes group discussions.

We suggest that instructors planning to teach DBT STEPS-A in their schools receive formal training. The training is optional, but it provides teachers with a more comprehensive understanding of the curriculum, a clear idea of what it looks like in the classroom, and chances to clarify issues of implementation and structure. In addition, the training demonstrates lessons according to a "tell, show, do" model: Selected skills are described, demonstrated, and then practiced by the teacher trainees in front of the other participants. Past participants have reported that the training was very helpful in providing concrete examples of the lessons and showing what certain skills look like when taught in a classroom setting. At this writing, training can be obtained by contacting the first two authors via email at *info@ dbtinschools.com*.

STANDARD LESSON STRUCTURE

All the DBT STEPS-A lessons follow a similar four-part structure: mindfulness exercise, homework review, teaching of new skill content, and lesson summary/homework assignment. The consistent structure not only aids classroom planning and implementation, but communicates to students what to expect in each lesson.

Brief Mindfulness Exercise (5 Minutes)

Each lesson begins with a brief mindfulness exercise. This is strategic because it helps students get into the right frame of mind (wise mind) to acquire and practice the new skill being taught. The practice of mindfulness also allows students to get more in tune with their senses, while freeing their minds from the distractions and/or stressors of the day. This type of exercise, when completed correctly, has been shown to enhance learning and regulate mood (Dimeff & Koerner, 2007).

Each lesson in Part II presents a different mindfulness exercise. The instructor, however, is free to implement one different from that described in the lesson plan or to repeat previous exercises. (A complete list of the different exercises can be found in the index.)

Homework Review (7–10 Minutes)

The homework review component of each lesson is often conducted in dyads or small groups, which should be changed frequently throughout the course to ensure different student combinations. Students check in with each other regarding the practice or implementation of the previous lesson. After students have reported their successes or struggles in implementing the particular skill, one member of each dyad or small group reports back to the larger group on another member's outcomes or his or her own. The design of the homework review helps students get used to sharing a peer's or their own successes and/or struggles in trying to implement the skills. Self-disclosure is difficult for most students, and the homework review helps students slowly gain comfort in with providing personal information to peers in a nonjudgmental environment. As part of a time management strategy, we recommend that the instructor model a brief homework report to the larger group, taking approximately 30–45 seconds to complete the report. This establishes the expectations for the group. Here is an example of such a report: "I was stuck in traffic driving to school the other day, and I started getting upset about being late. But then I remembered to use paced breathing [a TIP skill], and it really worked to calm me down."

The homework review also provides a structure for monitoring students' skill practice and implementation. Specifically, it gives the instructor necessary information on how well certain skills have been implemented and whether some skills need to be revisited. Discussions that occur in the larger group during homework review can also give the instructor a general idea of which students are making a concerted effort to apply the skills outside the classroom. This information can be used as part of the grading rubric for the DBT STEPS-A class, discussed later in this chapter.

Teaching of New Skill Content (25–35 Minutes)

The majority of time in each lesson is spent on teaching the new skill to the students. It receives 50–70% of the class time, so that the instructor and students have enough time to interact with the materials in teaching the new skills. Each lesson contains an explanation of the new skill (or skills), the reasons why the skill is needed, the components of the skill, and several examples that provide an appropriate application of the skill. Handouts describing the components of the skill are also reviewed.

This segment of the lesson often provides students with an interactive structure for practicing the skill and making it more tangible in their lives. The interactive structure varies; it may include students' reading out loud from their student handouts, practicing the new skills with each other, engaging in small-group discussions and activities, and/or participating through the use of posterboards (i.e., 2′ × 3′ poster or flipchart paper). The overall goal is to get the students involved and participating in the learning process. If students can gain some firsthand experience of what each skill includes and how to apply it, they are more likely to apply the skill successfully in settings outside the classroom (skill application and generalization).

Lesson Summary and Homework Assignment (3–5 Minutes)

During the last several minutes of each lesson, the instructor summarizes the main points and assigns homework due for the next class. This helps students remember the big picture—what the skill is, why they should use it, and when to use it.

The summary is followed by asking students to put the new skill into action through the homework assignment, which usually involves the application of the newly learned skill. At least one homework sheet is provided for each lesson from Lesson 2 onward in Part III. The instructor goes over the homework sheet and gives students a chance to ask questions and to get clarification on the assignment before the class ends. New diary cards (see p. 32) are also distributed, listing all the skills taught in the class. Students are encouraged to practice previously learned skills as well as new skills, and to record their practice on the diary cards.

MATERIALS FOR STUDENTS

Student Handouts

All of the student handouts for the DBT STEPS-A curriculum are provided in Part III of this book, paralleling the instructional guide provided to teachers in Part II. Students hear the instructions while being able to read and see the instructions in the handouts. The handouts give multiple examples of what the skills look like, while also providing useful advice on what *not* to do. The handouts can be used as resources after and between classes to help students remember the skills and how to practice them.

There are two types of handouts: those with student activities and skill explanations and those with homework assignments. (As explained further in the section on Homework, the latter contain practice exercises to be completed primarily outside the DBT STEPS-A class.) Each student should have a binder in which to keep all handouts, take notes on them during class instruction, and take completed homework sheets out for homework collection. In the Part II lesson plans, the phrase "student binder" is often used to refer to the student handouts it contains. The handouts are numbered according to the lesson and the sequence in which they are reviewed in the lesson. For example, the first handout in Lesson 10 is Handout 10.1. Homework sheets are numbered continuously with the informational/activity handouts but are called "Homework" rather than "Handout"; for example, the homework sheet assigned in Lesson 10 is Homework 10.4.

Homework sheets contain skills practice exercises and assignments and ask students to record the results of their practice. Students can then receive instructor and peer coaching for challenges they encounter in trying to implement the skills. Similar to the informational/ activity handouts, the homework sheets offer opportunities for students to practice skills and maintain their application beyond the semester and/or academic year. The number of homework sheets per lesson is limited to two, with most lessons assigning a single homework sheet.

Diary Cards

The diary card is an ongoing method for students to track their skills practice. The card is intended to function as a daily reminder to use skills in different environments outside the classroom. Students are asked to circle what skills were practiced on what day and to rate their skill use effectiveness for the week on a scale of 0–7. The card also provides an ongoing log of skill practice attempts. As the cards are completed each week, they provide a quantitative method for the instructor to evaluate which skills are working well for students and which are not. A new diary card is distributed to each student at each lesson, and the previous one is collected. Each new card shows all skills taught to that point in the course, including that lesson's new skill. A partial example of a filled-out diary card is shown in Figure 2.1 for a student who has completed the DBT STEPS-A class through the Distress Tolerance module. A reproducible blank diary card is provided at the beginning of Part III.

TEACHER ADMINISTRATIVE ISSUES

Assignments and Attendance

The rules for requiring homework and attendance should be consistent with school policy and with the rules for other courses taken by students. Because the DBT STEPS-A curriculum structure utilizes a "tell, show, do" procedure, missed classes are difficult for a student to make up because the student hasn't received the "show" or demonstration part of the skills covered in those classes. However, students do get sick or miss class from time to time, so having a plan in place to help students learn the missed skills and complete the missed homework is important. Consistent with DBT STEPS-A, students often learn best from one another, and

Scale for determining effectiveness of the skills used: **Name:** Joe Jones **Date started:** 5/15/2015

0 = Not thought about or used	4 = **Tried, could do it/them, but they didn't help**
1 = Thought about, not used, didn't want to	5 = **Tried, could use it/them, helped**
2 = Thought about, not used, wanted to	6 = **Didn't think about it, used it/them, didn't help**
3 = Tried but couldn't use it/them	7 = **Didn't think about it, used it/ them, helped**

NS = **Have not learned the skill**

Circle Days Practiced								DBT STEPS-A Skills	Weekly Skills Use Rating/Comments
								MINDFULNESS	
M	T	W	Th	F	Sa	Su		1. Wise mind (balance between emotion mind and reasonable mind)	5, worked
M	T	W	Th	F	Sa	Su		2. Observe (just noticing the experience)—one of the "what" skills	4, too distracted
M	T	W	Th	F	Sa	Su		3. Describe (putting words to the experience)—one of the "what" skills	
M	T	W	Th	F	Sa	Su		4. Participate (throwing yourself completely into it)—one of the "what" skills	
M	T	W	Th	F	Sa	Su		5. Nonjudgmentally (seeing but not evaluating; just the facts)—one of the "how" skills	3, always judging
M	T	W	Th	F	Sa	Su		6. One-mindfully (being completely present)—one of the "how" skills	4, distracted
M	T	W	Th	F	Sa	Su		7. Effectively (focusing on what works)—one of the "how" skills	
								DISTRESS TOLERANCE	
M	T	W	Th	F	Sa	Su		8. ACCEPTS (Activities, Contributing, Comparisons, Emotions, Pushing away, Thoughts, Sensations)	
M	T	W	Th	F	Sa	Su		9. IMPROVE (Imagery, Meaning, Prayer, Relaxation, One thing in the moment, Vacation, Encouragement)	
M	T	W	Th	F	Sa	Su		10. Self-Soothe (with five senses, plus movement)	
M	T	W	Th	F	Sa	Su		11. TIP (Temperature, Intense exercise, Paced breathing)	5, worked
M	T	W	Th	F	Sa	Su		12. Pros and cons	5, pretty helpful
M	T	W	Th	F	Sa	Su		13. Radical acceptance (freedom from suffering requires acceptance) ≠ approval	
M	T	W	Th	F	Sa	Su		14. Turning the mind (to the acceptance road); willingness (doing just what is needed)	
M	T	W	Th	F	Sa	Su		15. Mindfulness of current thoughts	

FIGURE 2.1. Partial example of a filled-out DBT STEPS-A Skills Daily Diary Card.

thus the teacher should assign a classmate who understands or has demonstrated the particular skills well to help the student who missed the material in class.

Grades

The grading for the DBT STEPS-A class should be consistent with the grading policies of the school and with those of similar classes (e.g., health). Because the DBT STEPS-A class focuses on skill acquisition and practice, it is recommended that the grading structure reflect the effort made in acquiring and practicing the skills. There are four distinct areas that lend themselves to grading: homework completion, scores on the tests given after each module, class participation, and weekly diary cards. Each of these areas is discussed next.

Homework Completion

Homework assignments primarily consist of practicing the skill (or skills) learned during class and recording that practice on the homework sheet (or sheets). Thus there are no right and wrong answers; rather, the emphasis is on trying the skills in different environments. There is a homework review section early in each lesson: As described earlier, the instructor asks about the previous lesson's assignment, and there are dyadic or small-group discussions of the successes and/or challenges of the homework, which are then shared with the entire class. Based on the regular homework review discussions and the successes or challenges each student reports, the instructor should be able to make a reasonable estimate of the effort each student has put into homework. This area of grading is relatively subjective.

Scores on the Module Tests

Tests are given at the ends of the Distress Tolerance, Emotion Regulation, and Interpersonal Effectiveness modules. These three tests, plus their answer keys, are provided at the end of Part II (following the lesson plans). Exam questions for the Mindfulness module are built into these three exams since mindfulness skills are taught throughout the course. These are knowledge-based tests, in which students are asked to describe some of the skills learned and the situations in which they can be used. The exams consist of questions with short answers, brief essays, fill-in-the-blank items, and multiple-choice items. The majority of the items have right and wrong answers, and guidance for what the short essays should include is provided in the answer keys. The tests are thus well suited for grading purposes.

Student Participation

Because DBT STEPS-A is a participatory curriculum, it is essential to get students involved and participating in the class exercises, homework, and small-group discussions, as well as in filling out their diary cards. Thus we believe that class participation should be weighted heavily in the overall course grade, even though it is subjective.

There are numerous places within DBT STEPS-A where participation is structured and allows for evaluation. These include the mindfulness exercises that begin each class, the homework reviews (which, again, are often done in dyads or small groups, with outcomes presented to the class as a whole), and the teaching of the new materials. In teaching new content, the instructor relies on class participation for reading handouts, conducting class exercises, providing personal examples, and asking clarifying questions. These different opportunities for student participation should give the instructor a good amount of information in this area for grading purposes.

Diary Cards

The diary cards are the last component in evaluating students taking the DBT STEPS-A class. As described above, the students use the diary cards to log their skills practice, along with their successes and challenges in implementing the skills, over the course of the class. Because diary cards are collected once a week (or twice a week if the class is taught twice per week), they allow the instructor to see what skills students are trying to implement and how successful they have been in implementing those particular skills. Continuous monitoring of diary cards tells the instructor how well students are developing and implementing skills outside the classroom.

Lack of Satisfactory Progress in DBT STEPS-A

When a student is making unsatisfactory progress in the DBT STEPS-A class, the procedures used should be similar to those used in other courses. However, learning and practicing skills in a DBT STEPS-A class are not as dependent on sequential learning as they are in a math or a language class. If a student didn't perform well in the first half of the DBT STEPS-A class, he or she can still become engaged and learn valuable information during the second half. Thus students should be encouraged to remain in the DBT STEPS-A class, with a reminder that it is likely to be the only class that allows them to set up their own personalized goals and receive course credit for practicing to make better decisions.

Credits Applied to Graduation

The DBT STEPS-A class should be viewed like other courses within the school curriculum, and therefore students completing this class should receive a designated course credit that is applied toward graduation. Schools have been recently criticized for equating education only with academics, as indicated by the sharply increased emphasis on high-stakes testing and statewide academic standards (Mazza & Hanson, 2014a). However, such a restricted definition of education ignores the relationship between academic learning and social–emotional well-being (CASEL, 2013; Cook et al., 2010). Thus providing credit for the DBT STEPS-A class helps schools broaden their impact by educating the "whole child"—that is, combining the teaching of academics with the development of good decision making, emotion regulation, and interpersonal skills. As discussed in Chapter 1, several states are recognizing the importance of SEL curricula as an integral part of education and are beginning to establish statewide standards in this area.

Schools have increased responsibilities to ensure the safety and well-being of their students. With the increased focus on bullying, school shootings, and student mental health, providing students with skills for surviving encounters with very difficult emotional situations and events needs to become part of the education process and deserves credit applied toward graduation.

SPECIAL RULES FOR DBT STEPS-A SKILLS CLASSES

Although the general classroom rules or guidelines for the DBT STEPS-A class should be consistent with those for other courses within the school, several rules that apply to this particular class are likely to be unique. Most of these guidelines are covered in the Orientation lesson (Lesson 1; see Handout 1.1), and they need to be enforced so that all students can feel safe and participate in the class. Some of the most important guidelines and related issues are discussed in detail below.

Being Nonjudgmental

An absolutely essential DBT STEPS-A guideline is this: "Be nonjudgmental: No put-downs. Abusive language and behavior will not be tolerated." The reason this guideline is so important is that one of the most challenging issues an instructor is likely to face in teaching the DBT STEPS-A curriculum is classroom-interfering behavior by students. Most instructors have experienced this before; however, the personal nature of the class and some of the likely disclosures make it important to stop or reduce any teasing or bullying. Students need to feel that the class environment is safe and nonjudgmental in order to share personal issues.

Addressing such behaviors is not as straightforward as it may appear. Because the DBT STEPS-A lessons are packed with content and have specified time allocations, reacting to and addressing every problem behavior will not be realistic or practical. In groups where DBT skills have been implemented, instructors report that they ignore roughly 90% of interfering behaviors. The other 10% are addressed by using more individualized strategies, such as a tap on the shoulder or a nonverbal gesture that does not draw the attention of the entire group. Alternatively, problem behavior can be used as an opportunity for the student to practice a skill—ideally, the skill being taught. This is where the experience of the instructor plays a major role in managing classroom-interfering behaviors. If in-class individualized strategies do not appear to be working, then it may be necessary to see the particular student or students after class.

Some student behavior may become so problematic that the skills are not getting taught to the other students. In such a case, the instructor needs to use his or her experience to determine whether the student exhibiting this behavior can remain in the class. The one exception may be that if the student's interfering behavior is due to a lack of skills or emotional dysregulation, then removing the student from the very class that is going to teach him or her the skills and allow for practice and coaching doesn't make a lot of sense. However, this decision will depend on the instructor's ability to minimize the interfering behavior until the student learns to use the skills. The instructor may want to consult with other instructors or administrators before making the decision to remove a student from the classroom because of behavioral issues.

Confidentiality

The confidentiality rule in DBT STEPS-A is as follows: "What is discussed in the class stays in the class. Information about other people in the class may be private and should be respected." This rule is intended to discourage students from disclosing other students' personal and private information to a third party. Confidentiality and respect are essential to students' being willing to share personal situations in the DBT STEPS-A class where the skills can be applied. Students will be less likely to share an emotional struggle if they know it will be shared with others not in the class—or, even worse, be put on a social media website like Facebook. The DBT STEPS-A curriculum is designed around, and depends upon, students' ability to rely on one another as supports and coaches when they are learning and applying their new skills to personal situations. Peer support builds trust, which facilitates a willingness to share further personal struggles. The more students can personalize the class, the more effective the skills and practice will be for them as individuals. Therefore, the belief that whatever a student shares in the class will be broadcast to everyone else in the school and beyond undermines a central foundation on which the DBT STEPS-A curriculum was developed.

However, it is important to note that confidentiality cannot be rigidly or completely enforced. Therefore, students are also encouraged to be mindful about what personal information they share in the class with peers, as there are no guarantees that other students will keep the information private. The instructor may highlight the dialectical nature of this situation, because the instructor is also encouraged to remind the students of the importance of respecting one another and keeping everyone's information private during each module. The instructor should emphasize that class confidentiality is a "win–win" situation for everyone in the class because it facilitates discussions, peer support, and peer coaching.

Use of the Term "Target Behavior"

There are three reasons for the guideline of asking students to use the term "target behavior." (The full guideline is as follows: "We will identify target behaviors for each of us that you are willing to work on increasing or decreasing in class. We will refer to these identified behaviors as 'target behaviors' in class, rather than naming the specific behaviors themselves.") As described in Lesson 1, this rule is intended to help students stay focused and pay attention. If one student's target behavior is different from those of other students, the other students may think that the discussion is not relevant for them. Yet different problem behaviors can have the same purposes in helping to increase or decrease emotions.

A second reason not to identify target behaviors is to prevent discussion of risky behaviors (e.g., substance use, sexual behaviors, self-harm or suicidal behaviors). This may make others in the class anxious and emotionally vulnerable—the opposite of what the DBT STEPS-A class is intended to do. The rule is based on research (Gould, Greenberg, Velting, & Schaffer, 2003; Miller, 2011) showing that adolescents appear susceptible to a contagion effect when they hear of peers' risky behaviors. This rule reduces the likelihood of such contagion. If a student does break this rule, the instructor should remind him or her (along with the entire class) that the rule exists because the skills can be applied to everyone's target behaviors, regardless of what these are. It is important to note that this rule only applies to class discussions. Students can list their specific target behaviors on Handout 1.2 in Lesson 1 because the individual handouts are not shared with the class. Finally, the third reason for this rule is to help maintain the students' confidentiality among peers by not having the students share problems that may be too personal for school. As mentioned above in the discussion of the confidentiality guideline, privacy cannot be guaranteed; therefore, this is another step toward assisting students in maintaining their own privacy.

SPECIAL ISSUES FOR DBT STEPS-A INSTRUCTORS

It is important that the instructor be aware not just of students' progress, but of the possibility that problematic student behaviors may emerge over the course of the class. There are several noteworthy behaviors that the instructor should monitor, and some of them are difficult to determine without directly asking the students. These behaviors include but are not limited to drug and alcohol use, suicidal behaviors, and self-harming behaviors. Each of these behaviors is discussed in greater detail in the following sections. Table 2.1 shows common warning signs for each behavior. All three of these types of at-risk behaviors require that a student trust the instructor enough to disclose them. Yet disclosing drug use, for example, usually results in disciplinary action, which would discourage further student self-disclosures. If students are going to be honest with the instructor, then providing them with support and as much reassurance as possible is warranted.

Alcohol and Drug Use

Most general school rules state that students are not to be in school under the influence of alcohol or drugs. This rule deserves mentioning here because the DBT STEPS-A class focuses on emotional stressors within each student's life. The personalized nature of the class and disclosure of difficult situations may raise a student's level of anxiety or feelings of being judged, for which the student may self-medicate through drinking or getting high before class. If a student does come to class drunk or high, a discussion between the instructor and the student should take place privately. School policy may require the student to be suspended or expelled; however, this type of consequence for poor decision making removes him or her from the one class dedicated to better decision making. One alternative to addressing a student's first offense is an "in-school" suspension, with the requirement that the student must attend his or her DBT STEPS-A class as part of the suspension. If a second offense occurs, standard school discipline rules should be applied.

The issue of dealing drugs is more problematic, as the student is encouraging or promoting the use of drugs by other students. This type of behavior makes it very difficult for individuals who have engaged in past drug use or who have current urges to use. In addition, selling drugs to other students reinforces poor decision making and creates opportunities for other students to become emotionally dysregulated—the exact opposite of what the DBT STEPS-A

TABLE 2.1. Common Warning Signs of Suicidal Behavior, Self-Harming Behavior, and Alcohol or Drug Use

Suicidal behavior	Self-harming behavior	Alcohol or drug use
1. Thoughts about suicide	1. Unexplained cuts, bruises, or burns	1. Severe mood swings
2. Drug/alcohol use	2. Drug and/or alcohol use	2. Extreme defiance
3. Withdrawal	3. Isolation from peers	3. Running away
4. Sudden change in behavior	4. Symptoms of depression	4. Engaging in self-harming behavior
5. Dramatic drop in school grades	5. Change in eating habits	5. Doing poorly in school
6. Anxiety	6. Low self-esteem	6. Sudden change in behavior and/or mood
7. Sense of hopelessness		7. Illegal behaviors
8. Feeling trapped		

curriculum is trying to teach. If a student is identified as dealing drugs, we recommend the removal of this student from the DBT STEPS-A class in order to foster a safe, nonjudgmental environment and to reduce the urges of other classmates to use drugs.

Suicidal Behaviors

Adolescent suicidal behaviors are much more prevalent than many instructors may think, and they may come to light over the course of a DBT STEPS-A class. Plans and strategies for how to handle a student's disclosure of suicidal or other self-harming behaviors should be in place at the beginning of the school year.

"Suicidal behavior" is an inclusive term for a continuum of behaviors: thoughts about death and suicide ("suicidal ideation"), suicidal intent, suicide attempts, and death by suicide (Mazza & Reynolds, 2008). Adolescents will disclose this information when being asked by a caring, nonjudgmental adult, and thus instructors should not be afraid to ask students direct questions about suicidal behavior. Asking questions about suicidal behavior does *not* increase suicidal behavior, nor does it put ideas in students' minds (Gould et al., 2005). If an adolescent does self-disclose recent suicidal behavior, then the next important step is to have an assessment conducted by a professional trained in suicide risk assessment. Most general education teachers do not receive this formal training; such teachers should check to see whether the school psychologist, school social worker, school nurse, or school counselor has completed this training. Some school policies require that school officials (i.e., teachers, school psychologists, counselors) call the local hospital for an immediate medical evaluation, and stipulate that the student cannot return to school until given medical clearance. It is important to know the specific school and district policies with regard to these behaviors. If the risk assessment indicates that the student's suicidal risk level is moderate to low, and if the student is being monitored by a mental health professional, then allowing him or her to participate in the class becomes very important. The DBT STEPS-A curriculum will teach at-risk students the skills and strategies to tolerate their distress and manage their emotions more effectively, which will probably lead to a decrease in suicidal behavior. If a student's risk level is determined to be high or imminent, then following the school procedures is the necessary course of action.

Self-Harming Behaviors

The issues with self-harming behavior are similar to those with suicidal behavior. If a teacher becomes aware that a student is engaging in self-harming behavior, the student should be referred to the school mental health professional for a suicide risk assessment and possible referral for mental health services. There is a strong relationship between self-harming behavior and suicidal behavior, and an adolescent may be engaging in both. As with suicidal behavior, adolescents engaged in self-harming behavior can benefit from the DBT STEPS-A curriculum, and should be encouraged to remain in the class and participate. Often adolescents who engage in nonsuicidal self-injurious behavior are trying to escape emotional pain by experiencing physical pain. Self-cutting and other forms of self-harm can function as forms of emotion regulation. The emotion regulation skills taught in DBT STEPS-A provide healthier alternatives.

CHAPTER 3

Teaching DBT STEPS-A
to Challenging Students

The DBT STEPS-A curriculum is designed to be taught at the universal level of general education, meaning that its content and structure are intended for all students. However, we know that some students require more structure and time than can be delivered at the universal level. These students may be already identified by the school as struggling with emotional and/or behavioral problems, and may be receiving services for academic or mental health issues. Others may be in separate programs or classes to meet their special education needs, and may learn new material more slowly than their peers do. In teaching the DBT STEPS-A curriculum, instructors need to account for these challenges. Such students may need additional support and strategies to help them acquire and practice the intended skills.

THE RESPONSE-TO-INTERVENTION FRAMEWORK

Many schools have structured their assessment and delivery of support and services according to a multi-tiered systems of support (MTSS) model, whether the students' needs are academic or social–emotional (Cook et al., 2015). Response to intervention (RTI) is one such MTSS model that is used in educational settings to meet academic and social–emotional needs. Within the RTI framework, different levels of support are provided, depending on the severity of the academic concerns involved. For example, students who may need some added support in math or reading are categorized as receiving Tier 2 services. In contrast, students who require individualized instruction or intensive support, such as an IEP, are categorized as receiving Tier 3 services. Figure 3.1 illustrates a continuum of educational services within an RTI delivery model. It is important to note that the continuum of services does not end in general education after Tier 3. Rather, it continues within the classification of special education, depending on the results of a comprehensive assessment. The first three tiers of intensified services within special education parallel the general education tiers; that is, these spe-

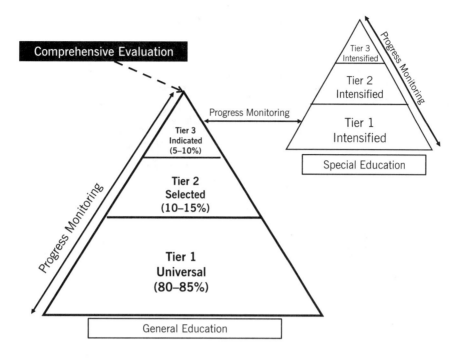

FIGURE 3.1. Continuum of educational services within an RTI delivery model. Adapted from Cook (personal communication, 2014). Used by permission of Clayton R. Cook.

cial education tiers are also numbered as Tiers 1, 2, and 3, ranked according to the intensity and level of support they provide.

BEYOND SPECIAL EDUCATION TIER 3

Although the system of educational support services does not end at special education Tier 3, most schools do not have the trained personnel and resources to provide services beyond Tier 3 within their buildings. Placements in alternative schools (considered Tier 4) and residential treatment schools (Tier 5) are also on the continuum of services, with hospitalization being the most intensive support service at Tier 6.

The continuum of special education support services within an RTI model provides a framework for developing a parallel model that can be applied to mental health services for students. The special education continuum has primarily focused on services for students' academic needs, yet recent work in the area of school-based mental health (SBMH) services along a similar continuum using an MTSS approach has shown great promise (Cook, 2015). Combining the special education tiered levels of supports that focus on academic needs with SBMH services addressing mental health and behavioral needs will provide a service delivery system that is balanced and serves the "whole child." Figure 3.2 shows an MTSS model that accounts for academic and social–emotional needs and services from Tier 1 to Tier 6. In addition, Figure 3.2 accounts for the relationships between academic and social–emotional difficulties, in a manner consistent with the literature (Cook, 2015).

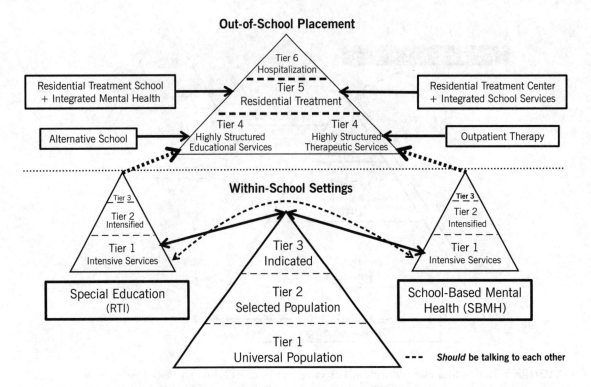

FIGURE 3.2. Overall continuum of services within an MTSS model.

DBT STEPS-A WITHIN AN MTSS

As discussed above, DBT STEPS-A is designed for students at the Tier 1 or universal level, and is intended to be delivered within general education settings. Approximately 80–85% of students are at Tier 1, meaning that they don't need any services other than those being provided in the general education curriculum. Students at the Tier 2 or selected level (10–15% of students) are those who need some additional support for their academic and/or social–emotional needs. Thus these students receive DBT STEPS-A in a smaller class setting, plus some additional services to supplement the DBT STEPS-A curriculum. Students at the Tier 3 or indicated level (5–10% of students) need much more intensive services and supports, and may be placed within the special education system or may have IEPs. These students receive DBT STEPS-A in the smaller class setting similar to Tier 2 students, plus additional support and intensified services.

According to the MTSS model, 15–20% of students may need additional supports with their emotion management issues, problem solving, interpersonal relationships, or decision-making skills even after receiving DBT STEPS-A. Thus we have provided supplemental strategies that can be used in conjunction with DBT STEPS-A for students who need Tier 2 or Tier 3 services within the general education framework. These supplemental strategies are discussed below.

STRATEGIES FOR WORKING WITH STUDENTS AT TIERS 2 AND 3 IN GENERAL EDUCATION

Before we discuss specific strategies in working with students at Tiers 2 and 3, we empha-size the importance of having the appropriate school personnel in place to teach the DBT STEPS-A curriculum at these levels, while also providing the necessary support services. Thus we recommend that the instructors for DBT STEPS-A classes of students at Tiers 2 and 3 be school counselors, school psychologists, social workers, or other school personnel with extensive training in adolescent mental health issues. This recommendation is in contrast to our recommendation for teachers of students at Tier 1, which is for general education teachers (e.g., health teachers) who have some mental health background. Because students who need services at Tiers 2 and 3 are already more likely to have been identified with mental health concerns or to have engaged in at-risk behaviors, having school professionals who are trained in working with such students teach these DBT STEPS-A classes and provide the supportive services and strategies is strongly recommended.

Strategies for Tier 2 Students

Support strategies to bolster the strength of the DBT STEPS-A curriculum for students at Tier 2 include but are not limited to the following. First, the size of the class should be smaller, probably no more than 10–15 students. A smaller class provides students with more oppor-tunities to practice and receive feedback on their skill practice. Because the instructor is monitoring fewer students during homework review, there is a greater likelihood that each student will receive feedback and coaching on his or her skill practice. In addition, a smaller class size will increase students' participation during the teaching of the lessons and will give them more opportunities to ask questions.

Second, the DBT STEPS-A curriculum may need to be adjusted to fit these students' needs. For example, slower learners may benefit from two cycles through the curriculum, rather than the one recommended for Tier 1 students. A second cycle through the curriculum gives students additional opportunities to learn all the skills, as well as additional practice time. The two-cycle strategy is sometimes used in DBT skills groups for adolescent outpatients (Rathus & Miller, 2015). A second alternative may be to slow down the pace of the class by splitting the content of one lesson over two or more class periods, depending on the students' needs.

Finally, we recommend that the instructor offer individual coaching as needed to stu-dents who are experiencing emotionally stressful situations. This recommendation, of course, is dependent on the instructor's availability. Such coaching can provide Tier 2 students with assistance regarding what skills to use during an emotionally stressful event, as well as oppor-tunities to role-play what to say or do. It is important for the instructor to inform each student when coaching is available during the school day and under what circumstances the student may ask for coaching.

Strategies for Tier 3 Students

Tier 3 students in the DBT STEPS-A curriculum need the same strategies as those described above for Tier 2 students: a smaller class size; an instructor with extensive training in adolescent mental health issues; a second cycle through the curriculum, or a slower pacing of lessons; and individual coaching. In addition, they need some further strategies that include but are not limited to the following.

First, unlike Tier 2 students (who receive as-needed coaching), every Tier 3 student should receive weekly in-school individual coaching, monitoring, and mentoring from the instructor. This strategy helps the instructor stay up to date on the specific issues and stressors each student is currently experiencing. This designated period is not for therapy, but rather for skill practice and individual coaching; it can range from 15 to 45 minutes, depending on the instructor's availability. It is important to emphasize that this individual coaching is not considered to be individual psychotherapy.

The second strategy is facilitating a group consisting of parents and their Tier 3 sons and daughters in the DBT STEPS-A class. This group should meet once or twice a month during the evening. The rationale behind this strategy is threefold. First, it can help parents understand the skills being taught in the DBT STEPS-A curriculum and the rationales for these skills. Second, it can teach parents how to support their children during difficult times, and can increase support in the home environment for both students and their parents. Finally, parents can have opportunities to support one another in the challenges of having children with social–emotional learning difficulties. Multifamily parent–child groups have been used successfully as part of comprehensive DBT for adolescent outpatients (Mehlum et al., 2014; Miller et al., 2007). For details on how to facilitate these parent groups, see Rathus and Miller (2015).

The third strategy is a DBT STEPS-A instructor/teacher consultation team, made up of all school personnel who are teaching and/or supporting DBT STEPS-A for students at Tier 3. This team should meet every 1–2 weeks to discuss students' progress or difficulty, as well as the skills and strategies particular students are learning; to enable instructors working with challenging students to support each other; and to provide a mechanism for sharing information about what has worked well and what has not. Team consultation is a formal component of comprehensive DBT and has been shown to keep treatment on track, to provide opportunities for collegial supervision and support, and to reduce burnout. The team consultation meetings can take place before or after school, if team members' schedules are so hectic that finding a suitable time during the school day is impossible. The meetings can last 45–90 minutes, depending on the needs of the team (Sayrs & Linehan, in press).

SERVICES WITHIN TIERS 1–3 OF SBMH

It is important to note that even with all the supportive DBT STEPS-A strategies we've described, there are likely to be students at Tier 3 in general education who need more intensive services. Fortunately, the MTSS model provides a continuum of services that can be applied specifically to DBT skills training and other DBT services with this high-risk population of students. Figure 3.3 illustrates a modified MTSS model with the different levels of DBT services at Tier 1–6. As mentioned earlier in this chapter and depicted in Figure 3.3, beyond the three tiers in general education is a second set of school-based services for social–emotional needs under the classification of SBMH, which parallels the special education classification on the academic side. Within the SBMH classification are intensified DBT services for Tiers 1–3. We recommend that instructors providing these services use Miller et

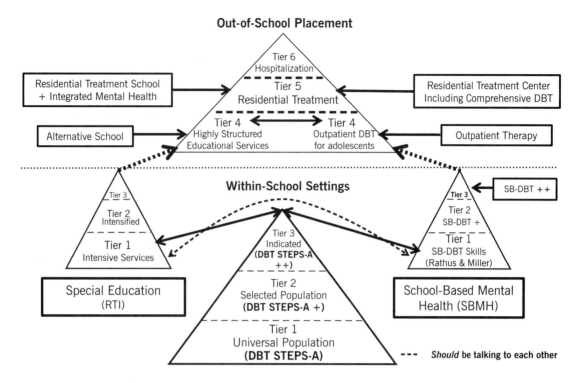

FIGURE 3.3. Continuum of DBT services within an MTSS model.

al.'s (2007) *Dialectical Behavior Therapy with Suicidal Adolescents* and Rathus and Miller's (2015) *DBT Skills Manual for Adolescents*, rather than the DBT STEPS-A curriculum.

The rationale for using the *DBT Skills Manual for Adolescents* (Rathus & Miller, 2015) within the SBMH tiers, instead of using DBT STEPS-A, has several components. First, the *DBT Skills Manual for Adolescents* allows for weekly meetings of 90–120 minutes, versus the 50-minute lessons for DBT STEPS-A. Second, an instructor of a DBT skills group within the SBMH tiers should be someone who is DBT-trained, and thus is able to provide more in-depth and possibly more precise strategies and support for students. Third, the diary cards in the *DBT Skills Manual for Adolescents* include the individualized target behaviors and goals, and thus become part of the individual DBT sessions between a mental health professional and a student. Finally, the *DBT Skills Manual for Adolescents* implements Walking the Middle Path, a fifth skills module that is also included in *Dialectical Behavior Therapy with Suicidal Adolescents* (Miller et al., 2007). This module includes parents and focuses on teaching students and parents alike ways to think and act more dialectically (e.g., less black-and-white thinking and acting); principles of reinforcement (e.g., positive and negative reinforcement and the use of effective punishment) for the purpose of effectively influencing the behavior of others; and ways to validate others and oneself more effectively.

It is beyond the scope of the present book to provide the comprehensive details of intensified DBT support services at SBMH Tiers 1–3. However, it is important to note that several schools and school districts around the United States have implemented school-based individual DBT treatment sessions/coaching and DBT skills training groups (collectively referred to as SB-DBT) successfully, and continue to do so. These include Lincoln High School (Portland, Oregon), Pleasantville High School (Pleasantville, New York), the City School District of New Rochelle (New Rochelle, New York), and the Ardsley Union Free School District (Ardsley, New York), to name a few.

These schools and school districts have successfully implemented SB-DBT with subgroups of their high-risk students who either were on the verge of being sent out of a district due to increasing emotional needs, or were requiring increasing amounts of time from school personnel (psychologists, social workers, and administrators) due to emotional and behavioral difficulties that were not being adequately addressed within the current school structure. The staff members at these schools received formal training and ongoing consultation from expert DBT therapists/consultants, who covered the different components of comprehensive SB-DBT: (1) skills training group, (2) individual therapy/counseling, (3) in-school coaching as needed, (4) DBT school staff consultation team meetings, and (5) parent skills training and family therapy/counseling sessions as needed. Studies investigating this comprehensive school-based DBT model are ongoing, with pilot data showing that high-risk students in these schools are responding well to this model and that staff members are reporting feeling empowered again in working with these high-needs students (Miller et al., 2014). These outcomes constitute a "win–win" situation for everyone.

DBT SKILLS AND SERVICES BEYOND SCHOOL SETTINGS

It is important for school psychologists, counselors, and social workers to recognize the limitations of their skills and training, especially if a student's identified needs are beyond what the general educational setting can provide. For schools with high-risk students, we suggest the use of a team approach to identify the students who require more intensive services in different areas, and then to determine which placement is most appropriate for each individual. If a referral is made for outpatient therapy to a community mental health agency or other outpatient provider (Tier 4), then providing supplementary support services at the school will be important. If the referral is for a residential treatment center/therapeutic boarding school (Tier 5) or hospitalization (Tier 6), a facility that provides comprehensive DBT for high-risk adolescents (Miller et al., 2007) will be ideal because the student already has been exposed to the skills and language of DBT. Such a placement will provide continuity of care for the student and will build on previous learning and successes. In addition, students who receive comprehensive DBT in their out-of-school placement can make the transition back into a regular school at Tier 3, using the same language and strategies for their behavior.

PART II

INSTRUCTOR INFORMATION, LESSON PLANS, AND TESTS

The information in Part II is provided for instructors or teachers of the DBT STEPS-A curriculum. Within this section are the 30 different lesson plans for the students, as well as the three module tests and their respective answer keys.

LESSON 1

Orientation

SUMMARY

The purpose of the first lesson is to have the students get to know each other and become oriented to the format, guidelines, and general underlying principles of the DBT STEPS-A class and curriculum.

MATERIALS

1. Handouts for this lesson:
   - Handout 1.1. General Guidelines
   - Handout 1.2. Goals of DBT STEPS-A
   - Handout 1.3. Options for Solving Any Problem
   - Handout 1.4. Class Schedule
2. Skills binder for each student and pens or pencils as needed or students to take notes.
3. Materials for the Word Scramble class cohesion-building exercise (see below): Letters on different colors of paper, plus the letter chart (see Figure L1.1).

PREPARATION

1. Review student handouts for this lesson (these may be put in the students' binders).
2. Review the class schedule on Handout 1.4, and make adjustments if necessary to meet the needs of your class.
3. Arrange the desks in the classroom, if possible, so that students are able to see each other.

LESSON OVERVIEW AND TIMELINE

- Introduction of class and DBT STEPS-A curriculum (30 minutes)
  - Review of Handout 1.1. General Guidelines (5 minutes)
    - Nonjudgmental classroom behavior

- o Confidentiality and respect
- o Definition/use of the term "target behavior"
  - ■ Review of Handout 1.2. Goals of DBT STEPS-A (10 minutes)
    - o Defining "dialectical"
    - o Difficulty managing emotions (emotion regulation skills)
    - o Confusion/distraction (mindfulness skills)
    - o Impulsiveness (distress tolerance skills)
    - o Relationship problems (interpersonal effectiveness skills)
    - o Identifying behavior goals
  - ■ Review of Handout 1.3. Options for Solving Any Problem (5 minutes)
  - ■ Review of Handout 1.4. Class Schedule (2 minutes)
  - ■ Review of grading criteria (3 minutes)
  - ■ Questions (5 minutes)
- • Class cohesion-building exercise: Word Scramble (20 minutes)
  - ■ Each student draws a letter from a bag or basket (refer to the class cohesion exercise chart, Figure L1.1).
  - ■ Students are placed in groups based on the color of paper in which their letter is printed. Students in each group introduce themselves and share one thing from their most recent school break or holiday.
  - ■ Students work together to unscramble their word or words.

DETAILED LESSON PLAN

Introduction of Class and DBT STEPS-A Curriculum (30 minutes)

Welcome students to the class. Put your name on the board. Have students introduce themselves, with each student saying his or her name, and what grade the student is in at school (if applicable and if he or she wishes).

Explain what the class will be about, saying something like this. (Note that here and throughout the Part II lesson plans, suggestions for what to say to students are given in italics.)

This class teaches practical decision-making and coping skills to use both inside and outside the classroom. Briefly, this means we are going to learn skills that we can use in order to be more effective in our lives, especially when our emotions are a part of the equation. Can any of you think of a time or situation when you had an intense emotion and you did something as a result of having that emotion? For example, you were really angry at one of your parents for not allowing you to stay out longer at your friend's house on a Friday, so in response you yelled at your parent, slammed the door, and walked out, or you hung up the phone on your parent. Do you think you would have responded that way if your anger was not so high or was in control?

Elicit other examples from students.

So these are examples of what we are going to learn in this class. We are going to learn how to be aware when our emotions are making our decisions. We call this "emotion mind," and we will learn a lot more about emotion mind in the next few weeks. As we go through the first few handouts today, I will explain in a lot more detail the topics we will address. This is also a class where we will expect everyone to participate a lot. This will include reading the handouts, doing the homework activities, and helping each other out.

Pass out the binders or sets of student handouts.

Review of Handout 1.1. General Guidelines (5 minutes)

Have students turn to Handout 1.1. Explain that general school rules and guidelines apply to this class, just as they do to other classes. Then read through items 1 and 2.

NONJUDGMENTAL CLASSROOM BEHAVIOR

Read item 3: "Be nonjudgmental: No put-downs. Abusive language or behavior will not be tolerated." Explain:

The same rules apply in this class as they do in all of your classes. However, here we are going to work specifically on being nonjudgmental and supportive of each other. This means respect for each other and no put-downs.

CONFIDENTIALITY AND RESPECT

Read item 4: "What is discussed in the class stays in the class. Information about other people in the class may be private and should be respected." Explain:

I hope you will use the skills you learn here in your lives outside this classroom. Much of the homework is about applying skills to help you solve problems and make better decisions. So when we discuss homework in class or otherwise use examples, you may discuss personal issues or problems you are having. We cannot ensure respect and confidentiality for anyone, but we can discuss it and explain reasons we would want both of these values for each other in this class.

You can state:

I am going to be asking all of you to participate and to provide examples of problems you may be working on as teaching examples. I want everyone to feel comfortable sharing information, but no one will be comfortable if what they share is going to be the next big thing on Facebook, Twitter, or any other social media site and be all over the school (and the world!). We expect courtesy, respect, and trust. We want to create a safe and nonjudgmental environment for being able to share personal struggles and successes, without fear of repercussions for sharing. Therefore, please do not talk about other students' individual examples outside this class. This does not mean that you need to refrain from discussing the skills we are learning in here with other people. If there is something you are worried about sharing about yourself, then it is OK to use your best judgment not to share that information, and to find examples that you are comfortable with other people knowing about.

DEFINITION/USE OF THE TERM "TARGET BEHAVIOR"

Read item 5: "We will identify target behaviors for each of us . . ." You can state:

> Each of you will identify "target behaviors" that you can work on increasing and decreasing throughout the course. We will use "target behavior" as a general term, rather than any specific behavior. Behaviors to increase can include things such as studying and going to school. Behaviors to decrease can include talking back to teachers or parents, fighting, self-injury, drug or alcohol use, risky sexual behaviors, or bullying behaviors.
>
> One reason why we use this term is to help everyone stay focused and pay attention. Although someone else's target behavior may be different from yours, often the behaviors have the same purpose. By this, I mean that we often do these behaviors as a way to change how we are feeling—to either increase or decrease an emotion. For example, you have a huge test in science tomorrow, and you are anxious about it. Every time you look at your books to start studying, you become overwhelmed. Next you decide to work on your math homework or to watch TV for a while, and your anxiety goes down. Avoidance helps with the anxiety, but it's not helping you prepare to pass the test. However, if someone else describes his or her struggle as "fighting with my parents every time I get angry because they won't let me go out on the weekends," we don't want you to stop paying attention in how to reduce your emotion just because someone else is talking about a different type of anxiety. The skills that person is using will probably be helpful to you too. In this class, you can learn other ways to reduce anxiety or other emotions, so it's easier to increase your ability to study or tolerate your urges to not yell at your parents. We are going to develop your list of behaviors to change in a few minutes, so I want you to start thinking about it.

Review of Handout 1.2. Goals of DBT STEPS-A (10 minutes)

DEFINING "DIALECTICAL"

Students should turn to Handout 1.2. Explain the full name of DBT STEPS-A: Dialectical Behavior Therapy Skills Training for Emotional Problem Solving for Adolescents. Then briefly define "dialectical":

> We will delve into what "dialectical" means next week. For now, I will just say that it means that there are different ways of looking at any situation, and no single view holds the complete truth. Another way of saying it is that thinking dialectically gets us out of being stuck in extremes, like black-or-white thinking. Anyone here ever get stuck in black-or-white, or all-or-nothing, thinking? Anybody ever tell their parents or friends that they "never listen to you" or "always make you do things their way"?

Ask for a show of hands.

> OK, we will talk more about this in the next class. I just wanted to give you a brief introduction, as it will help us move on to the next topic. There are four main areas where teenagers tend to have problems, and there are four sets of skills that we are going to learn to assist us in these areas.

DIFFICULTY MANAGING EMOTIONS (EMOTION REGULATION SKILLS)

You can ask:

What do you think it means to have difficulty managing emotions? Do you ever feel like your emotions are on a rollercoaster? Maybe you were really worried about a test, and then find out you got an A on it; all of a sudden you are jumping up and down with excitement. Or maybe you received an F on the test, and now you are walking out and slamming the classroom door. Emotions can happen so fast that you are not even sure what you feel, let alone able to think about them.

Difficulty managing emotions is when your emotions are up and down and you don't know how to change them—to get them to decrease or increase as needed. It is also when your emotions are controlling your actions. On the second page of Handout 1.2, place an X on the continuum between the two extreme behaviors: "I am completely in control of my emotions and never try to push them away or change them" on the left, and "My emotions control everything I do and I cannot change them, or I don't do/have emotions" on the right. It is OK if you think that sometimes you fall on both sides of the continuum and rarely in the middle. If that is true for you, you can place two X's on the continuum to represent that for yourself.

In this class, we are going to learn a variety of emotion regulation skills that are going to teach us not only how to identify and label the different emotions we have, but also how to change our emotions and how to tolerate and experience emotions without acting on them.

CONFUSION/DISTRACTION (MINDFULNESS SKILLS)

You can ask:

What do you think it means to be confused or distracted or to be unaware or not focused?

Gather examples and write them on the board. Then say:

At some times, we all lose our focus—are not aware of what emotions we are feeling or why we are feeling them. Not being able to focus is the same as being distracted. We all also become confused about who we are and who we want to be. This is a part of growing up and becoming an adult. Have you ever questioned yourself as to whether or not you did something because you really liked it, or because someone else told you to do it, or because everyone else was doing it so you thought you should too? Confusion about yourself is when you don't always trust yourself to decide what you should be doing, thinking, or feeling. You may turn to others to tell you what to feel, do, or think, or you may watch what others are doing and follow them. You want to fit in, but you are not completely sure if they are doing what you want to be doing.

Here's another example: Maybe your parents really want you to be studious, to be athletic, or to dress in a certain way. And every morning when you get dressed and ready for school, you just don't feel comfortable in your clothes or comfortable about the activities that lie ahead, but you have always listened to what your parents tell you, so you just keep doing it. Here's the thing that is really important about this. This is all normal; it doesn't mean something is wrong with you. You are just trying to figure out who you are. That's what teenagers are supposed to do. What do you think that means?

Elicit examples from students. Then continue:

> *The great thing is that we have an entire set of skills to help you become more comfortable listening to and finding yourself. These are called "mindfulness skills," or sometimes "core mindfulness skills" because they are so important. These skills also help us to stay focused in the present moment and do less thinking about what will happen in the future or about something in the past. Also, these skills help increase our awareness of our thoughts, feelings, and urges. As the second continuum in Handout 1.2 shows, confusion or distraction about yourself can range from "I am always completely comfortable with and aware of who I am, how I think, and how I feel" on the left, to "I am not at all comfortable or aware of who I am, how I think, or how I feel" on the right. On this second continuum, put an X on the line for where you would rate yourself. You don't have to share with the rest of the class where you fall on the continuum.*

IMPULSIVENESS (DISTRESS TOLERANCE SKILLS)

You can ask:

> *What do you think "impulsiveness" means? What are some impulsive behaviors, and what leads to them?*

Write examples down on the board. If the class is struggling with ideas, add some (calling out in class, skipping class, drinking, using drugs, yelling and screaming, slamming doors, self-injuring, etc.). Then continue:

> *Sometimes we act without thinking things through, or we think we have thought them through, but it is really our emotions running the show and we may not be making the best decisions. Sometimes problems can't be solved immediately, and we have to sit with the distress until we can solve the problem. On the third continuum on Handout 1.2, place an X where you think you may fall between the two extremes: "I am always in control of my behaviors; they are never impulsive or emotion-based" versus "My behavior is always out of control and impulsive or emotion-based." You don't have to share where you marked yourself.*
>
> *We are going to learn a set of skills called "distress tolerance skills" that will help to us get through difficult crises without acting impulsively and making the situation worse. Distress can feel intolerable; these skills help make distress easier to tolerate in the moment when the problem can't be solved immediately, and also help us to accept things in our lives that we can't change either now or in the long term. As we get to each of these modules of skills, we will go into a lot more depth as to what all these skills are.*

RELATIONSHIP PROBLEMS (INTERPERSONAL EFFECTIVENESS SKILLS)

You can ask:

> *What do we mean by "relationship problems"?*

Elicit examples from students. Then continue:

> *Sometimes it can be really difficult figuring out relationships. How do you balance how much you give with what you receive from a relationship? Do any of you ever feel like you are giving too much in a relationship and then feel bad about yourselves for it?*

Elicit examples. Then go on:

> *Ever wonder if you have the right to ask for something or say no if someone asks you a favor? Maybe you're not sure how strongly to ask someone for something. How do you know when to give up and accept no? Here's the thing: All of us struggle with these issues. In this class, we'll learn a set of relationship skills called "interpersonal effectiveness skills" to give us some guidance to help get what we want from people, to help maintain healthy relationships, and to keep our self-respect. So on the fourth continuum on Handout 1.2, put an X where you fall between the two extremes: "I have great relationships; I feel great about myself in all my relationships; and I always feel comfortable asking for things and saying no" versus "My relationships are all over the place; I don't think I ever have the right to ask other people for things; and I always give people what they want because I am a bad person if I don't."*

Ask whether students have any questions up to this point. Point out:

> *All of this will make more sense when we get into learning the actual skills.*

IDENTIFYING BEHAVIOR GOALS

Identifying behavior goals can help students recognize areas where the skills can be helpful to them. At the bottom of the first page of Handout 1.2, under "Goals for DBT STEPS-A: What are your goals?", ask each student to write down at least one (and up to five) behaviors to work on increasing, and from one to five behaviors to work on decreasing. Explain that students do not have to change all of these behaviors tomorrow and that these are behaviors they can focus on over the course of the year (or semesters). They should look back on the list every so often to monitor their progress.

Review of Handout 1.3. Options for Solving Any Problem (5 minutes)

Have students turn to Handout 1.3 in their binders. You can walk the class through the following example and elicit feedback.

> *So here is what may seem like a radical idea: When you have a problem in life, there are four choices or options for how to respond to <u>any</u> problem. Those four choices or options are listed at the top of Handout 1.3. Let's walk through the four options with a couple of examples, and then if we have time, we can walk through these options with one of your examples. Here's the first example: You are failing a class, and you are very anxious about it. Let's look at the four options.*

Read through the choices.

EXAMPLE 1

The first option is that you could solve the problem. One way to do that would be to talk to your teacher about extra credit or about finding another way to bring your grade up. Any other ways you can solve this problem?

The second option is to feel better about the problem. You could tell yourself that this class is an elective and you didn't need the credit for graduation, if that is the case. With that, you may not be so worried about failing the class.

The third option is to tolerate the problem. In this option, you are accepting and tolerating that you didn't do the work, and that failing is just the natural consequence of your effort. Yes, you are worried, and you decide you are going to tolerate being worried about how failing this class will affect you over the long term.

The fourth option is to stay miserable and possibly make the situation worse. In this option, you feel so awful about failing the one class that you get angry at your teacher, you let your other grades slip, and pretty soon you are failing the whole semester.

EXAMPLE 2

It may appear in the first example that option 1, or maybe option 2 if the course really is an elective, is the best way to go. But now let's consider a different example. What if you just found out that one of your parents got a great job offer somewhere else and that you have to move to a different city and school? Let's assume that you have already tried option 1 and your parents have said no to all of your problem-solving ideas—staying with a friend so you can finish high school here, and so on. You could try option 2, but it's hard to feel better about the fact that you will need to leave all of your friends and start over in a new city. This is a situation where option 3 might be your best option—to accept and tolerate that this is where you are right now. Option 4 would be telling yourself and anyone who will listen over and over again that this is unfair and should be changed. If you continue with option 4 in the face of no chance that your parents will change their minds, you may continue to suffer and feel more miserable for the rest of your life. Plus, eventually, everyone may stop listening to you, even when things you have to say are valid and important. Although option 3 doesn't mean you won't feel any pain, it means that your long-term suffering may become less severe once you accept the situation. When we learn the skills about accepting reality, this is all likely to make more sense.

So this is really just a preview of what's to come. This is how we are going to apply all the skills we learn to our problems. This class is all about understanding the options you have and deciding how best to respond by using skillful behavior when you have a problem. Or, more specifically, this class teaches the skills you need to decide and to implement any of these options as listed at the bottom.

Review of Handout 1.4. Class Schedule (2 minutes)

Have students turn to Handout 1.4. This is a list of what skills will be taught each week. Students can use this information to read ahead to next week's material or to catch up if they missed a class. You can point out to the class that each of the four skills areas discussed earlier is listed and will be covered in a module: Mindfulness, Distress Tolerance, Emotion Regulation, and Interpersonal Effectiveness. Because mindfulness skills are the "core" skills and important components of each of the other skills, the Mindfulness module will be reviewed before each subsequent skills module is started.

Review of Grading Criteria (3 minutes)

If students are being graded or evaluated for the DBT STEPS-A class, go over the grading criteria at this time. Note when tests will be given, as shown on Handout 1.4.

Questions (5 minutes)

Give students an opportunity to ask questions. You can explain to the class that normally homework will be assigned at the end of each class, but there is none for today, other than to think more about the goals for decreasing and increasing behaviors and to identify a few more.

Class Cohesion-Building Exercise: Word Scramble (20 minutes)

Identify the number of students in your class. Then find the corresponding word (or words) on the class cohesion exercise chart (see Figure L1.1) for the number of students in your class.

Write the letters of each word on single sheets of paper (one letter per page). For some of the larger classes, there is more than one word. In these cases, the letters for each word should be written on a different color of paper. For example, the words for the number 12 are PEER COACHING. The letters P-E-E-R should be on one color of paper, and the letters C-O-A-C-H-I-N-G should be on another color of paper.

Pass out one letter to each student in the class. Once all the letters are passed out, have students who have the same color sheets of paper group together. Provide the following instructions:

> This exercise is called Word Scramble. Your job is to unscramble the jumbled DBT STEPS-A word [or words].

For single-word classes, say:

> Before you can begin working on your word, each person is to introduce him- or herself to the group and name one thing that the person enjoyed over the summer/holidays. Remember that what you say needs to be within the classroom rules we discussed earlier.

For multiple-word classes, say:

> Form into a small group with other members of the class who have sheets of paper in the same color. Before your group begins to unscramble the word, each person is to introduce him- or herself to the group and name one thing that the person enjoyed over the summer/holidays. Remember that what you say needs to be within the classroom rules we discussed earlier.
> If your group completes the Word Scramble, then you are to join another group. However, you must first introduce yourself to the group members and share with them

Class Size																						
5	G	O	A	L	S																	
6	S	K	I	L	L	S																
7	E	M	O	T	I	O	N															
8	D	I	S	T	R	E	S	S														
9	T	O	L	E	R	A	N	C	E													
10	D	I	A	L	E	C	T	I	C	S												
11	M	I	N	D	F	U	L	N	E	S	S											
12	P	E	E	R	C	O	A	C	H	I	N	G										
13	I	N	T	E	R	P	E	R	S	O	N	A	L									
14	D	E	C	I	S	I	O	N	M	A	K	I	N	G								
15	T	A	R	G	E	T	B	E	H	A	V	I	O	R	S							
16	S	K	I	L	L	A	C	Q	U	I	S	I	T	I	O	N						
17	E	M	O	T	I	O	N	R	E	G	U	L	A	T	I	O	N					
18	N	O	N	J	U	D	G	M	E	N	T	A	L	C	L	A	S	S				
19	D	I	A	L	E	C	T	I	C	A	L	B	E	H	A	V	I	O	R			
20	M	I	N	D	F	U	L	N	E	S	S	E	X	E	R	C	I	S	E	S		
21	I	N	T	E	R	P	E	R	S	O	N	A	L	P	R	O	B	L	E	M	S	
22	E	M	O	T	I	O	N	A	L	D	Y	S	R	E	G	U	L	A	T	I	O	N
23	D	E	C	I	S	I	O	N	M	A	K	I	N	G	A	B	I	L	I	T	I	E	S
24	N	O	N	J	U	D	G	M	E	N	T	A	L	E	N	V	I	R	O	N	M	E	N	T
25	S	K	I	L	L	A	C	Q	U	I	S	I	T	I	O	N	&	P	R	A	C	T	I	C	E
26	I	N	T	E	R	P	E	R	S	O	N	A	L	E	F	F	E	C	T	I	V	E	N	E	S	S

FIGURE L1.1. Class cohesion exercise chart.

one thing you enjoyed over your most recent school vacation. You may also share with the group what your group's word was, and this may help them decipher the current word.

Once all the words are solved, bring the groups back together, and have the whole class figure out the word order. After the students have completed this last task, congratulate them, and say that this course will provide many opportunities for them to get to know each other, to work together, and to help each other out.

Dialectics

SUMMARY

In order to understand the DBT STEP-A skills, which have been adapted from the second edition of the *DBT Skills Training Manual* (Linehan, 2015a) and the *DBT Skills Manual for Adolescents* (Rathus and Miller, 2015), it is important for the students to have a basic understanding of dialectics. Understanding dialectics allows the students to realize that there is more than one way to see a situation.

MAIN POINTS

1. Dialectics assumes that there is always more than one way to see a situation and that two things that seem opposite can both have truth in them.
2. Dialectics helps students to move away from "either–or," "always–never," or "black-or-white" thinking to more balanced thinking.

MATERIALS

1. Handouts for this lesson:
   - Handout 2.1. Dialectics: What Is It? What's the Big Deal?
   - Handout 2.2. Dialectical Thinking: "How To" Guide
   - Homework 2.3. Practice in Thinking and Acting Dialectically
2. Extra student skills binders or handouts, with pens or pencils, for students who attend class without materials.
3. Dry-erase markers or chalk for writing on the board.

PREPARATION

1. Arrange desks in the classroom, if possible, so students are able to see each other.
2. Review the lesson plan as well as handouts for this lesson.

LESSON OVERVIEW AND TIMELINE

- Introduction of main ideas (7 minutes)
- Discussion: Dialectics (35 minutes)
  - Review of Handout 2.1. Dialectics: What Is It? What's the Big Deal? (15 miuntes)
    - Class exercise: Finding synthesis—The middle path (10 minutes)
  - Review of Handout 2.2. Dialectical Thinking: "How To" Guide (10 minutes)
- Lesson summary (3 minutes)
  - Dialectics tells us there is more than one way to see a situation and helps us to get unstuck from black-and-white/all-or-nothing thinking.
- Homework assignment (5 minutes)
  - Homework 2.3. Practice in Thinking and Acting Dialectically
    - Go through a step-by-step process of helping students figure out how to honor the dialectic.

DETAILED LESSON PLAN

Introduction of Main Ideas (7 minutes)

Welcome the class and begin with a brief review of Lesson 1:

In the first lesson we talked about four problems teens often have and the skills we will be learning to help solve those problems. Who remembers what those are? You can refer to Handout 1.2 if you can't remember.

If necessary, prompt the students to reply: difficulty managing emotions (emotion regulation skills); confusion about self or distraction (mindfulness skills); impulsiveness (distress tolerance skills); and relationship problems (interpersonal effectiveness skills). Then ask the students if they have any questions about any of the material that was covered in Lesson 1.

Now write "DBT STEPS-A" and "Dialectics" on the board. Explain:

Today we are going to talk about a concept that underlies everything we are going to learn throughout the year: "dialectics." As I told you in Lesson 1, the full name of DBT STEPS-A is Dialectical Behavior Therapy Skills Training for Emotional Problem Solving for Adolescents. For the most part, the origins of the skills are not relevant, but having an understanding of the term "dialectics" and how it can affect our ways of thinking and acting is very important. So that is what we are going to focus on today.

Underline the word "Dialectics" on the board.

Discussion: Dialectics (35 minutes)

Review of Handout 2.1. Dialectics: What Is It? What's the Big Deal?
(15 minutes)

Explain:

> *Dialectics is a philosophy, a way of thinking, or a world view. Has anyone in the class ever heard of dialectics? Does anyone know what it means?*
>
> *"Dialectics" is a method of examining and discussing opposing ideas in order to find a synthesis." Basically, what dialectics teaches us is that no one has the absolute truth in a situation, so we need to allow ourselves to see truth in both sides of an argument.*
>
> *So to start, we are going to discuss how this way of thinking can be a useful skill for us. It's not unusual for us to get stuck in "black-or-white" or "all-or-nothing" thinking. Or we may find ourselves using the words "always" or "never" when we get into a discussion or argument. When we do that, we wind up taking one extreme position, digging our heels in, on the side that we believe is completely right—and believing that other people are completely wrong. What usually happens then is an argument that nobody wins. Everyone just digs deeper into his or her position. We find we are stuck. Sound familiar to anyone? Dialectical thinking will show us how to get unstuck with ourselves and with others.*

Read through (or ask a student to read) the first five bullet points on Handout 2.1. Elicit examples from the class with each point (or part of a point).

> ***"There is always more than one way to see a situation . . . ":*** *It is important to look at a situation from multiple perspectives. This does not mean you will automatically agree with the other person or perspective. It simply allows you to hold two or more perspectives at the same time.*
>
> ***" . . . and more than one way to solve a problem":*** *Again, if we can see a situation from multiple perspectives, we can begin to identify different ways to solve the problem.*
>
> ***"All people have unique problems and different points of view":*** *We are increasing our ability to understand other people's experience in a situation, even if it is different from our experience. Neither we nor the other people are wrong or right; we are simply different.*
>
> ***"Change is the only constant":*** *Can you think of anything that remains the same in your life? Every day, every moment, things are changing. We are constantly learning new things. Our bodies are constantly changing, even if only on a molecular level. Change is constant. For some people, change is a really difficult thing to deal with. Dialectical thinking helps to remind us that nothing in life remains the same. This doesn't mean that things always get worse; that would be nondialectical thinking. It means that things simply change, whether for the better or for the worse, and then they will change again.*
>
> ***"Two things that seem like (or are) opposites can both be true":*** *Isn't that like your relationship with your parents? Some days you love them, some days you can't stand them, and both are true: You can both love and hate your parents even in the same moment for the same situation. Similarly, you can understand someone's perspective and disagree with that person at the same time. This is where the saying "We can agree to disagree" comes into play.*

"Trying to honor the truth on both sides of a conflict is the best approach. . . . Avoid seeing the world in 'black-or-white,' 'all-or-nothing' ways. . . .": Thinking in the extremes is often what gets people stuck or rigid in situations. So how can dialectics get us unstuck? It's by trying to find and honor the truth in two opposites. We call this "finding the synthesis" or "finding the middle path." The middle path is not a compromise; a compromise between black and white would be gray. Instead, the middle path we are searching for looks like black-and-white polka dots or a checkerboard. Some examples are "I am doing the best I can, AND I need to try harder," "You can accept yourself for who you are now, AND you want to change."

CLASS EXERCISE: FINDING SYNTHESIS—THE MIDDLE PATH (10 MINUTES)

So how does getting unstuck actually work? Let's look at an example: You want to stay out until midnight, and your parents want you home by 10 P.M. How do you find a synthesis?

Help guide the class discussion by first eliciting the teen's views (write these down on one side of the board); then having the students generate what they think might be the parents' perspective (write these down on the other side of the board); and finally having the class work together to find a synthesis that honors both sides of the dialectic (write this in the center). For example:

Teen's view: "I want to hang out with my friends and not miss out on activities/socializing."

Parents' view: "We want you safe; we don't know where you are, who you are with, or what you will be doing; we'll stay awake worrying until you get home; and we both have early morning appointments."

Possible syntheses: Teen has friends over at his or her house and everyone can stay late; teen carries a cell phone; teen's parents speak to the other kids' parents; teen comes home at 10 P.M., and parents validate how angry or sad teen may be and figure out how teen can spend time with friends another time when parents don't have early morning appointments.

Explain:

The key here is that we are not just looking for ways to compromise (such as getting the parents to let the teen stay out until 11:00). We are trying to recognize each person's concerns and find a solution that could meet the needs of each person. So with this example, if you were the teen, you could go home and work through this with your parents so you could both understand each other's side. This does not automatically mean you are going to get to stay out later. The goal here is to see that there are multiple ways to get unstuck by honoring and understanding both sides.

If time allows, the class can work through an example offered by a student in the classroom who is stuck and is having a difficult time seeing another perspective (e.g., upcoming family move; recent punishment or loss of privileges; disagreement with an adult or a peer who is not in the classroom; personal conflict in making a decision such as colleges, jobs, or after-school activities).

Read through the four bullet points at the bottom of Handout 2.1 with the students, and give them a moment to add their own examples of dialectics. Then ask for volunteers to share their examples, providing much encouragement. Other examples of dialectics include any two seeming opposites (e.g., shy and friendly, scared and tough, being studious and a partier, lazy and motivated).

Review of Handout 2.2. Dialectical Thinking: "How To" Guide (10 minutes)

Tell students:

> *Now we are going to go through some specific ways in which you can actively practice being more dialectical in your thinking. Let's read through them one by one.*

Read through each of the first seven numbered points on Handout 2.2, or ask for volunteers to read out loud. Highlight points as noted below. Ask for additional examples.

> **1. "Move to 'both–and' thinking and away from 'either–or' thinking. . . . "** *The first step toward this goal is to become aware of extreme ways of thinking. Another helpful way to do this is to notice when you use the word BUT: "I appreciated your help yesterday, BUT what you were saying didn't make sense to me." What do you think the person is going to hear? He or she is likely only to hear, "What you were saying didn't make sense to me." The person may quickly become defensive and not register at all that you were appreciative. The word BUT can sometimes function as a giant eraser to anything that came before it. A more effective and dialectical way to communicate is by replacing the word BUT with the word AND: "I really appreciated your help yesterday, AND what you were saying didn't make sense to me."*

Have students generate other examples of how AND can replace BUT.

> **2. "Practice looking at all sides of a situation and all points of view. . . . "** *What does it mean to find a "kernel of truth," even if it is small, on the other side of an argument? For example, your parents won't let you get that piercing because they are afraid of infection. You know lots of people who have gotten piercings and they have not had an infection, and yet there is truth to their worry; it could happen.*
>
> **3. "Remember: No one has the absolute truth. Be open to alternatives."** *What this means is that there are always alternative ideas and thoughts. There is no one right way or answer. You can always ask, "What's being left out?" or "How can I bring up the other side?" Acknowledging the other side does not mean that you have to agree with it. It allows you to look at each perspective. This is similar to finding the kernel of truth in all sides of the argument.*
>
> **4. "Use 'I feel . . .' statements, instead of 'You are . . . ,' 'You should . . . ,' or 'That's just the way it is' statements."** *It is important to practice using nonblaming language. This will decrease the other person's level of defensiveness and make him or her more able to hear what you are saying. There's a difference between saying, "You always*

ignore me and are rude and make me feel like crap," and saying, "I feel like I am not listened to, and I feel ignored and hurt." See whether you can recognize the difference in how these statements affect the other person.

If time permits, conduct the following exercise: Have each student quickly identify a partner to work with. Instruct students to say something to their partners similar to the example just used (e.g., "You never listen to me, and I can't stand it!"), and then have them say the same thing again using 'I feel . . .'" statements (e.g., "I feel frustrated when I try to talk to you and it seems as if you are not paying attention to me because you are looking at your phone"). Elicit feedback from the students regarding whether they noticed any difference in their own reactions to the two statements. If there is still time, have students switch roles and repeat.

> **5. "Accept that different opinions can be valid, even if you do not agree with them. . . ."** *This is another example of replacing the word BUT with AND. Notice the importance of leaving out the word BUT in these types of statements: "I can see your point of view, BUT I do not agree with it" versus "I can see your point of view, AND it is OK that I do not agree with it."*
>
> **6. "Check your assumptions. Do not assume that you know what others are thinking. . . ."** *One of the biggest mistakes people make is that we assume we know exactly what someone else was thinking or intended, despite what they may have said or done. It is important to check the facts with other people, rather than make assumptions about meaning or intent.*
>
> **7. "Do not expect others to know what you are thinking. . . ."** *We should communicate our own thoughts and intentions when we think these may be misunderstood.*

Have students complete the practice exercise at the bottom of Handout 2.2, and then ask for volunteers to share their answers.

Lesson Summary (3 minutes)

Praise the class: Tell the students how proud you are of them for coming up with such great examples and working hard to learn new concepts. Then review the main points of dialectics:

> *There is more than one way to see a situation or solve a problem, and accepting different opinions can be legitimate, even if you don't agree with them. Dialectics helps us to get unstuck from black-or-white/all-or-nothing thinking.*

Homework Assignment (2 minutes)

Homework 2.3. Practice in Thinking and Acting Dialectically

Homework 2.3 asks students to identify two situations in which they did not think or act dialectically. Students are then to answer the corresponding questions about each situation. Read through the sheet with the students, asking whether it makes sense to them and whether there are any questions. Then say:

It is important that you complete the homework and arrive to class with your information written down. You will be expected to share what you did with the class. In general, you can practice your homework on as many different things as you like, but you must do at least one that you are willing to share with the class.

Finally, do some troubleshooting: Ask students whether they have any questions about the homework or any obstacles to completing it. If so, answer the questions and address the obstacles. Obstacles may include, but are not limited to, the following: Students have no intention of doing the assignment, have too much other homework this week, are likely to forget, or don't understand the assignment. Help students to identify their obstacles, and work with them to make a plan to overcome them. Examples include encouraging a student to write down the assignment and set a reminder in a cell phone or calendar to complete it; discussing why a student has no intention of doing the homework, and working on increasing his or her motivation and the relevance of the assignment (e.g., grades); or clarifying any other points. Troubleshooting should be done each week after the homework is assigned.

Mindfulness
Wise Mind

SUMMARY

Mindfulness skills are essential to the DBT STEPS-A curriculum and support all other skills taught. The core ideas are to bring awareness to our everyday living, and learn to be in control of our minds instead of letting our minds be in control of us—to live our lives mindfully rather than mindlessly. There are three states of mind: reasonable mind, emotion mind, and wise mind. Wise mind is the synthesis of emotion and reasonable mind. Everyone has inner wisdom.

MAIN POINTS

1. Learning to live just this one moment is freedom from the past and the future.
2. There are three states of mind: reasonable mind, emotion mind, and wise mind.
3. All people have a well of wisdom within them.

MATERIALS

1. Handouts for this lesson:
   - Handout 3.1. Mindfulness: Taking Hold of Your Mind
   - Handout 3.2. Mindfulness: Why Bother?
   - Handout 3.3. Mindfulness: Three States of Mind
   - Handout 3.4. Practicing Wise Mind
   - Homework 3.5. Practice Observing Yourself in the Three States of Mind
2. Extra student skills binders or handouts, with pens or pencils, for students who attend class without materials.
3. Dry-erase markers or chalk for writing on the board.
4. DBT STEPS-A diary cards.

PREPARATION

1. Review the lesson plan as well as handouts in student skills binder.
2. Arrange desks in the classroom, if possible, so that students are able to see each other.

LESSON OVERVIEW AND TIMELINE

- Homework review (10 minutes)
  - Homework 2.3. Thinking and Acting Dialectically?
    - Sharing with partners
    - Sharing with class
- Introduction of main ideas: What is mindfulness, and why bother? (9 minutes)
  - Review of Handout 3.1. Mindfulness: Taking Hold of Your Mind (4 minutes)
    - Mindlessness
    - Mindfulness takes practice
    - Mindfulness is how we access Wise Mind
  - Review of Handout 3.2. Mindfulness: Why Bother? (5 minutes)
    - Benefits of being mindful
      - Increase control and choices
      - Reduce suffering
      - Increase focus
      - Increase compassion
      - Improve health
- Discussion: States of mind (26 minutes)
  - Review of Handout 3.3. Mindfulness: Three States of Mind (18 minutes)
    - Emotion mind
    - Reasonable mind
    - Wise mind
  - Class exercise with Handout 3.4. Practicing Wise Mind (8 minutes)
- Lesson summary (1 minute)
  - Mindfulness is being aware of the present moment and putting your mind where you want it.
  - Briefly review the three states of mind.
- Homework assignment (4 minutes)
  - Homework 3.5. Practice Observing Yourself in the Three States of Mind
    - Identify times this week when you are in emotion mind, reasonable mind, and wise mind.
  - Handout 3.4. Mindfulness: Practicing Wise Mind
    - Choose two wise mind practices from Handout 3.4 to do between now and the next class.
  - DBT STEPS-A diary card
    - Introduce students to the diary card and explain how to complete it during the week.

DETAILED LESSON PLAN

Homework Review (10 minutes)

Homework 2.3. Thinking and Acting Dialectically?

SHARING WITH PARTNERS (5 MINUTES)

Divide the students into pairs for homework review. Orient students:

> *You will be doing a lot of group and partner work throughout the year, and at one point or another, you will all get a chance to work with everybody in the class.*

Briefly review dialectics and dialectical thinking. Ask students:

> *Who can share what we learned last week about dialectics and thinking dialectically?*

Provide feedback and correct answers as needed. Now instruct pairs of students to share with each other what they did for their homework assignment, thinking and acting dialectically. After 4 minutes, instruct each dyad to pick one example from one partner's homework that they would like to share with the class.

SHARING WITH CLASS (5 MINUTES)

Have the students come back together as a whole class, and go around asking students to share examples of the situations they experienced in which they had to practice being dialectical in their thinking. Ask specifically what steps were used, troubleshoot, and correct as needed. Reinforce any student who shares by saying that he or she really tried hard or by simply saying thank you. If appropriate, ask students for things that they might do differently if they were to try this activity again. Depending on the class size, you may not be able to elicit examples from each group. Collect homework sheets from students to review, and provide further feedback if needed.

Introduction of Main Ideas: What Is Mindfulness, and Why Bother? (9 minutes)

Review of Handout 3.1. Mindfulness: Taking Hold of Your Mind (4 minutes)

Have students turn to Handout 3.1. Explain:

> *Mindfulness has two elements to it, and we will briefly go through each.*

Write the following points on the board:

1. Opened mind: Being present and participating fully in the moment (being "in the zone").
2. Focused mind: Intentionally focusing your attention on one thing in the moment.

Continue:

> *Overall, "mindfulness" is focusing the mind in the present moment, without judgment and without trying to change it. Being mindful is being alert and aware to what is happening inside you and around you. It is experiencing reality as it really is. Most important, mindfulness practice is the continual task of bringing the mind back to the present moment without judging it.*
>
> > • *It is about learning to be in control of your own thoughts, emotions, and behaviors, instead of them being in control of you.*
> > • *It is about putting your mind where you want it to be. Doing this can lead to freedom from worries about the future or regrets about the past, such as worrying all day every day for weeks about a big test coming up, or feeling sad all of the time about a friendship that ended 3 months ago.*

Ask:

> *If you can't focus on the present, why could that become a problem?*

Discuss responses. Then ask:

> *Can anyone describe a time when you realized that you were making decisions or doing things without fully thinking about them? Maybe it seemed like your emotions were making all the decisions?*

Allow students to provide one or two examples. Emphasize:

> *Mindfulness will help us to be aware of when things like that are happening. When you are fully aware of the present moment, you are aware both internally (that is, of your physical sensations, thoughts, feelings, and urges) and externally (of what is going on around you). You are able to put your mind, your attention, where you want it.*

Review of Handout 3.2. Mindfulness: Why Bother? (5 minutes)

BENEFITS OF BEING MINDFUL

Ask students to turn to Handout 3.2. Then ask:

> *Does anyone remember a time when you were unable to control your attention and this caused problems? For example, having to take a test after breaking up with a boyfriend or a girlfriend?*

Refer students to the points listed on Handout 3.2. Ask a student to read through each point, and discuss. You can say:

What points 1 and 4 tell us is that being mindful can help us to be in control of our minds, rather than our emotions' being in control, or our being so unaware that we don't even realize what we are doing or where we are. The more in control we are, the more choices we have.

What point 2 tells us is that by being more mindful, we can decrease how much time we spend with our emotions in control, and can therefore decrease our emotional suffering.

What point 3 tells us is that as we learn the mindfulness skills, we will learn how to make decisions mindfully.

What point 5 tells us is that the more mindful we are, the less judgmental we will be. This can help us to be more compassionate rather than judgmental of ourselves and others.

What point 6 tells us is that being mindful also means focusing on the present and not the past or the future. This in itself can help to decrease stress, and less stress can lead to better overall health.

MINDLESSNESS

Ask:

Have you ever noticed times when you arrive at your next class or arrive home from school, and you do not remember how you got there? You don't remember turning down the hallway or crossing the street? These are examples of "mindlessness"—of not being aware of the present moment, of doing things on automatic pilot. This is the opposite of our goal in mindfulness. Can anyone provide examples of when or how this might be problematic?

Ask students for examples, or use the following:

1. *You are 3 days late on an assignment, and you have been avoiding your teacher so you don't have to discuss it with him. If you are mindlessly walking around and not paying attention to him, you might walk right into him in the halls or walk past his office. Or it could be an ex-boyfriend or ex-girlfriend you are trying to avoid.*
2. *You just learned that you have to eat gluten-free food, and while you are at the store grabbing a snack with your friends, you mindlessly grab your usual snack or eat your friends' snack, and before you know it you are sick to your stomach.*

THE IMPORTANCE OF MINDFULNESS PRACTICE

Emphasize:

The skills of mindfulness take practice. Because this is such an important set of core skills, and it is needed for all of the other skills, we will return to it several times over the course of the class. Plus, like any skills, the more you practice mindfulness the better you get at it!

Discussion: States of Mind (26 minutes)

Review of Handout 3.3. Mindfulness: Three States of Mind (18 minutes)

State:

> *A goal of mindfulness is to learn how to access and use our "wise mind." Wise mind is the inherent wisdom that is within all of us. All people have wisdom inside them, but for some, finding that wisdom can be very difficult.*

Draw two overlapping circles on the board, resembling the circles in Handout 3.3. Continue:

> *There are three states of mind. "Wise mind" is a synthesis or balance between "reasonable mind" and "emotion mind." The goal is not to get rid of reason or emotions; the goal is to hold or visualize the two simultaneously and respond to both sides.*

Label and fill in each area as you describe it below.

EMOTION MIND

> *Emotion mind is your state of mind when your emotions are in control; they influence and control your thinking, behavior, and urges to act or say things. Facts, logic, and reason are not important. They are dismissed.*

As an exercise, have students generate a list of emotions. Ask the students to get into pairs. Instruct each pair to generate a list of emotions—all kinds of emotions (e.g., happy, joyful, loving, contented, excited, surprised, proud, sad, angry, jealous, envious, scared, anxious, ashamed, guilty). When students are done, instruct them to count the number of positive or neutral emotions and then the number of negative or painful emotions they generated. Then have them count up the total number of emotions and write two fractions (e.g., 7/15 positive, 8/15 negative).
Discuss:

> *What did you notice about your emotion lists?*

Have students provide feedback. Then say something like this:

> *Often when people are asked to generate a list of emotions, it is common that they list many more negative or painful emotions than they do joyful or positive emotions. People also often pay more attention to painful emotions in themselves and in others. If we want to see more positive emotions in ourselves and in the people around us, we want to be sure we are noticing and commenting on them. Being mindful of all our emotions is helpful in doing so.*

Ask students to share their emotion lists and generate a list on the board next to the "emotion mind" circle. Then continue:

Emotions can be beneficial. Without emotions, we would not have great art, poems, love stories, and movies that we all enjoy. If a woman on her wedding day is highly emotional, that's acceptable and expected. Being emotional is not what we mean by emotion mind. Emotion mind is what happens when all reason vanishes and the emotions are in total control. That's when you see "Bridezilla." Another example may be after your team lost the big soccer game at regionals, and everyone's emotions are high. The players are angry and sad. After the game, your mom or dad comes up to you and says, "Good game. If you could have just blocked a few more of those passes, we would have had a chance." This makes you feel even angrier, and you start yelling at your mom or dad right in the middle of the parking lot and throw your water bottle at the car. Your emotions are running the show.

Elicit other examples of when it would not be good to be in emotion mind. Or use the examples of a pilot flying a plane or a student taking a math test. Go on:

Emotion mind is problematic when the emotions take control of us and we start acting on the urges that go along with the emotions. Every emotion has an "action urge" that goes along with each. We will spend a lot of time learning about this when we start the Emotion Regulation module. Briefly, let's just talk about what action urges go with some of our emotions. When you are angry, what do you have the urge to do?

Elicit: Attack, yell, scream . . .

When you are sad, what do you have the urge to do?

Elicit: Sleep, withdraw, hide . . .

When you are anxious, what do you have the urge to do?

Elicit: Avoid, distract . . .

When these emotions occur, do you always act on them? Sometimes you may and sometimes you may not. When you do, it is possible that you are in emotion mind and not even aware that your emotions are connected to and guiding your behavior.

An example of negative emotions' taking control may be getting very angry at your parents and throwing something across the room or walking out of the room and slamming the door. You are not thinking; you are just acting on your anger. Positive or joyful emotions can also become problems if they take control. For example, you are at a party and having such a great time, you may decide to start [drinking, using drugs, smoking cigarettes, dancing on furniture, posting inappropriate pictures on social media, playing extremely loud music, running away] without thinking about the consequences.

Under what situations do you think you may be more susceptible to getting into emotion mind?

Ask for examples. Answers may include being sick, tired, high, drunk, hungry, stressed; bingeing; or winning a big game/match.

Instruct students to write down on Handout 3.3 their own definitions of emotion mind and to describe how they behave or think when they are in emotion mind.

REASONABLE MIND

Explain:

> *On the other side of the dialectic is "reasonable mind." Reasonable mind is cool, rational, logical, calculated, and task-focused.*

Write these words on the board next to the "reasonable mind" circle.

> *When you are in reasonable mind, feelings, desires, and needs are not important.*

Now ask:

> *Why is reasonable mind important?*

Gather examples from students (e.g., without reason, people would not be able to solve logical problems, do science, build homes).

> *What professions do you think would require someone to be in reasonable mind?*

Discuss professions that rely on reason (e.g., airplane pilot, engineer, and air traffic controller). Gather examples from students about other roles and situations in which it may be important to be in reasonable mind.

> *Is there anything wrong with being in reasonable mind all the time? Are there times when it's not good to be in reasonable mind? Remember, when you are in reasonable mind, you do not take your emotions into account at all.*

Again, ask for examples from students (e.g., making decisions such as where to go to college, whom to marry).

Instruct students to write down on Handout 3.3 their own definitions of reasonable mind and to describe how they behave or think when they are in reasonable mind.

WISE MIND

Continue:

> *Ultimately, the goal is to find "wise mind," where there is a balance between your emotions and your reason. Wise mind is discovering within you the natural, intuitive wisdom that is a part of every person. Wise mind is the part of each person that knows and experiences truth. It is almost always quiet and peaceful.*

Put these words next to the "wise mind" area in the overlap between the "reasonable mind" and "emotion mind" circles.

> *It is where a person knows something in a centered way. When in wise mind, you experience reality as it is in the here and now.*

Ask for examples of wise mind decisions. These examples can be big decisions, such as where to go to college, whether to try out for the football team or soccer team, whether to marry someone when the time comes, or whether to stay in a current relationship or end it. Wise mind decisions can also be smaller decisions about day-to-day activities, such as whether to go to a house party, whether to sneak out in the middle of the night, whether to stay up late chatting online, or whether to study for a test now or later.

> *Every person has a wise mind within, although no one is in wise mind all the time. Other ways to think of wise mind include what you know as your "heart of hearts" or your "true self." It is the part of you that knows what is true. Wise mind practice is finding and listening to our inner wisdom. For some of us, it is a gut feeling; others feel it in their chests; still others feel it as the part of themselves that is in tune with faith or God. Where do you feel wise mind?*

Have students define wise mind for themselves and describe how they may know when they are in wise mind on Handout 3.3. Have students share examples of times when they think they may have been in wise mind.

Now put it all together with an example:

> *It is the homecoming football game, and the whole school is excited for a big win. The players on the field are all very excited and motivated to win the game. And the team is down by 10 points. The quarterback has been sacked four times already and has one interception. What happens to the quarterback if he is only in emotion mind?*

Allow students to make suggestions. Or say:

> *He may become frustrated and worried about being sacked again, so he throws the ball again just to get rid of it, which may produce another interception.*

Then ask:

> *What happens if the quarterback is only in reasonable mind?*

Again, allow students to make suggestions. Or say:

> *He focuses only on the logic of the play and where the ball is supposed to go, without thinking about the defenders. This can also lead to a sack because he has no fear in him to get away from the defenders, and he may also not have as much motivation to win the game.*

Now go on:

> *So what do we want from our quarterback in this big game? We want him in wise mind. In wise mind, he can find a balance between his emotions and his logic, so that he can be most effective on the field. What do you think the quarterback would do if he was in wise mind?*

Once more, allow students to make suggestions. Or say:

> *He knows the play and reads the defenders so he doesn't get sacked, and he doesn't let his fear take over so he just throws away the ball or runs backward for a loss of yards. He quickly decides to follow the planned play or to make a change based on the defenders' coverage. He probably doesn't get sacked or throw an interception.*

CLASS EXERCISE WITH HANDOUT 3.4. PRACTICING WISE MIND (8 MINUTES)

Remind students that getting into wise mind is a skill, and that, like any skill, it takes practice. Tell the students:

> *So the next question is this: How do we get into wise mind? The answer is with practice. So we are going to review a variety of different mindfulness practices we can do to help us get into wise mind. Turn to Handout 3.4. We are going to practice together as a class the exercise numbered 3 on Handout 3.4: breathing "Wise" in, "Mind" out.*

Direct the students to think of a decision that they have coming up in their lives. It could range from high school or college choices, to what to do this weekend, to which friends to eat lunch with this afternoon. Remind them that accessing their wise mind will help them to make an effective decision. Ask students to clear their desks of their binders or turn them over, if they think that the binders will be a distraction. Tell students:

> *I am about to give you all a set of directions for our mindfulness exercise. These are instructions we will use each time we do a mindfulness practice. We are going to start off by getting into a "mindful" position; this means that you are sitting in your chair with both feet on the ground and your hands on your lap. Keep your eyes open with a soft gaze; this means looking down but not focusing on any one thing in particular.*

You should be sitting in a chair as well, modeling this position to the students. Go on:

> *Pay attention to your breath as you are breathing in and breathing out. Breathe naturally, not either deeply or in shallow, rapid breaths. As you practice, your breath will find its own rhythm. As you breathe, let your attention settle to your center. If you get distracted during the exercise, just bring yourself back to what you were doing. Notice any thoughts and judgments that come up, let them go, and bring your attention back to your breath. Noticing that you are distracted and bringing yourself back to the practice is the practice. Let's begin now.*

In a soft, slow, steady voice, read the instructions for the mindfulness exercise.

As you breathe in, say to yourself, "Wise." As you breathe out, say to yourself, "Mind." After a while, see if you can sense yourself settling into wise mind.

After another minute or two, say:

You can now bring yourself back to the room.

Go around the room and ask students to share one comment on the experience. Remind them that the exercise is not for the purpose of calming them down or making them feel better. If time permits, ask students to pick a second exercise from Handout 3.4 to practice. Follow the same instructions as before.

End this exercise with a discussion of how to know the difference between wise mind and emotion mind. Explain:

It can be difficult to know the difference right away. But if you give it time, letting the decision sit for a while, like a day or two, and you still feel certain, calm, and secure that it is a wise mind decision, then it probably is. If your decision has changed with time, it was likely an emotion-minded decision.

Lesson Summary (1 minute)

Begin summarizing Lesson 3 by saying:

Mindfulness may seem abstract at first and hard to grasp, but don't worry, because it will be reviewed several times before the course is over. Furthermore, over the next two lessons we will focus on what we need to do and how to practice being mindful.

Repeat:

Mindfulness is being aware of the present moment and putting your mind where you want it.

Briefly review the three states of mind. Remind students:

Everyone has a wise mind and inner wisdom. It just takes practice to be able to find it.

Homework Assignment (4 minutes)

Note: There are a total of three assignments for this week's homework.

Homework 3.5. Practice Observing Yourself in the Three States of Mind

Tell students:

> *Identify times this week when you are in emotion mind, reasonable mind, and wise mind, and then fill out Homework 3.5.*

Handout 3.4. Practicing Wise Mind

Tell students:

> *Choose two wise mind practices from Handout 3.4 to do between now and the next class, and put a check on Handout 3.4 by the ones you practiced.*

DBT STEPS-A Diary Cards

Hand out diary cards. Explain:

> *This is what we call a "diary card." It is a way for you to keep track of all the skills that you are going to learn and practice during this course. It also provides you with a summary of the skills you have learned in this class, as well as a way to monitor what skills you are using on a weekly basis and their effectiveness. In addition, the diary cards will show me how often you are using the skills and which ones, plus how you perceive their effectiveness.*
>
> *First, fill out your name and today's date at the top. Next, let's look at the list under the heading "DBT STEPS-A Skills." The skills in this list are all of the skills we are going to learn during this class. As you learn a new skill (or skills) in each lesson, you will be able to circle the skills you used and rate the usefulness of these skills.*
>
> *There is a column at the far right of the diary card headed "Weekly Skills Use." You will use this column to rate your "average" use of each skill during the week, plus how helpful you thought it was. The 0–7 scale listed at the top of the card is the scale you will use to make these ratings.*

Read through the scale with the students. Then continue:

> *The diary card will allow us to track how often you are using skills, whether they are helpful to you, and whether you have to think about them before using them or they come auto- matically. The expectation is that at the beginning they will be more difficult to use, so at first you may find yourself ranking skill use for the week at a 0 (you didn't think about them or use them). Your short-term goal may be to get to a 5 (you thought about using skills and they helped), and your long-term goal may be to reach a 7, where using the skills is more automatic (you didn't have to think about using skills, you did use skills, and they helped).*
>
> *For example, as of today you know the skill of wise mind. So this week you should circle each day in which you used wise mind, and then for the week you should rate your overall skill use on the 0–7 scale at the top of the card. Next week, and each week after that, I will collect these cards from you, so be sure to fill them out daily. There should be*

a number by each skill that you have learned in the far right-hand column. As you learn more skills, you will be rating the different skills you know. Our goal is to have you practice the skills daily until they become automatic in your life.

Elicit questions from the class about the diary card.

Ask students if they have any questions about any of the homework or any obstacles to completing it. If so, address the obstacles. Ask for a verbal commitment from students to complete both the mindfulness homework and the diary card this week. It is often helpful to ask students where they plan to keep the diary card, so that they can remember to fill it out each day. It is more difficult and takes more time to fill it out once a week or every few days; the goal is to complete it daily. Problem-solve with students as needed in regard to completing both the mindfulness homework and the diary card.

Finally, do some troubleshooting: Ask students whether they have any questions about the homework or any obstacles to completing it. If so, answer the questions and address the obstacles. Obstacles may include, but are not limited to, the following: Students have no intention of doing the assignment, have too much other homework this week, are likely to forget, or don't understand the assignment. Help students to identify their obstacles and work with them to make a plan to overcome them. Examples include encouraging a student to write down the assignment and set a reminder in a cell phone or calendar to complete it; discussing why a student has no intention of doing the homework, and working on increasing his or her motivation and the relevance of the assignment (e.g., grades); or clarifying any other points. Troubleshooting should be done each week after the homework is assigned.

Mindfulness
"What" Skills

SUMMARY

This lesson begins with a mindfulness exercise, as will all subsequent lessons. Briefly review the definitions of "mindfulness" and "wise mind" from Lesson 3, and link these to this lesson on the three mindfulness "what" skills: observing, describing, and participating. These skills are what to do when practicing mindfulness. The lesson includes practice exercises with the class on how to observe and describe mindfully.

MAIN POINTS

1. Mindfulness skills are divided into the "what" and "how" skills.
2. The "what" skills are observing, describing, and participating.
3. Only one "what" skill is done at a time.
4. The "how" skills will be covered in Lesson 5.

MATERIALS

1. Handouts for this lesson:
   - Handout 4.1. Mindfulness: "What" Skills
   - Handout 4.2. Mindfulness: Observing Practice
   - Homework 4.3. Mindfulness: Practicing "What" Skills
2. Extra student skills binders, with pens or pencils, for students who attend class without materials.
3. Dry-erase markers or chalk for writing on the board.
4. Diary cards: Have new diary cards ready to distribute at the end of class. If possible, highlight the three "what" skills on them.

PREPARATION

1. Think of personal examples of "what" skills that you can use or examples that may have occurred at your school, to help make the "what" skills understandable to your students.
2. Write the three different "what" skills on the board, leaving room to add words that describe them as part of the lesson
3. Review the lesson plan, as well as handouts in student skills binders.
4. Arrange desks in the classroom, if possible, in order for students to be able to see each other.

LESSON OVERVIEW AND TIMELINE

- Mindfulness exercise (5 minutes)
  - Observing the breath (3 minutes)
  - Describing observations of the exercise (2 minutes)
- Homework review (10 minutes)
  - Handout 3.4. Mindfulness: Practicing Wise Mind
  - Homework 3.5. Practice Observing Yourself in the Three States of Mind
    - Sharing with partners
  - Diary cards
- Introduction of main ideas (2 minutes)
  - Mindfulness is awareness in the present moment without judgment.
  - The "What" skills are used to achieve wise mind: Observe, Describe, and Participate.
- Discussion: Observe (8 minutes)
  - Review of Handout 4.1. Mindfulness: "What" Skills (first part)
    - Observing outside
    - Observing inside
    - Thoughts: Only thoughts, not facts
    - Observing: Noticing present reality
    - Class exercise with Handout 4.2. Mindfulness: Observing Practice
    - Observing without describing
- Discussion: Describe (10 minutes)
  - Review of Handout 4.1. Mindfulness: "What" Skills (second part)
    - Class exercise: Observing versus describing hands on desk
    - Describing only what has been observed
    - Class exercise: Describing an "angry" face
    - Describing thoughts as thoughts
    - Class exercise: Observing and boxing thoughts on a conveyor belt
- Discussion: Participate (9 minutes)
  - Review of Handout 4.1. Mindfulness: "What" Skills (third part)
    - Class exercise: Examples of participating
- Doing only one "What" skill at a time (1 minute)
- Lesson summary (2 minutes)
  - Define mindfulness
  - Review the three "What" skills
- Homework assignment (3 minutes)

- Handout 4.3. Mindfulness: Practicing "What" Skills
- Diary cards

DETAILED LESSON PLAN

Mindfulness Exercise (5 minutes)

Observing the Breath (3 minutes)

Introduce the exercise as follows:

> *We are continuing with mindfulness skills this week, and, we will start every class from now on with a mindfulness exercise. Today we are going to observe our breath. Focusing on our bodily sensations helps anchor us in the present moment. Since we always have our breath with us, it is something we can always use as a focusing point. So today we are going to practice focusing all of our attention on only our breath.*
>
> *Begin by sitting in a mindful position. This means that we have our feet flat on the floor; we are sitting up straight, as if a string was pulling us from the top of the head; and our hands are in our laps. For this exercise, our eyes are open with a soft gaze, which means looking forward and down, but focusing on nothing in particular. If you notice that your mind is drifting away from your breathing, gently bring it back. If you find yourself having judgmental thoughts, notice them and then let them go.*
>
> *I will start the practice by counting to 3. When I say 1, this is the signal to get yourself into the mindful/wide-awake position. When I say 2, this is the signal to take a deep breath. And 3 is the signal to begin the practice.*
>
> *When I say 3, start the practice by simply watching your breath. Feel the air in your nose, feel your lungs expand, feel the change in your diaphragm. Then breathe out, noticing the experience of breathing out. Continue until I say, "Stop."*

Now start the practice by counting to 3.

> *1: Get yourself into the mindful/wide-awake position. 2: Take a deep breath. 3: Begin the practice.*

Do the exercise for 2 minutes and then say, "Stop."

Describing Observations of the Exercise (2 minutes)

Ask several students to share one observation of their experience of the exercise. (Depending on the number of students in the class, you may not be able to call on each student every time.) Provide feedback about observations as needed, ensuring that each statement consists of something a student can observe and has described nonjudgmentally.

Homework Review (10 minutes)

Handout 3.4. Practicing Wise Mind
Homework 3.5. Practice Observing Yourself in the Three States of Mind

Ask students to take out their completed copies of Handout 3.4 (with two wise mind practices checked off) and of Homework 3.5. Ask which students have completed their homework.

Reinforce these students by having them each share an example of their wise mind practice and their descriptions of the different states of mind from the week. You may review several students' homework at once by asking whether any other students did the same practice as the first student you call on. Ask for similarities or differences in experiences. Ask who did a different wise mind practice. Continue in a similar fashion with as many students as possible.

Next, ask who didn't complete the homework. Briefly ask these students what got in the way of their doing the homework and how they will get it done next time.

SHARING WITH PARTNERS

Have each student turn to the student sitting next to him or her and share what the student thinks wise mind is and where he or she feels it. Walk around listening to students' responses and interjecting when necessary.

Diary Cards

Ask all students to turn in their diary cards and homework sheets in to be reviewed by you. If you are not able to review homework with each student each lesson, then be sure to get to each student over the course of several lessons.

Introduction of Main Ideas (2 minutes)

Tell the students:

> In Lesson 3, we learned about wise mind. Today we are learning some of the skills for balancing emotion mind and reasonable mind in order to achieve wise mind. There are three mindfulness "what" skills, which are what we do, and three mindfulness "how" skills, which are how to do them. Today we are learning the "what" skills.

Remind students that mindfulness is awareness of the present moment without judgment; it is being in control of our own minds, instead of our emotions and thoughts being in control of us; and it is about putting our minds where we want them to be.

Now continue:

> There are three "what" skills: observe, describe, and participate. You can only do one of these at a time. These are what we do in order to reach wise mind and be mindful.

Write these three skills on the board.

Discussion: Observe (8 minutes)

Review of Handout 4.1. Mindfulness: "What" Skills (First Part)

Have students turn to Handout 4.1. Go around the class and have students read aloud each bullet point in the first section of the handout ("Observe"). Explain:

Observing is paying attention on purpose, without reacting. It is the process of focusing the mind on one thing—what you sense or experience. You are just noticing the experience; it's wordless watching.

Write "wordless watching" and "just noticing" next to "observe" on the board. Then go on:

Being able to control your attention means that you can control your mind. Most important, it is about observing what reality is, not what we think about reality.

OBSERVING OUTSIDE

Explain:

We can only observe the outside world through our five senses: seeing, hearing, smelling, tasting, and touching.

OBSERVING INSIDE

Explain:

We observe our inside worlds through sensing our thoughts, emotions, and internal bodily sensations. We can just watch our thoughts go by as if they are individual cars of a train or items on a conveyor belt. We can just notice and watch them pass, even when they are painful. We don't want to avoid or suppress the thoughts and emotions we are observing. Trying to block a thought or emotion is a sure way to keep having it. The more you try to block thoughts, the more they will keep coming back. The best way to get rid of a thought is just to observe it. It will go away on its own.

THOUGHTS: ONLY THOUGHTS, NOT FACTS

Continue:

The experience of a thought is an experience of a mental event. In this way, all thoughts are the same. A thought about sitting in an easy chair is not the experience of sitting in an easy chair. We could think right now about being on a beach on a tropical island or fighting in a battle somewhere around the world. The experience of these thoughts is not the same as experiencing the reality of a beach or a battle. We are still sitting here in our classroom. We could all try imagining that our chairs are plush recliners, but that won't make it so.

OBSERVING: NOTICING PRESENT REALITY

Go on:

Observing is about just noticing what is going on around us in this moment, without putting labels on it or trying to change it. Just as you wouldn't try to cross a busy street with your eyes closed, you do not want to go through life not seeing reality as it is. Believing that if we don't look at the cars they won't hit us will not make it true. We need to be observing and paying attention. And part of that is paying attention to the real world around us.

CLASS EXERCISE WITH HANDOUT 4.2. MINDFULNESS: OBSERVING PRACTICE

Tell the students:

It's good to practice observing, because it's very easy not to see things that are there. It's also easy to see things that are not there.

To make this point, have students turn to Handout 4.2. Ask:

What shapes do you see?

Discuss participants' experiences. Have students share what they observed. Explain:

It's clear that there are three black circles and that each has a notch, like a missing pie piece. In addition, many people see a triangle when they look at the shapes in this handout. But there is no triangle in the box. The notches in the three circles happen to line up with each other. If there were lines that connected the notches, then there would be a triangle. But there are no lines connecting the notches, and so there is no triangle shape. Our minds, however, can provide these "missing" lines so that we "see" a triangle even though it isn't really there. The mind has the ability to fill in blanks so that we "see" something we expect, even when it's missing. When the mind is not fully paying attention, it can also erase something unexpected even though it's there. In fact, most people stop paying attention when they think they know what something is. This can be useful and save us a lot of time. But it can cause lots of problems when what we think we see doesn't line up with what's really out there.

OBSERVING WITHOUT DESCRIBING

Say:

It can be hard to observe without describing. From when we were babies, people named everything we saw, heard, touched, and tasted. Soon everything had a label, and now it can be nearly impossible for us to hear a "meow" and not think "cat." But in reality, that "meow" could be a child playing. You cannot observe and describe at the same time.

Discussion: Describe (10 minutes)

Review of Handout 4.1. Mindfulness: "What" Skills (Second Part)

Have different students read each of the bullet points in the second section of Handout 4.1 ("Describe"). Explain:

Describing is putting what you have observed into words. Describing is labeling what is observed; it is wordful watching.

Write "wordful watching" next to "describe" on the board.

CLASS EXERCISE: OBSERVING VERSUS DESCRIBING HANDS ON DESKS

Have the students place their hands on their desks. Say:

Experience the sensation of your skin on the desk surface. Just observe and notice it, without putting any words or labels on the experience.

Wait a few seconds to allow students to register the experience.

Now put words to the experience. Label the sensations.

Again, give students a few seconds before going on.

When we were first just noticing our hands on our desks, that is observing. We were paying attention to the sensory experience. When we put words to the experience, that is the skill of describing. We were identifying what is—what we directly observed.

Ask students to describe the sensations of their hands on the desk (e.g., cool, smooth, flat, hard). Then ask:

Did any of you notice an immediate urge to describe what the desk felt like as soon as you put your hands on it?

Elicit reactions. Then say:

Mindfulness is about slowing down and doing just one thing at a time. We can't observe and describe at the same time.

DESCRIBING ONLY WHAT HAS BEEN OBSERVED

Continue:

Describing is labeling what we have observed, as if explaining it to a blind person or to an artist who is going to draw on the basis of our description. We can only describe something if we observed it. We cannot observe the thoughts, feelings, or intentions that are inside other people. This is a key point that we often forget.

CLASS EXERCISE: OBSERVING AN "ANGRY" FACE

Tell the students that you want them to observe and then describe your face. Then make a very angry face. Most will describe it as "angry." Point out to the students that they did not observe an emotion; what they observed was your eyebrows furrowed, your mouth frowning, your teeth gritting, and so on.

DESCRIBING THOUGHTS AS THOUGHTS

Explain:

> *Our brains are constantly sending us thoughts, but these are just thoughts, not facts. Just because you think, "Everyone hates me," or "I'm stupid," this doesn't mean it's true. If I were to hand out a pop quiz right now, you might observe your stomach tightening and your heart racing, and you might have the thought, "I'm going to fail." But that is just a thought, and all thoughts are mental events, not facts in the world. The trick is to be able to observe a thought as just a thought and label it as such.*

Give an appropriate personal example of having misinterpreted thoughts as facts, such as the following:

> *When I walked into school today, I saw Principal [last name here]. I smiled at him, and he turned the other way without smiling back. I had the thought, "Uh-oh, he must be angry with me because I left the faculty meeting 5 minutes early yesterday, and now I am going to get in trouble and have to do detention duty for 2 weeks." I decided to apologize to him when I saw him in the main office later that morning, and he said that he was in such a rush this morning he didn't even see me come in, and that he hadn't even noticed that I left the meeting early.*

Ask students for examples of when they have misinterpreted thoughts:

> *When have you incorrectly "described" the emotions or intentions of a friend, parent, or teacher?*

CLASS EXERCISE: OBSERVING AND BOXING THOUGHTS ON A CONVEYOR BELT

Tell the students:

> *I want you all to close your eyes and imagine that your mind is a conveyer belt, and that thoughts are coming down the belt. Put each thought in a box near the belt. You could have one box for thoughts of things that happened in the past, one box for thoughts about sensations in your body, one box for urges to do something. Noticing the thoughts is using the skill of observing; putting them into the labeled box is the skill of describing. Notice if you get distracted, and gently bring your mind back to the task.*

Practice with the class for 1 minute. Then say:

> *The take-home point is this: If you didn't observe it, you cannot describe it. We cannot observe someone else's thoughts, emotions, or intentions. For example, "My brother is trying to push my buttons and get me mad" is impossible to observe.*

Discussion: Participate (9 minutes)

Review of Handout 4.1. Mindfulness: "What" Skills (Third Part)

Go back to Handout 4.1 and have a student read each of the bullet points in the third section ("Participate"). Explain:

> *Participating is entering wholly into an activity—spontaneously becoming one with the activity. It is throwing yourself into something.*

Write "throwing self completely into present experience" on the board. Continue:

> *Participating wisely in the present moment without judgment is the goal of mindfulness. We will learn more about being nonjudgmental in the next lesson, with the "how" skills.*
> *Participating is being fully present to our own lives, without self-consciousness, effortlessly in flow—forgetting ourselves and becoming what we are doing. Watch young children play. Whether they are running through a park, splashing in puddles, or dancing to music, children are great examples of participating.*
> *Participating is not thinking about yesterday or tomorrow. It is not worrying about what other people are thinking or feeling about us right now. It is about jumping into the current activity 100%.*

CLASS EXERCISE: EXAMPLES OF PARTICIPATING

Have students break into pairs. Ask students to share examples of when they think they may have been fully participating in an activity. Examples may include playing a sport, dancing and singing with friends, or taking an algebra exam where a student had studied really hard and knew how to do all the problems.

Ask students how they knew they were participating. Were they thinking about their emotions, or what other people were thinking about them, or about how they acted in the past? If so, they may not have been fully participating.

If some students don't think they were fully participating, ask them what would have needed to be different in order for them to be fully participating 100%.

After the dyads have completed the activity, have them share their examples with the entire class.

Doing Only One "What" Skill at a Time (1 minute)

Say to students:

> *The "what" skills can only be done one at a time. For example, if you are learning an instrument, you might first observe the sounds or how another person plays it. Then you would put words on the experience (describing and labeling where you put your fingers, and so on). When you put words on the experience, you are then describing. Eventually, you may reach a point where you can play without having to describe the individual steps. You may experience completely forgetting yourself as you play the music. That is participating.*

Explain that the next lesson will include a practice of participating after the "how" skills are introduced. The "how" skills are the ways in which we observe, describe, or participate.

Lesson Summary (2 minutes)

Congratulate students for learning the "what" skills and for giving personal examples in class. Remind them:

> We will come back to mindfulness and learn about the "how" skills in the next class. We will begin every class with a mindfulness exercise, so you will have more time to learn and practice these core skills.

Repeat, or ask students to define, what mindfulness is:

> Mindfulness is being aware of the present moment and putting our minds where we want them.

Add:

> It is a skill that you will get better at over time. Right now your mind may feel like it is jumping all over the place, but with practice you will begin to notice when your attention wanders and bring it back to the present.

Review the three "what" skills.

Homework Assignment (3 minutes)

Homework 4.3. Mindfulness: Practicing "What" Skills

Explain:

> Using the "what" skills takes practice. The more we practice them, the easier it will become over time to be mindful and access our wise mind.

Students will practice at least one "what" skill over the next week and briefly describe their experience. Students may practice all three of the skills if they choose. Students who do not complete the practice will explain what interfered with the practice at the bottom of the page.

Diary Cards

Pass out the new diary cards. The students have now learned how to observe, describe, and participate. They should practice these skills for homework, as well as wise mind, and rate their use of these skills on the diary card.

Finally, do some troubleshooting: Ask students whether they have any questions about the homework or any obstacles to completing it. If so, answer the questions and address the obstacles. Obstacles may include, but are not limited to, the following: Students have no intention of doing the assignment, have too much other homework this week, are likely to forget, or don't understand the assignment. Help students to identify their obstacles, and work with them to make a plan to overcome them. Examples include encouraging a student to write down the assignment and set a reminder in a cell phone or calendar to complete it; discussing why a student has no intention of doing the homework, and working on increasing his or her motivation and the relevance of the assignment (e.g., grades); or clarifying any other points. Troubleshooting should be done each week after the homework is assigned.

Mindfulness
"How" Skills

SUMMARY

This lesson covers the mindfulness "how" skills—that is, how to observe, describe, and participate. The "how" skills are taking a nonjudgmental stance, focusing on one thing in the moment, and being effective (which is doing what works). Doing things nonjudgmentally is taught by distinguishing two types of judgment: "evaluation" (to be avoided) and "discrimination" (to be kept). Additionally, judgments can act as "fuel" for our emotions. Doing things one-mindfully means no multitasking. Doing what works means choosing to act in ways that further long-term goals. The lesson ends with a class exercise in participating.

There is a lot of information in this lesson about the three "how" skills. It is important to note that you will be reviewing these skills two more times in the curriculum. You will be able to refer back to this lesson to cover any areas where you think the students may need more time. We believe it is very important to give the students the opportunity to practice the participation exercise at the end of this lesson.

MAIN POINTS

1. Build on the mindfulness "what" skills by doing them with the "how" skills.
2. The "how" skills are nonjudgmentally, one-mindfully, and effectively.
3. Unlike the "what" skills, the "how" skills can be used together simultaneously.

MATERIALS

1. Handouts for this lesson:
   - Handout 5.1. Mindfulness: "How" Skills
   - Homework 5.2. Mindfulness: Practicing "How" Skills
2. Extra student skills binders, with pens or pencils, for students who attend class without materials.

3. Dry-erase markers or chalk for writing on the board.
4. Diary cards: Have new diary cards ready to distribute at the end of class. If possible, highlight the three "how" skills on them.

PREPARATION

1. Think of personal examples you can use to help make the "how" skills understandable to the students.
2. Arrange desks in the classroom, if possible, in order for students to be able to see each other.
3. In advance, write on the board a list of the three different "what" skills, adding the three "how" skills under each one. This will emphasize that although a student can do only one "what" skill at a time, that "what" skill can be done by using the three "how" skills simultaneously. The following is an example of such a list.

> Observe
>> Nonjudgmentally
>> One-mindfully
>> Effectively
>
> Describe
>> Nonjudgmentally
>> One-mindfully
>> Effectively
>
> Participate
>> Nonjudgmentally
>> One-mindfully
>> Effectively

4. In advance, on a different part of the board, draw a two-column table with the column headings "Judgments That Discriminate" and "Judgments That Evaluate." This will be used for the class exercise on distinguishing discrimination (and description) from evaluation and can save time in teaching the lesson.

LESSON OVERVIEW AND TIMELINE

- Mindfulness exercise (5 minutes)
  - Counting the breath (3 minutes)
  - Describing observations of the experience (2 minutes)
    - The importance of catching distraction
- Homework review (10 minutes)
  - Handout 4.3. Mindfulness: Practicing "What" Skills
    - Sharing with class
  - Diary cards
- Introduction of main ideas (2 minutes)
  - Mindfulness is awareness of the present moment, without judgment and being in control of your own mind, instead of it being in control of you.

- Introduce the three "How" skills
  - Discussion: Nonjudgmentally (10 minutes)
    - Review of Handout 5.1. Mindfulness: "How" Skills (first part)
      - Two types of judging
      - Example: Calling a person "a "jerk"
      - The problem with evaluative judgments
      - Class exercise: Distinguishing discrimination (and description) from evaluation
      - Being nonjudgmental, step by step
  - Discussion: One-mindfully (5 minutes)
    - Review of Handout 5.1. Mindfulness: "How" Skills (second part)
      - Examples: How not being one-mindful can be harmful
      - Sets of behaviors
      - Multitasking: Not as effective as people think
  - Discussion: Effectively (10 minutes)
    - Review of Handout 5.1. Mindfulness: "How" Skills (third part)
      - Doing what works
      - Knowing our long-term goals
      - Class exercise: Long-term goals and "playing by the rules"
      - Obstacles to effectiveness
      - Participating effectively
  - Participating exercise: Throwing sounds (5 minutes)
  - Lesson summary (1 minute)
    - Review the "How" skills
  - Homework assignment (2 minutes)
    - Homework 5.2. Mindfulness: Practicing "How" Skills
      - Choose three "How" skills to practice
    - Diary cards

DETAILED LESSON PLAN

Mindfulness Exercise (5 minutes)

Observe: Counting the Breath (3 minutes)

Welcome the class and say:

> We are going to start with a mindfulness exercise, as we will do every week. Each mindfulness practice will focus on at least one of the seven mindfulness skills. So far we have learned four of the mindfulness skills. What four mindfulness skills have we learned so far?

Elicit: Wise mind, observe, describe, and participate. Continue:

> Today we are going to do an observing and describing practice called "counting the breath." Last time we did "observing the breath"; this time we will "count our breath."

Introduce the exercise as follows:

As I said last time, focusing on our bodily sensations helps anchor us in the present moment. Since we always have our breath with us, it is something we can always use as a focusing point.

For this practice, we are going to count 1 on the in-breath, then 2 on the out-breath, 3 on the in-breath, and 4 on the out-breath, all the way up to 10. When you get to 10, stop and begin counting at 1 again. If you lose count, just notice it and begin back at 1. If you notice that all of a sudden you are at 11, 17, or 38, just notice it, let it go, and begin back at 1 again. If you notice that your mind is drifting away from your breathing, notice it, and gently bring your attention back to your breath and counting. If you find yourself having judgmental thoughts, notice them, let them go, and return to your breath. If you notice any urges to move, other than blinking or swallowing, notice each urge without acting on it, and return your focus to your breath.

When I say 1, that's the signal to sit in a mindful position, also called a wide-awake position. We did this for our exercise last time. This means that we have our feet flat on the floor; we are sitting up straight, as if a string was pulling us from the top of the head; and our hands are in our laps. For this exercise, again, our eyes are open, but with a soft gaze, which means looking forward and down, but at nothing in particular. We don't want to practice mindfulness all the time with our eyes closed, because we don't live our lives with our eyes closed. When I say 2, that's the signal to take a deep breath. When I say 3, that's the signal to begin the practice. I'll say, "Stop," to end the practice.

Now start the practice by counting to 3.

1: Get yourself into the mindful/wide-awake position. 2: Take a deep breath. 3: Begin the practice.

Do the exercise for 2 minutes and then say, "Stop."

Describing Observations of the Exercise (2 minutes)

Ask students to describe and share one observation of their experience of the exercise. (Depending on the number of students in the class, you may not be able to call on each student every time.) Ask whether any students lost track of their counting, and if so, how often.

THE IMPORTANCE OF CATCHING DISTRACTION

End the exercise by saying to students:

It is just as important to notice when we are distracted as it is to stay focused on counting the breath. By noticing when we are distracted and bringing our attention back to our breath, we are strengthening our "observing muscles." This is important, because when we are in emotion mind, we need to notice this in order to get back to wise mind. When we are daydreaming in class and not paying attention to the lecture, we want to observe that we are daydreaming, so we can bring our attention back to the present moment. Over time and with a lot of practice, these skills will get stronger.

Homework Review (10 minutes)

Homework 4.3. Practicing "What" Skills

SHARING WITH THE CLASS

Ask students to take out their completed copies of Homework 4.3. Ask which students have completed their homework. Reinforce these students by having them each share an example of their use of the "what" skills. You may review several students' homework at once by asking whether any other students did the same practice as the first student you call on. Ask for similarities or differences in experiences. Ask who did a different "what" skill. Continue in a similar fashion with as many students as possible.

Next, ask who didn't complete the homework. Briefly ask these students what got in the way of their doing the homework and how they will get it done next time.

Diary Cards

Ask all students to turn in their diary cards and homework sheets in to be reviewed by you. If you are not able to review homework with each student each lesson, then be sure to get to each student over the course of several lessons.

Introduction of Main Ideas (2 minutes)

Tell the students:

> *In Lessons 3 and 4, we have learned wise mind and the mindfulness "what" skills of observing, describing, and participating. Remember that mindfulness is awareness of the present moment and being in control of your own mind, instead of it being in control of you. It is about putting your mind where you want it to be. This week we are going to learn the "how" skills for balancing emotion mind and reasonable mind to achieve wise mind. Just as there are three "what" skills, there are also three "how" skills: nonjudgmentally, one-mindfully, and effectively. Unlike the "what" skills, which can only be done one at a time, the "how" skills can all be done at the same time.*

Refer to the lists of skills you have written on the board.

Discussion: Nonjudgmentally (10 minutes)

Review of Handout 5.1. Mindfulness: "How" Skills (First Part)

Have students turn to Handout 5.1. Go around the class and have students read aloud each bullet point in the first section of the handout ("Nonjudgmentally"). Explain:

> *The way to observe, describe, or participate mindfully is to take a nonjudgmental stance. In other words, do not judge anything as good or bad, as valuable or not valuable, as worthwhile or worthless, as how things should or should not be.*

TWO TYPES OF JUDGING

> *There are two types of judgments: judgments that "discriminate" and judgments that "evaluate."*

Discriminating/Differentiating Judgments

> *A judgment that discriminates determines whether or not two or more things are the same or different, or whether or not something meets a predetermined set of standards. The word "differentiate" can be used instead and works equally well. For example, a judge discriminates by stating whether something was within the boundaries of the law or outside the law. A teacher discriminates (differentiates) or judges whether an answer on a test is correct or incorrect. This is not a judgment of "good or bad"; it is a statement about whether or not something fits within certain predetermined parameters. Discrimination is based on facts and is essential to life. We do not want to get rid of discriminating judgments. However, this type of discriminating judgment does not refer to discriminating between people as if one person or type of person is better than another. Discriminating judgments that lead us into good versus bad are the type of judgments we are working to decrease. If discriminate seems too loaded for you, it may help to use the word "differentiate" instead, which has the same meaning and often without the good versus bad judgment.*

Ask students to generate other types of judgments that are used to discriminate (e.g., fish is fresh and safe to eat, or rotten and unhealthy to eat; milk is spoiled, or safe to drink; clothes fit, or are too small/too big . . .).

Evaluating Judgments

> *Judgments that evaluate are based on opinions, ideas, and values, and are not based on facts or reality. These judgments often categorize things as "good or bad," "valuable or not valuable," "right or wrong." These thoughts are based on our perceptions rather than based in reality. Therefore, one person's perception may be different from another person's.*
>
> *Some evaluative judgments can be considered a shorthand way of describing something. For example, we might describe a piece of fruit as "bad" instead of explaining that it is rotten, brown, and full of bugs. We might also describe a piece of fruit as "good" when we mean that we like the way the fruit tastes. A different person may think that your "good" fruit is not ripe enough.*

EXAMPLE: CALLING A PERSON A "JERK"

Ask students to explain what they mean when they say a person is a "jerk." Elicit multiple non-judgmental descriptions. Highlight that calling someone a jerk doesn't really tell another person what the jerk did. Discuss the consequences of labeling a person as a jerk, versus giving a nonjudgmental description of what the person's behavior is or how the behavior is affecting others. Point out that there are many opinions about what makes someone a jerk (e.g., ignoring people, slamming doors in people's faces, calling people names, bullying someone, smiling in a certain way). In order to communicate what the person actually did, we need to be more specific, rather than using "jerk" as a form of shorthand.

THE PROBLEM WITH EVALUATIVE JUDGMENTS

Say to students:

> *One main problem of evaluative judgments is that over time, people forget they are short-hand descriptions or based on opinion, and begin to take them as statements of fact. Over time, these judgments begin to affect our emotions. Judgments can be "fuel" for our emotions. The more judgmental we are, the more intense our emotions can become, and we can end up in emotion mind. By being nonjudgmental, we can practice staying in wise mind.*

CLASS EXERCISE: DISTINGUISHING DISCRIMINATION (AND DESCRIPTION) FROM EVALUATION

If you haven't prepared in advance a two-column table like that in Table L5.1, write such a table on the board now. Label one column "Judgments that discriminate." Label the second column "Judgments that evaluate." Go through several examples with the class, such as those in Table L5.1, and have them determine which column each example belongs in and what the corresponding statement for the other column may look like.

Emphasize to the students:

> *Being nonjudgmental does not mean giving approval. It also does not mean denying consequences. Actions have consequences, regardless of how we think things "should" be.*

Instruct students to fill in the appropriate blanks on Handout 5.1 with their own definitions of discriminating and evaluating judgments.

TABLE L5.1. Discriminating Judgments versus Evaluating Judgments: Examples

Judgments that discriminate	Judgments that evaluate
"I am overweight according to the body mass index."	"I am fat and ugly, and I look disgusting."
"I failed the science test because I studied the wrong chapter."	"I failed the science test because I am an idiot and studied the wrong chapter."
"I am angry at myself because I studied the wrong chapter."	"I feel like such a jerk and so stupid because I studied the wrong chapter."
"My mother repeatedly came into my room this morning to wake me up, and when I wouldn't get out of bed, she poured cold water on me. It made me really angry."	"My mother was being such a jerk this morning. I hate her and don't want to ever be around her."

BEING NONJUDGMENTAL, STEP BY STEP

Say to students:

> *Being judgmental is a natural thing that many people do. However, we are now learning that it can also cause pain and difficulty for us. So we are going to start practicing being nonjudgmental in our descriptions of things. There are three steps to becoming more nonjudgmental.*

Notice Your Judgments

> *The first step is to notice your judgments. Begin just by noticing when you have a judgment. Just notice it and let it go. Don't judge yourself for judging; this is a natural thing, and you are now learning how to change it.*

Count Your Judgments

> *The second step is to count your judgments. You may want to start counting your judgments on a daily basis. One way to do this is to get a counter that you can keep in your pocket (like one that is used in golf or that an umpire uses to count pitches in baseball), and click it each time you notice a judgment. Another option is to track judgments on your phone or to keep a piece of paper with you and make a tally mark each time you notice a judgment. If you think you are someone who is judgmental all the time, then maybe just choose an hour a day to start counting your judgments.*

Restate Your Judgments in a Factual Way

> *The third step is to restate your judgments by describing facts. Let go of evaluating people, emotions, or things as good or bad. Recognize your preferences without judging. Describe what you observe without placing opinions or emotions on the observations. The goal is to be nonjudgmental; therefore, we don't want to switch from judging something bad to judging it good. If we allow judging something as good or valuable, it can also be judged as bad or worthless. Our goal is to get rid of "good" and "bad," and replace them with the facts.*

Discussion: One-Mindfully (5 minutes)

Review of Handout 5.1. Mindfulness: "How" Skills (Second Part)

Have students turn back to Handout 5.1. Go around the class and have students read aloud each bullet point in the second section of the handout ("One-Mindfully"). Explain:

> *One-mindfully means doing only one thing at a time, in the moment, with awareness and alertness. It is about the quality of awareness. Focusing attention on only one thing helps bring the whole person to the activity without expectations. It means focusing on what is immediately present, and not the past or the future. The past is over, and the future is not here yet. Remember the examples we talked about in Lesson 3: not worrying for weeks about a test that is a month away or continually being sad about a friendship that ended 3 months ago.*

Continue:

> *When we practice our mindfulness exercises, we practice doing one thing in the moment. However, sitting in this class while thinking about what to do after class, or thinking about the fight you had with your mother this morning, is not doing one thing in the moment. To be one-mindful, you need to think entirely about other things, or be entirely in class.*

EXAMPLES: HOW NOT BEING ONE-MINDFUL CAN BE HARMFUL

Determine which of the following sets of examples to use, based on age-appropriateness. For classes with mostly students below the driving age, say to the students:

> *Doing more than one thing at a time can get you in trouble or hurt you. How do you think this can happen?*

Elicit examples, or use this one:

> *You are walking down the street while you are looking at your phone or reading a book. You don't see a car coming around the corner, and you get hit by the car or force the car to swerve out of the way and crash.*

> For classes with mostly students of driving age, say to the students:

> *Doing more than one thing at a time can ruin your life. It can even lead to manslaughter charges and going to jail. How can this happen?*

Elicit an answer like this:

> *Texting while driving is not driving one-mindfully. It is doing more than one thing at a time. It can cause fatal accidents.*

Add:

> *Think about this—and the possible consequences—the next time you "observe" the urge to text, eat, or do something else while you are driving.*

SETS OF BEHAVIORS

Clarify the difference between doing one thing at a time in the moment and doing a set of behaviors that function together:

> *One-mindfully does not mean that you don't take notes while you are in class because you are only listening to the teacher. Or that you don't talk to friends in the hall between classes because you are walking to class. Some behaviors can function together as a set.*

Taking notes and listening to the teacher is "classroom behavior"; talking to friends and walking to class is "between-class hallway behavior."

MULTITASKING: NOT AS EFFECTIVE AS PEOPLE THINK

Tell students what research on multitasking (Rubinstein et al., 2001) has shown:

Experiments have been completed where people were given a list of tasks to complete as quickly as possible. The results showed that people who completed the tasks one at a time, as opposed to multitasking, had greater levels of accuracy and completed the tasks faster.

Emphasize this point by asking:

How many of you try to study or do your homework at night while you are watching TV? Does your homework or studying take longer when you do it that way? How well do you complete your homework while watching TV?

Discussion: Effectively (10 minutes)

Review of Handout 5.1. Mindfulness: "How" Skills (Third Part)

Have students turn back to Handout 5.1. Go around the class and have students read aloud each bullet point in the third section of the handout ("Effectively").

DOING WHAT WORKS

Say to students:

Doing something effectively means going along and playing the game. It is being skillful, not just "giving in." It means not getting caught up in what is right versus wrong, fair versus unfair. For example, it means being respectful and polite to your teacher even when you think that the teacher gave you an unfair response. The teacher still controls your grades to some extent in the class.

KNOWING OUR LONG-TERM GOALS

Continue:

To be effective is to do what works to reach our goals. Once we can identify our objectives, then we can begin to determine the most effective route to obtaining them.

Provide your own example of a long-term objective, or use the following. Tell the students that you want to go on a family vacation over winter break in order to have some quality family time and relax. You want to go somewhere sunny and warm with a beach, but the rest of your family wants to go skiing in the mountains. Ask the students what they think your objective is: to take a sunny vacation, or to have some quality family time?

CLASS EXERCISE: LONG-TERM GOALS AND "PLAYING BY THE RULES"

Group the students into pairs, and ask the students to take a few moments to identify some of their long-term goals (e.g., graduating from school, extending curfew at home, going on a spring break vacation with friends, making the football team, running for class president, getting a job, helping family more at home). Write some of the goals on the board.

1. Have the students in each pair discuss things that they might do that could get in the way of their obtaining their goals.
2. Explain that "playing by the rules" is another example of being effective. Ask the pairs of students to generate examples of how they may have to "play by the rules" in order to reach their goals.
3. Have pairs share with the larger class.

OBSTACLES TO EFFECTIVENESS

Being Right versus Being Effective

> There are two major sets of obstacles to being effective. The first is needing to be "right" rather than effective. Effectiveness is about letting go of doing something to prove a point, and instead doing what will move us toward our goals.

Elicit examples from students of times when they have focused on being right rather than effective. Then continue:

Emotions versus Being Effective

> The second set of obstacles to being effective consists of emotions and "shoulds." Our emotions can get in the way of accomplishing our goals. For instance, we can mistake the fear of going toward a goal for not really wanting that goal. Sometimes other negative feelings, such as anger or vengeance, can get in the way of reaching our goals. Or we may think others "should" act differently or that we have to act in a certain way based on principle even though it may take us away from our goals.

Give examples of being ineffective because of "shoulds" and ask students to generate additional examples:

> Some people might start a fight with a person who accidentally bumps them in the hall between classes, because they want to show that they can't be pushed around and the other person "should" be more respectful. This can be a big problem if you have already been in two fights this year and a third will get you suspended. Another example is tailgating a slow car in the left lane because that person "should" be going faster, instead of just passing on the right or slowing down.

PARTICIPATING EFFECTIVELY

As a transition to the exercise in participating that comes next, say to students:

When you throw yourself 100% into an activity, you need to do it effectively—which means knowing your goals, objectives, and the actual situation. A person could be fully partici- pating but not be doing it effectively. For example, you are playing in the homecoming football game, and the other team keeps making rude comments about your school and your team. Do you go after the other players, pushing them around after the play or pil- ing on a tackle that has been already made, and thus causing a penalty? Or do you get your team to focus on being in wise mind and mindful of the objective to win the game? Ask yourself, "Is getting into a fight to prove they need to respect our team in line with my long-term goal of winning the game and being able to continue playing?" If it is not in line with your long-term goal, it is not effective.

Participating Exercise: Throwing Sounds (5 minutes)

Explain:

This exercise involves playing "catch" with sounds. One person "throws" a sound as if it were a ball, using voice and body to throw the sound to another person. That person catches the sound by repeating it and the body movement. The person who caught the sound now throws a new sound and movement to another person, and the exercise con- tinues.

This is an exercise in participating effectively, where you will practice throwing yourself completely into the activity. We will also practice being nonjudgmental of ourselves and others; this includes both positive and negative judgments. If you notice a judgment, let it go, and come back to the exercise. In addition, we will focus on one-mindfully being in just this moment, not thinking about what sound will be thrown next or the sound that we just heard.

After 2 minutes or so, have all students stop and stay where they are. Ask:

Think about how you participated in the exercise. On a scale from 1 to 10, with 1 being "not at all" and 10 being "totally," rate how much you participated in this exercise. How many of you were at 1, 2, 3 . . . 8, 9, 10? OK, if you weren't at a 10, I want you to close your eyes and imagine what would be different if you were at a 10. What would you be doing differently, and what would that look like? Can you all see yourselves participating at a 10? OK, now we are going to do the exercise again with all of you participating at a 10, just like you imagined.

Repeat the exercise for another 2 minutes or so. Notice whether there is a change in volume and energy in the practice. As the teacher, it is very important that you are at a 10 for participation during these exercises, so you can model what this is like for the students. Prac- ticing at home or with colleagues is a great way to increase your participation.

Lesson Summary (1 minute)

Congratulate students for completing the "how" skills. Remind students:

> *We will come back to mindfulness skills at the start of each new module of skills because these are "core" skills—foundational to all the other skills. We want to make sure you really understand them and are practicing them. As we did today, we will begin every class with a mindfulness exercise, so you will have more time to learn and practice these core skills.*

Repeat:

> *Mindfulness is being aware of the present moment and putting your mind where you want it. It is a skill that you will get better at over time. Right now your mind probably jumps all over the place, or you have a hard time getting yourself to focus your attention when you need to, but with practice you will begin to notice when you are distracted and bring your attention back.*

Review the "how" skills.

Homework Assignment (2 minutes)

Homework 5.2. Mindfulness: Practicing "How" Skills

Explain:

> *This homework focuses on the "how" skills. Choose any of the three "how" skills to practice at least one time over the next week. You may practice all three. Then answer the questions on the homework sheet to describe your experience of using each skill.*

Diary Cards

Pass out new diary cards, and collect the previous week's cards if you have not yet done so. Note that the students have now learned observing, describing, participating, nonjudgmentally, one-mindfully, and effectively. When the students practice these skills for homework, or practice wise mind, they should rate whether they used the skill each day and provide an overall weekly skill use rating on the diary card.

Finally, do some troubleshooting: Ask students whether they have any questions about the homework or any obstacles to completing it. If so, answer the questions and address the obstacles. Obstacles may include, but are not limited to, the following: Students have no intention of doing the assignment, have too much other homework this week, are likely to forget, or don't understand the assignment. Help students to identify their obstacles, and work with them to make a plan to overcome them. Examples include encouraging a student to write down the assignment and set a reminder in a cell phone or calendar to complete it; discussing why a student has no intention of doing the homework, and working on increasing his or her motivation and the relevance of the assignment (e.g., grades); or clarifying any other points. Troubleshooting should be done each week after the homework is assigned.

Distress Tolerance
Introduction to Crisis Survival Skills, and ACCEPTS

SUMMARY

This is the first of six lessons covering the distress tolerance skills, which emphasize learning to bear pain skillfully. This lesson briefly introduces the Distress Tolerance module, as well as the two types of distress tolerance skills: crisis survival and reality acceptance. It then focuses on the first set of crisis survival skills: Distracting with Wise Mind ACCEPTS.

MAIN POINTS

1. Distress tolerance skills teach how to tolerate the urge to act from emotion mind when experiencing intense emotions.
2. Crisis survival strategies are used to get through a bad situation without making it worse.
3. When there is no immediate solution to a highly stressful situation, reality acceptance skills are used.
4. The first set of crisis survival skills is to distract oneself by using Activities, Contributing, Comparisons, Emotions, Pushing away, Thoughts, and/or Sensations (ACCEPTS).

MATERIALS

1. Handouts for this lesson:
   - Handout 6.1. Distress Tolerance: Why Bother Coping with Painful Feelings and Urges?
   - Handout 6.2. Distress Tolerance: When to Use Crisis Survival Skills
   - Handout 6.3. Distress Tolerance: Crisis Survival Skills
   - Handout 6.4. Distress Tolerance: Distract with Wise Mind ACCEPTS
   - Homework 6.5. Distress Tolerance: Practicing Wise Mind ACCEPTS
2. Extra student skills binders, with pens or pencils, for students who attend class without materials.
3. Dry-erase markers or chalk for writing on the board.

4. Small sticky note pads (one for each student).
5. Diary cards: Have new diary cards ready to distribute at the end of class. If possible, highlight the "ACCEPTS" skills on them.
6. Pennies for the mindfulness exercise (enough pennies so that you and each student can choose one).

PREPARATION

1. Review the lesson plan, as well as handouts in student skills binders.
2. Arrange desks in the classroom, if possible, in order for students to be able to see each other.
3. In advance, prepare a table with two columns and seven rows on a large piece of posterboard. As shown later in this lesson in Figure L6.1, write the title "Wise Mind ACCEPTS" at the top. In the left column, write each of the ACCEPTS distraction methods: Activities, Contributing, Comparisons, Emotions, Pushing away, Thoughts, and Sensations. Leave the right column blank for the class activity.

LESSON OVERVIEW AND TIMELINE

- Mindfulness exercise (7 minutes)
  - Observing and describing a penny (5 minutes)
  - Describing observations of the exercise (2 minutes)
- Homework review (10 minutes)
  - Homework 5.2. Mindfulness: Practicing "How" Skills
    - Sharing with partners
    - Sharing with class
  - Diary cards
- Introduction of main ideas (4 minutes)
  - Review of Handout 6.1. Distress Tolerance: Why Bother Coping with Painful Feelings and Urges?
    - Two types of distress tolerance skills: Crisis Survival and Reality Acceptance Skills
- Discussion: Crisis survival skills (25 minutes)
  - Review of Handout 6.2. Distress Tolerance: When to Use Crisis Survival Skills (10 minutes)
    - What is a crisis?
    - Crisis survival skills
    - The emotional thermometer
  - Review of Handout 6.3. Distress Tolerance: Crisis Survival Skills (1 minute)
    - Brief overview of 5 Crisis Survival skills
  - Review of Handout 6.4. Distress Tolerance: Distract with Wise Mind ACCEPTS (14 minutes)
    - What does it mean to distract?
    - When to distract
    - Class exercise: Generate examples of Wise Mind ACCEPTS using posterboard.

- Lesson summary (2 minutes)
  - Review ACCEPTS mnemonic by randomly calling on students.
- Homework assignment (2 minutes)
  - Homework 6.5. Distress Tolerance: Practicing Wise Mind ACCEPTS
    - Identify and practice two ACCEPTS skills this week.
  - Diary cards

DETAILED LESSON PLAN

Mindfulness Exercise (7 minutes)

Observing and Describing a Penny (5 minutes)

Welcome the class and introduce the exercise. Pass out one penny to each student as you do so. Say:

> *We are going to begin with a mindfulness activity that involves observing and describing. I want you each to take one penny and put it on the desk in front of you. We are going to start with observing the penny—just noticing it.*
>
> *Begin by sitting in the mindful/wide-awake position. As we know by now, this means we have our feet flat on the floor; we are sitting up straight, as if a string was pulling us from the top of the head; and we have our hands in our laps. For this exercise, we will keep our eyes open. During the practice, if you notice that you have become distracted by thoughts, judgments, or body sensations, just notice it without acting on the urge; let it go and bring your attention back to the penny.*
>
> *Begin observing, just noticing the penny.*

Do this for 1 minute. After 1 minute, instruct the students:

> *Now put words to what you are observing. In your own mind, describe the penny to yourself.*

After 1 more minute, tell the students to continue their mindful describing to themselves, while you collect all of the pennies.

Then pass the handful of pennies to a student, instructing each student to try to find his or her own penny. Once that penny has been found, the pile should be passed to the next student and that student should look for his or her penny, continuing on to each person in the class. If the class is large, collect the pennies by the row and then redistribute them to that row only. Remind students to look for their pennies quietly, noticing any thoughts or judgments that may come up; when a student finds his or her penny, the student should turn his or her attention back to the penny.

After the pile has gone around, ask if each student was able to find his or her own penny. Point out that some may not have found their penny if it was taken before the pile reached them.

Describing Observations of the Exercise (2 minutes)

Highlight how challenging and involved the skill of observing can truly be, and how there are so many things around us each day that we just don't notice. Ask each student for what he or she noticed while observing the penny or for any other observations about the exercise. Provide feedback about observations as needed, ensuring that each statement consists of something a student can observe and describe nonjudgmentally. For example, you can help students to restate their observations by saying:

> *I noticed an increase in tension and frustration when I could not find my penny. I noticed the urge to tell my neighbor to give me my penny. I noticed stopping with each pause. I noticed a thought about how this was different from last week's exercise. I noticed a thought . . . , I noticed the sensation . . . , I noticed my mind wandering to other thoughts.*

If necessary, note how this differs from the following:

> *I thought, "How could this be helpful to me?" I liked last week's practice better. I was uncomfortable, so I had to move.*

Homework Review (10 minutes)

Homework 5.2. Mindfulness: Practicing "How" Skills

SHARING WITH PARTNERS

Divide the students into pairs for homework review. Have one student restate what the homework was last week. Then have the students share with their partners one of the situations in which they practiced the homework. Instruct them to share how it helped or did not help with the situation.

SHARING WITH THE CLASS

Have the students come back together as a whole and share with the class which skills they practiced to indicate whether they found them helpful, unhelpful, or neutral and to explain the second answer. Ask whether there is anything else about the skill use they would like to share with the class.

   If students are reporting that the skills were not at all helpful, encourage them to think of ways the skills could be done differently to have a different effect. Also ask whether they "noticed" that the skills were not helpful. Then ask how could they have noticed this without using the skills.

Diary Cards

Ask all students to turn in their diary cards and homework sheets to be reviewed. If you are not able to review homework with each student each lesson, then be sure to get to each student over the course of several lessons.

Introduction of Main Ideas (4 minutes)

Explain:

> Today we start a new skills module called Distress Tolerance. All the skills in this module are about how to cope with distress and pain.

Review of Handout 6.1. Distress Tolerance: Why Bother Coping with Painful Feelings and Urges?

Read the three numbered points on Handout 6.1 aloud, or ask one or more students to do so. Discuss these as follows:

> *"Pain is part of life and can't be avoided."* Now nobody wants distress and pain. Maybe you don't even want to think about it, much less how to cope with it. But can we get rid of <u>all</u> pain in our lives? No, we all experience pain.

Elicit examples (e.g., parental divorce, death of a loved one, a chronic medical problem, relationship breakups, struggling to do well in certain classes).

> *"If you can't deal with your pain, you may act impulsively."* Has anybody in here ever acted impulsively when they experienced intense emotions, like you were really angry or scared?

Again, elicit examples.

> *"When you act impulsively, you may end up hurting yourself, hurting someone else, and not getting what you want."* But have you ever been so intensely emotional and upset that you just couldn't stand it? What do you do when that happens? Maybe you do something you'll later regret, like trashing your things or your relationships.
>
> Because pain is unavoidable, and we want to make sure we don't cause more pain in our lives by our lack of ability to tolerate pain, we are going to learn the distress tolerance skills.

TWO TYPES OF DISTRESS TOLERANCE SKILLS

Explain:

> There are two categories of distress tolerance skills: crisis survival skills and reality acceptance skills.

Crisis Survival Skills

> The goal of crisis survival skills is to help you get through a short-term crisis situation without making it worse. Often when a crisis arises, we can act from emotion mind and cause more problems than where we started. Crisis survival skills help us tolerate our distress so we don't act on our emotions.

Reality Acceptance Skills

> *Reality acceptance skills are for longer-term distressing situations. When you are in a bad spot, and there's no way to change or fix it any time soon, that's when you need reality acceptance skills. Has anyone in the class ever thought that things "should" be different than they actually are? Maybe you felt angry, like you were fighting the way things are, refusing to accept the reality. This is a normal reaction, but it actually adds suffering to pain. In the second half of this module, we are going to learn a set of skills to use when we can't change those things in our lives that are painful, either because they happened in the past or they are out of our control.*
>
> *In a nutshell, crisis survival skills are about tolerating our distress for short-term problems, and reality acceptance skills are about tolerating our distress for long-term problems. Most important, distress tolerance skills do not solve the problem causing the distress. Their goal is not to get rid of the pain and make us feel good. Sometimes we might end up feeling better after using the skills, but their goal is to make the pain more tolerable.*

Have students fill in the definitions of crisis survival and accepting reality skills on Handout 6.1.

Discussion: Crisis Survival Skills (25 minutes)

Review of Handout 6.2. Distress Tolerance:
When to Use Crisis Survival Skills (10 minutes)

Have students turn to Handout 6.2. Tell them:

> *We will learn crisis survival skills first. These are skills to use in a crisis.*

WHAT IS A CRISIS?

Write the following on the board: "What is a crisis?" Then have students get into groups of two or three to discuss answers to this question. Instruct students to read through the top box on Handout 6.2 together and to generate examples of crisis situations.

After 2–3 minutes, have a brief class discussion about the definition of a crisis. Highlight for the students how, in such a situation, using skills that will help them to get through the situation without making it worse for themselves or others would be an effective thing.

Now ask a student to read the next two boxes on Handout 6.2. Emphasize:

> *Crisis survival skills are not for everyday use to solve all problems or for making life worth living. They are to help us carry on and stay functional, to avoid making things worse, or to stop impulsive behavior. They are for when emotion is high and problem solving is difficult or not possible right now.*
>
> *It is important that we know when to use our crisis survival skills and when not to. One of the skill sets we are going to learn about today teaches us that distracting from our emotions can be helpful at times. Do you think it would be effective or even possible to distract all of the time? No. So here is how we can gauge when to use our crisis survival skills.*

THE EMOTIONAL THERMOMETER

Draw a picture of a thermometer on the board, with 0 at the bottom and 100 at the top. Explain:

This is your emotional thermometer. The 0 means you are so calm you are practically sleeping, and the 100 means you are the most distressed you have ever been or could imagine being. You need crisis survival skills when a situation is intense. On a scale of 0–100, this would be around a 65 or higher. The situation can't be resolved right now; there is no immediate solution; you are in emotion mind; and you can't afford to make it worse.

Refer back to the examples provided earlier in small groups, and add some of the examples listed below if these are not already listed. Then have students rate their emotional temperatures for the different situations. Highlight that people have different levels of tolerance, so what may be a 40 for one person may be a 75 for another. (Here are some additional examples of crises you can use: "being swept up in the undertow at the ocean," "your parents saying that you cannot go out Friday night with your friends because you have a family obligation," "taking a test unprepared," or "someone saying something negative about you on social media.")

Now explain:

The goal of crisis survival is to stay effective. It can be hard to stay effective and not make the situation worse in a crisis because the stress and emotions are so high that the ability to problem-solve and cope can be lost. Crisis survival skills do not take away the crisis and the stress, but being effective and not making things worse are not small things in a crisis.

Have students think about a difficult situation or crisis that they needed to tolerate (e.g., being in trouble with their parents, being yelled at). Ask them what the difference was between tolerating the crisis and making it worse (e.g., by yelling back). Ask for examples of times when they responded poorly to a crisis and made the situation worse.

Review of Handout 6.3. Distress Tolerance: Crisis Survival Skills (1 minute)

Have students turn to Handout 6.3. Briefly highlight that there are five sets of crisis survival skills, which they will be learning over the next few lessons, and that today they have learned when to use crisis survival skills. Don't teach or review skills in this section. Move next to the first set of skills: distracting with wise mind ACCEPTS.

Review of Handout 6.4. Distress Tolerance: Distract with Wise Mind ACCEPTS (14 minutes)

Have students turn to Handout 6.4.

WHAT DOES IT MEAN TO DISTRACT?

Explain that distracting means:

1. Getting away from the urges to act on an emotion . . .
2. by doing something else . . .
3. while waiting for urges to come down on their own.

WHEN TO DISTRACT

Discuss with students times when distracting would be an appropriate way to deal with an emotional response to a situation. Examples could include these: "getting in a fight with a friend who now won't answer the phone, and you have the urge to leave a flaming message"; "not being able to find your wallet, which you think you left in your locker at school, but you cannot check until tomorrow and you have the urge to sneak back into the school building"; or "being grounded, and your parents are done talking to you, so you want to run away." Remind students:

Distracting does not fix any of these situations. It does not make you feel better about the situations. But it can get you through a situation without acting in ways that make the situation worse. So these skills really focus on helping you tolerate the urge to act on the emotion. For example, they can help you tolerate the urge to attack or yell at your parents when you are angry about being grounded or the urge to break into the school building and look for your wallet.

CLASS EXERCISE: EXAMPLES OF WISE MIND ACCEPTS

Bring out the sticky note pads, and either put up the "Wise Mind ACCEPTS" poster prepared before class (as shown in Figure L6.1), or draw it on the board now. Note that by using a posterboard, you will be able to save the students' ideas and leave it in the classroom for the students to see regularly, and it will be a reminder for them to use their ACCEPTS skills when needed. Finally, instruct students to take out Homework 6.5. Distress Tolerance: Practicing Wise Mind ACCEPTS.

Explain:

The word ACCEPTS is a "mnemonic"—that is, a memory helper. Each of the seven letters stands for a different way that you can distract yourself. The key to making these skills work is that you have to do them mindfully. This means participating fully in a skill, while being nonjudgmental and doing only that one thing in the moment.

Pass out a sticky note pad to each student, and have the students write each letter of ACCEPTS on a separate sheet. Instruct the students:

As we go through each of the letters and what they stand for, I want you to think about one or two examples that could work for you, and write them down under the corresponding letter. What we are about to do is very similar to your homework, so if you hear something that fits for you, then you should write it on Homework 6.5 as well.

Wise Mind ACCEPTS	
<u>A</u>ctivities	
<u>C</u>ontributing	
<u>C</u>omparisons	
<u>E</u>motions	
<u>P</u>ushing Away	
<u>T</u>houghts	
<u>S</u>ensations	

FIGURE L6.1. Template for a "Wise Mind ACCEPTS" poster.

Now go through each letter of ACCEPTS, explaining each distraction method and giving examples. Then have students write down on the sticky notes their own examples that they can use.

> **<u>A</u>ctivities:** *Distract your attention by doing something really engrossing, like reading a good book, watching TV, surfing the web, doing homework, working out, or any of the other activities listed on Handout 6.4. The key is that you become fully engaged and participate mindfully in the activity.*
>
> **<u>C</u>ontributing:** *Distract yourself by refocusing attention from yourself to others. This may also enhance self-respect. Handout 6.4 lists such things as helping a friend or volunteering. Another example might be talking to a store clerk and asking how his or her day is going.*
>
> **<u>C</u>omparisons**: *Distract yourself by refocusing attention from your current self and recasting yourself in a more positive light. This can be done by comparing yourself to those less fortunate or in worse situations than you, such as peers, guests on talk shows, or other people who seem unlucky. Another form of comparison is comparing your present self to a time when you were doing worse, knowing that you were able to get through that situation. Or compare yourself to a time when you coped effectively and were capable of getting through difficult moments. However, be aware that comparisons don't always work, and if you find yourself judging yourself or feeling guilty, then you should stop.*
>
> **<u>E</u>motions**: *Distract your attention by generating opposite emotions to change the current painful emotion. We have all been really sad, listened to heartbroken music, and felt worse. Or we have all been really pissed off, listened to angry music, and felt even more pissed off. That is* <u>not</u> *this method. The key is to evoke a different emotion. When you are angry, watch a funny movie or read a comic book. When you are sad, listen to happy music or watch a scary movie.*

Pushing away: Distract your attention by leaving the situation or blocking it from your mind. This decreases contact with the thing that is making you upset. In a crisis, denial is not always a bad thing; the secret is not overusing it. As Handout 6.4 says, build an imaginary wall between you and the situation. Put the situation in an imaginary safe or behind an imaginary locked door. You can even write down what is bothering you and put that piece of paper in a drawer or in a box on a shelf in the closet.

Thoughts: Distract your attention by filling your mind with other thoughts, so that negative or upsetting thoughts cannot get in. You can read, do crossword puzzles, count to 10, count or name the colors in the room, plan the rooms in your dream house, count the words when you are being yelled at, or translate the yelling into a foreign language.

Sensations: Distract your attention with physical sensations. Handout 6.4 suggests holding ice, listening to loud music, taking a hot or cold shower, or squeezing a ball.

After going through all the ACCEPTS skills, ask several students to come up and stick their ideas on the posterboard next to the corresponding letter of the mnemonic. Once all the sticky notes are on the posterboard, comment on how many different ways people were able to generate to distract from urges to act on their emotions. Add:

Now your goal is to be mindful enough to notice when you have intense urges, be effective and choose to use a crisis survival skill, and mindfully distract your attention from the urges.

After class, transcribe the ideas onto the posterboard and hang it in the room for the remainder of the course (without any identifying information about the students who provided the ideas).

Lesson Summary (2 minutes)

Tell the students how proud you are of their great examples. Ask for a volunteer to briefly review the main purposes of distress tolerance. Go around the room and call on different students to state what each letter in ACCEPTS stands for. Do this three or four times, getting faster each time.

Homework Assignment (2 minutes)

Homework 6.5. Distress Tolerance: Practicing Wise Mind ACCEPTS

Students will practice at least two of the ACCEPTS skills and write down each skill and the situation on the worksheet, as well as whether it helped.

Diary Cards

Pass out new diary cards, and collect the previous week's cards if you have not already done so. Highlight that the students have now learned the ACCEPTS skills. In each lesson, the students learn at least one new skill or set of skills; the skill or skills are added to the list of skills they are to monitor daily for whether they practiced it or not. Remind students that the only way to learn a new skill is to practice the skill over and over. Therefore, as they learn new skills, they are to practice these along with all the previously learned skills.

Finally, do some troubleshooting: Ask students whether they have any questions about the homework or any obstacles to completing it. If so, answer the questions and address the obstacles. Obstacles may include, but are not limited to, the following: Students have no intention of doing the assignment, have too much other homework this week, are likely to forget, or don't understand the assignment. Help students to identify their obstacles, and work with them to make a plan to overcome them. Examples include encouraging a student to write down the assignment and set a reminder in a cell phone or calendar to complete it; discussing why a student has no intention of doing the homework, and working on increasing his or her motivation and the relevance of the assignment (e.g., grades); or clarifying any other points. Troubleshooting should be done each week after the homework is assigned.

LESSON 7

Distress Tolerance
Self-Soothe and IMPROVE the Moment

SUMMARY

This lesson covers the next two sets of crisis survival skills: self-soothe and IMPROVE the moment. These skills continue the message from Lesson 6: Crisis survival skills are used to tolerate urges to act on intense emotions, in order to get through an emotional situation effectively and without making it worse by acting impulsively. This lesson also uses two posters, similar to the "Wise Mind ACCEPTS" poster created in Lesson 6 for classroom activities.

MAIN POINTS

1. Crisis survival strategies are used to get through a bad situation without making it worse.
2. Self-soothe is using movement plus the five senses (vision, hearing, smell, taste, and touch) to do something comforting, kind, and gentle for oneself.
3. IMPROVE the moment means replacing negative events with Imagery, Meaning, Prayer, Relaxing actions, One thing at a time, Vacation, and Encouragement.

MATERIALS

1. Handouts for this lesson:
   - Handout 7.1. Distress Tolerance: Self-Soothe Skills
   - Handout 7.2. Distress Tolerance: IMPROVE the Moment
   - Homework 7.3. Distress Tolerance: Practicing IMPROVE the Moment
   - Homework 7.4. Distress Tolerance: Creating Your Crisis Survival Kit
2. Extra student skills binders, with pens or pencils, for students who attend class without materials.

3. Dry-erase markers or chalk for writing on the board.
4. Diary cards: Have new diary cards ready to distribute at the end of class. If possible, highlight the "Self-soothe" and "IMPROVE" skills on them.
5. Small sticky note pads (one for each student).
6. Several small everyday objects (paper clips, keys, etc.; see the Detailed Lesson Plan for other suggestions). You will need one item for each student in the class.

PREPARATION

1. Review the lesson plan as well as handouts in student skills binder.
2. Arrange desks in the classroom, if possible, in order for students to be able to see each other.
3. In advance, prepare two tables with two columns each on two large pieces of posterboard. One will have six rows, and the other will have seven rows. As shown later in this lesson in Figures L7.1 and L7.2, title the tables "Self-Soothe Skills" and "IMPROVE the Moment," respectively. Down the left column, write each of the self-soothe or IMPROVE methods, as shown in those figures. Leave the right columns blank for the class activity.

LESSON OVERVIEW AND TIMELINE

- Mindfulness exercise (5 minutes)
  - Observing and describing an object (3 minutes)
  - Describing observations of the exercise (2 minutes)
- Homework review (10 minutes)
  - Homework 6.5. Distress Tolerance: Practicing Wise Mind ACCEPTS
  - Diary cards
- Introduction of main ideas (2 minutes)
  - Crisis survival skills help to tolerate acting on emotion urges.
- Discussion: Self-soothe skills (12 minutes)
  - Review of Handout 7.1 Distress Tolerance: Self-Soothe Skills
    - Class exercise: Generate examples of self-soothe skills using Self-soothe posterboard.
- Discussion: IMPROVE the moment (16 minutes)
  - Review of Handout 7.2. Distress Tolerance: IMPROVE the Moment
    - Class exercise: Generate examples of IMPROVE the moment using IMPROVE posterboard.
- Lesson summary (2 minutes)
- Homework assignment (3 minutes)
  - Homework 7.3. Distress Tolerance: Practicing IMPROVE the Moment
    - Practice two IMPROVE skills.
  - Homework 7.4. Distress Tolerance: Creating Your Crisis Survival Kit
    - Assemble items for each of the five senses plus movement to use to soothe yourself.
  - Diary cards

DETAILED LESSON PLAN

Mindfulness Exercise (5 minutes)

Observing and Describing an Object (3 minutes)

Welcome the class and introduce the exercise. For this exercise, you will need one object for each student. Suggestions for objects include (but are not limited to) markers, pens, pencils, stapler, paper clips, string cheese, candy wrappers, balls, bars of soap, feathers, pom-pom balls, washcloths, or fabrics of different textures. Say:

> *We are going to begin this lesson with another mindfulness activity that involves observing and describing. We have more senses than just our eyes, but so often we rely on our sight for our observation. Today you are going to close your eyes and be handed a common everyday object. Will you be able to describe the object by observing the object with senses other than your eyes?*

Explain:

> *After we begin the exercise, I will put an object in your hand. First, you are to practice observing the object, without looking at it—the way it feels, the texture, the shape, the weight, perhaps even the smell. After about 1 minute, I will tell you to describe the object to yourself—to put words to your observation.*

If necessary, clarify that the first step is simply to notice and observe. Then continue:

> *The next step is to take a mindful posture. When I say 1, that's the signal to sit in the mindful/wide-awake position we have learned. This means keeping our feet flat on the floor, sitting up straight, and putting our hands in an open position on your lap or desk. This time, also, close your eyes.*

Go on:

> *When I say 2, that's the signal to take a deep breath. When I say 3, that's the signal to begin the practice, and I will begin handing out the objects. I'll say, "Stop," to end the practice.*

> Now start the practice by counting to 3. Hand out the objects to students when you reach 3.

> *1: Get yourself into the mindful/wide-awake position. 2: Take a deep breath. 3: Begin the practice.*

Do the exercise for 2 minutes. Prior to saying, "Stop," instruct students to keep the object in their hands and place their hands under the desk or table, so that they do not see it when they open their eyes.

Describing Observations of the Exercise (2 minutes)

Go around the room and have students try to guess what their object is. At this time, allow them the opportunity to describe their observations about the activity. Model the correct usage of "I notice . . ." by noticing something successful about the exercise. Provide feedback about observations as needed, ensuring that each statement consists of something a student can observe and describe nonjudgmentally. For example, you can help students to restate their observations by saying:

> *I noticed the thought that my object is rough and soft. I don't know what this is. I noticed the urge to open my eyes and see the object. I noticed stopping with each pause. I noticed a thought about how this was different from last week. I noticed a thought . . ., I noticed the sensation . . . , I noticed my mind wandering to other thoughts.*

As in Lesson 6, if necessary, note how this observation differs from the following and help students to restate their observations as described above:

> *I thought, "How could this be helpful to me?" I liked last week's practice better. I was uncomfortable, so I had to move.*

Homework Review (10 minutes)

Homework 6.5. Distress Tolerance: Practicing Wise Mind ACCEPTS

Explain:

> *Because the homework was so similar to what was done last week in class, we aren't going to go into a lot of detail on it. I want us to focus on how you practiced the ACCEPTS strategies last week and how effective they were. If you came up with any additional ways to practice distracting, we want to hear those too, and we will add them to our list.*

Ask several students to share with the class the ACCEPTS skills that they practiced last week. When students share a situation, ask how effective the skill was, and whether they noticed a difference in their emotions before and after practicing the skill. Write any new ACCEPTS skills on the "Wise Mind ACCEPTS" poster.

Finally, ask who didn't complete the homework. Briefly ask these students what got in the way of their doing the homework and how they will get it done next time.

Diary Cards

Collect diary cards and homework sheets to be reviewed before the next class.

Introduction of Main Ideas (2 minutes)

Briefly review that distress tolerance skills are skills for getting through a difficult situation without making it worse; that crisis survival skills are for tolerating the urge to act when responding to short-term problems; and that the ACCEPTS skills are methods of mindfully distracting oneself in the short term. Remind students that the goal of crisis survival skills is not to solve problems or make us feel better, the goal is to get through the situation without acting on our emotion urges and possibly making the situation worse.

Then say to students that during this lesson two new sets of skills will be learned: how to self-soothe by using the five senses plus movement and how to IMPROVE the moment.

Discussion: Self-Soothe Skills (12 minutes)

Review of Handout 7.1. Distress Tolerance: Self-Soothe Skills

Have students turn to Handout 7.1. Say:

> *As this handout tells us, a good way to remember these skills is to think of soothing your five senses—vision, hearing, smell, taste, and touch—plus movement. These are skills for comforting, nurturing, and being kind and gentle to ourselves. By doing kind things for ourselves, we can reduce our vulnerability to negative emotions and increase our resistance to acting on our emotions. Again, and most important (and as with all of our skills), in order to be effective, we have to participate in each of these activities one-mindfully and without judgment.*

Ask students:

> *How many of you do nice things for yourself when you are experiencing intense emotions? How many of you think that you don't deserve soothing or nice things when you have intense emotions, especially painful emotions like anger, guilt, shame, or sadness?*

Discuss the students' responses. Some people believe that they do not deserve soothing, kindness, and gentleness; they may feel guilty or ashamed when they self-soothe. Emphasize to students that these are judgments. Since the goal is to practice these skills mindfully, it is important to be nonjudgmental and do what works in order to be effective in using the skills. Some students may believe that they should get soothing from others. Again, this may not be effective, so it is important for everyone to learn to self-soothe. However, these skills should not be overused; a problem should be solved, if it is solvable.

CLASS EXERCISE: EXAMPLES OF SELF-SOOTHING SKILLS

Bring out the sticky note pads, and either put up the "Self-Soothe Skills" poster prepared before class (as shown in Figure L7.1), or draw this figure on the board now. Note that by using a posterboard, you will be able to save the students' ideas and leave the poster in the room for the students to see regularly, and it will be a reminder for them to use their self-soothe skills when needed.

For each of the five senses and movement, read through the examples listed on Handout 7.1, and encourage students to call out their own ideas for things that would work for them. Write appropriate answers on the posterboard to be displayed in the classroom. Highlight

Self-Soothe Skills	
Vision	
Smell	
Touch	
Hearing	
Taste	
Movement	

FIGURE L7.1. Template for a "Self-Soothe Skills" poster.

that part of their homework will be to create their own kits for self-soothing, so if they hear an idea that fits for them, they should write it down.

Now pass out a sticky note pad to each student, and have the students write each of the five senses and movement on a separate sheet. Instruct the students:

As we go through the five senses plus movement, I want you to think about one or two examples for each one that could work for you, and write them down on the corresponding sticky note. For homework, you will create your own self-soothe kit. So if examples seem like they will be effective for you, be sure to write them down on your handout, so you can remember to put that item or similar items in your kit.

Go through each of the five senses and movement, giving examples and assisting students in generating further examples. Then have students write down on their sticky notes their own examples that they can use.

*   **Vision:** Soothe yourself by finding something pleasant to focus your sights on. This may include things like watching the flame of a candle dance, watching a picture slide show of your last family vacation or fun time with friends, or watching your dog run around the park.*

*   **Hearing:** Find something soothing to listen to. This can be music, laughter, sounds of nature, or even someone reading to you. If you listen to music, be sure it is not music that is going to make you feel worse or keep the emotion around. Listen to slow and calming music to soothe yourself. It is effective as long as it is not sad or depressing music. You can also combine the skill of distracting with other Emotions (the E in ACCEPTS) with*

self-soothing by listening to music that both is soothing and elicits a different emotion. For example, if you are sad, listen to peaceful and joyful music.

Smell: Soothe yourself by focusing on smells, such as lighting scented candles, using scented lotions, baking favorite foods, walking through a field of freshly mowed grass or fresh flowers, or visiting a rose garden.

Taste: As with all of these things, it is important that we do them mindfully, focusing only on one thing. Imagine what it would be like to eat your favorite food mindfully. Do you think you would enjoy that and find it soothing? Sometimes we eat so fast that we don't even fully enjoy our favorite foods. This skill is about doing the opposite: tasting one of your favorite foods and not missing any moment of it. What are some of your favorite things to eat?

Touch: This skill involves focusing completely on the sensation of touch. What are things that you find soothing to touch? This could be petting your cat, dog, or hamster, or rubbing a lucky rabbit's foot or something else soft you can keep in your pocket and keep with you wherever you go (unlike your pets). Or put on lotion and focus on the sensation of touch. You can combine this one with smell by using a scented lotion. What other types of things would be soothing to the touch for you?

Movement: Sometimes the most effective way to soothe ourselves and to be kind is by moving. This could be turning on music and dancing around, rocking in a hammock, slowing down and doing yoga or pilates, or going for a walk.

Emphasize to students:

It is important that whichever one you decide to do, do it mindfully. Eating your favorite food while stewing over the thing that has distressed you doesn't help you to feel better about the situation. Focus completely and mindfully on whichever of your five senses or movement you are soothing yourself with.

After going through all of the self-soothe skills, have students come up and stick their ideas on the posterboard next to the appropriate methods. After class, transcribe the ideas onto the posterboard and hang it in the room for the remainder of the year (without any identifying information about the students who provided the ideas).

Complete this part of the lesson by asking for questions or comments from students.

Discussion: IMPROVE the Moment (16 minutes)

Review of Handout 7.2. Distress Tolerance: IMPROVE the Moment

Have students turn to Handout 7.2. They should also pull out Homework 7.3. Practicing IMPROVE the Moment. Explain:

Just like the word ACCEPTS, the word IMPROVE is a "mnemonic"—that is, a memory helper. Each of the seven letters stands for a different skill for replacing immediate negative events with more positive ones. A negative event can range from things like fights with your parents, feeling overwhelmed with homework, or being sick and having to miss a dance, to events such as the death of a grandparent or being arrested for shoplifting. We are going to do an exercise as we go through the IMPROVE skills, similar to the exercises we did for the ACCEPTS and self-soothe skills. Our goal is for you to be able to remember these activities and then be able to do them when you find yourself with intense urges to act on your emotions.

CLASS EXERCISE: EXAMPLES OF IMPROVE THE MOMENT

Bring out more sticky note pads, and either put up the "IMPROVE the Moment" poster prepared before class (as shown in Figure L7.2), or draw this figure on the board now. Again, by using a posterboard, you will be able to save the students' ideas and leave it in the room for the students to see regularly, and it will be a reminder for them to use their IMPROVE skills when needed.

Pass out a sticky note pad to each student (if they don't have any remaining from previous exercise), and have the students write each letter of IMPROVE on a separate sheet. As you go through each letter of IMPROVE, describe the skill and assist students in generating examples. Emphasize to students before beginning:

It is important to balance improving the moment with staying in the present. Just as with the self-soothing skills, we don't want to overuse these skills, and we have to do them mindfully.

Now read through the examples listed on Handout 7.2, and encourage students to call out their own ideas for things that would work for them. After you go through each item have students write their examples on their sticky notes, as well as on Homework 7.3. Highlight that part of their homework will be to create their own list of items for improving the moment, so

IMPROVE the Moment	
Imagery	
Meaning	
Prayer	
Relaxation	
One thing in the moment	
Vacation	
Encouragement	

FIGURE L7.2. Template for an "IMPROVE the Moment" poster.

if during the discussion they hear an idea that works for them, they should write it down. You can give examples as follows:

Imagery: Imagery can be used to distract, soothe, or create different situations, or as practice for coping effectively with a crisis—that is, as mental rehearsal. Imagery creates safe spaces that you can temporarily go to. The key to using imagery is to practice using it during noncrisis situations. Imagine yourself being effective; imagine yourself in a safe place; imagine the painful emotions draining out of you like water out of a pipe.

Meaning: Finding or creating meaning helps many people in crisis. Adolescents whose parents get divorced often find themselves searching for meaning in their lives, while suffering intense emotion over the divorce. Finding meaning while experiencing a difficult situation can become a survival skill in this situation: It is finding the silver lining, making lemonade out of lemons, or focusing on whatever positive aspect you can find. For example, your parents' divorce may result in your getting closer to your siblings or grandparents, or in your spending more quality time alone with each parent and improving what may have been a distant relationship.

Prayer: This skill is about asking for strength and wisdom to tolerate the pain of the moment, rather than praying for the pain to go away. A person does not have to be religious or believe in a higher power to use this skill.

Practice: Have the students say out loud together: "Please make this stop happening to me. Please make it go away." Instruct the students to notice what they experienced while they said this. Now have the students say out loud together: "Please help me have the skills and strength to tolerate this difficult situation." Again, instruct the students to notice their experience while they said it. Did anybody notice a difference between the two experiences? Have a couple of students share their observations.

Note that the goal here is not to encourage all students to use prayer. You can say:

Prayer is something that works for some people. If you are not someone who believes in prayer, than this may not be a skill for you. This is similar to the Comparisons skill in ACCEPTS, which may not be for everyone, because some people feel worse after using it.

The goal of the practice above is to have students experience the difference between the two different ways of asking for help. If students choose to use prayer, have them generate different types of prayer they could use, and write them down on a sticky note under the corresponding letter.

Relaxation: This is finding activities that relax you. This is changing how the body responds to stress and crisis. Often people tense their bodies to try to control the situation; accepting the situation enables the body to communicate acceptance to the mind.

One Thing at a Time: This is the same skill we learned as part of the mindfulness skills. At times of intense emotions, we can begin to think that our entire lives are crises, rather than experiencing just this one crisis right now. We may have multiple problems occurring in the past and/or in the future, but the key to tolerating right now is remembering that we only have to survive this one moment. We do not have to relive the pain of the past or the pain of the future. Furthermore, when we might become overwhelmed with a big task we have to complete or a problem we have to solve, we can break it into small tasks and start with the easiest, doing one thing at a time. Here are a couple of examples: "When I am distracting with an activity, I am only doing that one activity," "I don't have to figure out how to pass all of my classes, just this one class right now," or "I don't have to figure out how to get my mother to stop yelling at me forever, just during this one interaction.

__Vacation:__ Sometimes everyone needs a vacation—but, unfortunately, a real vacation is not always possible. So our goal with this skill is to take a brief vacation. There are two key points to taking any type of vacation. First, it needs to have a planned end date or time. And second, it needs to be planned for an effective time. It is not effective to take a vacation the day before a major test or project is due. So the vacation may be 10 minutes or 2 hours, but usually not a whole day or 2. It is taking a brief time out to regroup. Examples might include closing your eyes and putting your head down on your desk for 5 minutes, or crawling into bed and pulling the covers over you for 5 minutes. Some of you may be quite good at taking vacations, and the key for you is to learn how to take them responsibly. Eventually you need to return to your regular life and begin to problem-solve.

__Encouragement:__ This skill involves talking to yourself the way you would talk to someone you care about who is in crisis, or the way you wish someone would talk to you. It is cheerleading yourself.

Practice: Have students raise their arms up in the air so they are perpendicular with their bodies. Instruct students to keep their arms up, and after about 30 seconds or a minute, have them say: "This is really hard. I can't do this. I need to put my arms down. I can't do this." Have students put their arms down and observe and describe their experience to themselves.

Now have students raise their arms again in the same position. This time, after about 30–60 seconds, have students begin to say: "I can do this. I can keep my arms up forever. I can tolerate this. Nothing can bring my arms down. I am doing a great job and working really hard." Then have students take their arms down, and again observe and describe their experience to themselves. Have a few students share their observations of the two types of experiences.

After you have gone through all the IMPROVE items, have students come up and stick their ideas on the posterboard next to the appropriate methods. After class, transcribe the ideas onto the posterboard and hang it in the room for the remainder of the year (without any identifying information about the students who provided the ideas).

Lesson Summary (2 minutes)

Congratulate the students for their hard work and for coming up with such great examples for the posterboards that will be put up in the classroom.

Review the purposes of self-soothing and IMPROVE. Then go around the class, having students say out loud what the five senses are plus one, and what each letter of IMPROVE stands for.

Homework Assignment (3 minutes)

Homework 7.3. Distress Tolerance: Practicing IMPROVE the Moment

Read through Homework 7.3 with students, and see whether they have any questions about this sheet. Students will identify two IMPROVE skills they will practice during the week. This practice could be in response to a distressing situation or not; the goal is to practice the skills. Students will describe each situation, identify whether the skill was helpful, and rate their level of distress and ability to manage urges to act on emotions. If students do not practice the skills, they will describe the obstacles to practice that occurred.

Homework 7.4. Distress Tolerance: Creating Your Crisis Survival Kit

Have students turn to Homework 7.4, and explain that each student will also put together a crisis survival kit for home and one for school. Instruct students:

> As another part of your homework, each of you will use some type of container (for instance, a shoebox, basket, or bag) and fill it with items that represent the types of crisis survival skills you have learned so far: ACCEPTS, IMPROVE, and self-soothe . These are items you can use during times of high distress to help you tolerate your emotions. Examples might include your favorite comedy movie and a bag of microwave popcorn; crayons/markers and coloring pages; candles; pictures of your favorite pet or best friends; or lotions. You will complete one kit for home and a smaller one for school that you can keep in your desk or locker. You can choose to bring in your kit next week, take a picture of your kit, or simply write down a list of included items to share during homework review next class.

Diary Cards

Hand out new diary cards to the students. Highlight that they have now learned the self-soothe and IMPROVE skills. When they practice these skills for their homework, they should rate whether they used the skills each day and provide an overall weekly skill use rating on the diary card, along with any other skills that they practice during the week.

Finally, do some troubleshooting: Ask students whether they have any questions about the homework or any obstacles to completing it. If so, answer the questions and address the obstacles. Obstacles may include, but are not limited to, the following: Students have no intention of doing the assignment, have too much other homework this week, are likely to forget, or don't understand the assignment. Help students to identify their obstacles, and work with them to make a plan to overcome them. Examples include encouraging a student to write down the assignment and set a reminder in a cell phone or calendar to complete it; discussing why a student has no intention of doing the homework, and working on increasing his or her motivation and the relevance of the assignment (e.g., grades); or clarifying any other points. Troubleshooting should be done each week after the homework is assigned.

Distress Tolerance
TIP Skills for Managing Extreme Emotions

SUMMARY

Today's lesson focuses on the impact of activating the parasympathetic nervous system (PNS) as a means of quickly reducing intense emotions for a brief amount of time. The PNS is part of the autonomic nervous system (ANS); the ANS consists of the PNS and the sympathetic nervous system (SNS). The SNS is the "fight-or-flight" system, which calls the body into action. The PNS is the body's physiological emotion regulation system, which calls the body into rest. The lesson includes a very brief overview of the PNS and SNS: and focuses on three skills that students can use to activate the PNS, using the mnemonic TIP (Temperature, Intense exercise, and Paced breathing). Students will practice using the T and P skills.

MAIN POINTS

1. Changing physiology can decrease the intensity of emotions.
2. TIP skills (Temperature, Intense exercise, Paced breathing) are to be used when a person is too aroused to do anything else.
3. TIP skills are used to avoid making a situation worse.

MATERIALS

1. Handouts for this lesson:
   - Handout 8.1. Distress Tolerance: TIP Skills for Managing Extreme Emotions
   - Homework 8.2. Distress Tolerance: Using TIP Skills for Managing Extreme Emotions
   - Extra student skills binders, with pens or pencils, for students who attend class without materials.
2. Dry-erase markers or chalk for writing on the board.

3. Play-Doh for the mindfulness exercise (enough for each student to make a 1- to 2-inch ball).
4. Diary cards: Have new diary cards ready to distribute at the end of class. If possible, highlight the "TIP" skills.
5. Zipper-lock bags of ice, or cold compresses, and paper towels for each student. These will be used for the practice exercise with Temperature.

PREPARATION

1. Review the lesson plan as well as handouts in student skills binder.
2. Arrange desks in the classroom, if possible, so that students are able to see each other.

LESSON OVERVIEW AND TIMELINE

- Mindfulness exercise (5 minutes)
  - Participating: Throwing sound (3 minutes)
  - Describing observations of the exercise (2 minutes)
- Homework review (10 minutes)
  - Homework 7.3. Distress Tolerance: Practicing IMPROVE the Moment
  - Homework 7.4. Creating Your Crisis Survival Kit
    - Sharing in small groups
    - Sharing with class
  - Diary cards
- Introduction of main ideas (7 minutes)
  - What is a crisis?
  - Autonomic Nervous System
    - Sympathetic Nervous System (SNS): Body's "fight or flight" system
    - Parasympathetic Nervous System (PNS): Body's natural emotion regulation system
- Discussion: TIP skills (23 minutes)
  - Review of Handout 8.1. Distress Tolerance: TIP Skills for Managing Extreme Emotions
    - Temperature (9 minutes)
      - Class exercise: Using cold to TIP temperature
    - Intense exercise (5 minutes)
    - Paced breathing (9 minutes)
      - Class exercise: Paced breathing
- Lesson summary (3 minutes)
  - Need to quickly bring emotions down in order to determine what other skills to use.
  - Briefly review TIP skills.
- Homework assignment (2 minutes)
  - Homework 8.2. Distress Tolerance: Using TIP Skills for Managing Extreme Emotions
    - Practice each TIP skills at least one time.
    - Practice intense exercise for 20 minutes since this is not done in class.
  - Diary cards

DETAILED LESSON PLAN

Mindfulness Exercise (5 minutes)

Participating: Throwing Sounds (3 minutes)

Welcome the class and state:

> *We are going to begin with a mindfulness activity that involves participating. We have already practiced today's exercise once before during Lesson 5. We are going to partici-pate mindfully participate in throwing sounds, or playing "sound ball," today.*
>
> *As you may recall, this exercise involves playing catch with sounds. One person throws a sound as if it were a ball, using voice and body, to another person. That person catches the sound by repeating it and the body movement. The person who caught the sound now throws a new sound and movement to another person, and the exercise continues.*
>
> *This is an exercise in participating: You will practice throwing yourself completely into the activity. We will also practice being nonjudgmental of ourselves and others; this includes both positive and negative judgments. If you notice a judgment, let it go, and come back to the exercise. In addition, we will focus on one-mindfully being in just this moment, not thinking about what sound will be thrown next or the sound that we just heard.*
>
> *This time we will not stop and evaluate how much we are participating on the scale of 1–10. Right now, I want you all to imagine yourselves participating 100%, at a level of 10. Do you see it? Now, when I say to begin, I want you to participate 100%.*

Instruct students to stand up and form a circle (or more than one circle, as necessary; there should be about five people per circle). Tell them:

> *When I say 1, that's the signal to stand up and mindfully get into a circle. When I say 2, that's the signal to take a deep breath. When I say 3, that's the signal to begin the practice the exercise. I'll say, "Stop," to end the exercise and let you return to your seats.*

Now start the practice by counting to 3.

> *1: Stand and move mindfully to a circle. 2: Take a deep breath. 3: Begin the practice.*

After 2 minutes, say, "Stop," to end the practice.

Describing Observations of the Exercise (2 minutes)

Go around the room and allow students to share any observations made about the activity. Provide feedback about observations as needed, ensuring that each statement consists of something that a student can observe and describe nonjudgmentally (e.g., I noticed stopping with each pause, I noticed a comparison thought about how this was different from last time, I noticed a thought . . . , I noticed the sensation . . . , I noticed my mind wandering to other thoughts. I had lots of thoughts about how this could be helpful to me, I noticed I liked last week's practice better, I noticed I was uncomfortable so had to move . . .).

Homework Review (10 minutes)

Homework 7.3. Distress Tolerance: Practicing IMPROVE the Moment
Homework 7.4. Distress Tolerance: Create Your Crisis Survival Kit

SHARING IN SMALL GROUPS (5 MINUTES)

Depending on the class size, break students into groups of three. Instruct the members of each group to start off by sharing some of the items in their crisis survival kits with each other, followed by how they practiced the IMPROVE skills over the week. Preferably, each student should describe the IMPROVE skill that he or she found to be most effective or one that was not used as an example in the previous lesson.

SHARING WITH THE CLASS (5 MINUTES)

Have the students come back together as a whole class, and ask each group to share with the class one item from each person's crisis survival kit that the group members found interesting and thought would be helpful. As you go around the class, have the students explain why each item meets the criteria for self-soothe.

Finally, ask who didn't complete their homework. Briefly ask these students what got in the way of their doing homework and how they will complete it next time.

Diary Cards

Ask all students to turn in their diary cards and homework sheets to be reviewed. If you are not able to review homework with each student each lesson, then be sure to get to each student over the course of several lessons.

Introduction of Main Ideas (7 minutes)

Review by asking students to share what constitutes a crisis: a stressful, short-term event that a person wants to resolve now but cannot. Then say:

> *Remember, we talked about when our emotions get into the "red zone," at about a 65 or higher on the distress scale of 0–100. At that point, it is helpful to use the crisis survival skills we have learned so far: ACCEPTS, IMPROVE, and self-soothe. However, there are times when our emotions are so intense that our ability to use skills such as distracting or self-soothing breaks down: We cannot think about what to do because our emotions are so extreme that they are getting in the way. We call this the "fight-or-flight" mode, when we are too aroused to practice skills. This might happen if you fail a test that you needed to pass in order to participate in the school play or go out with your friends this weekend, or if you learn that your boyfriend or girlfriend has cheated—anything that gets you "amped up" emotionally and puts you in emotion mind and the extreme red zone. When emotions get really intense and the other crisis survival skills don't work, or when you can't even focus enough to use the other skills, these are the times to use the TIP skills we are going to learn today to get intense emotions down fast by changing your body chemistry.*

The key to remember here, though, is that the effects of these skills usually only last about 5–20 minutes so they are not a long-term solution or answer. They will just buy you enough time, in a more calmed state, to mindfully determine what additional skills you need to use.

Continue:

Extreme emotions can be changed quickly by changing your body chemistry. So we are going to learn and practice the TIP skills in order to decrease our emotions quickly. Our focus will be on learning skills that will activate the parasympathetic nervous system, or PNS for short—the body's natural emotion regulation system. So, first, it will help us to understand the PNS.

This is an opportunity to teach students *briefly* about the ANS and its two components, the SNS and PNS. Some students may have learned about this in other classes, so you can ask them to participate in the discussion.

*The **sympathetic nervous system**, or SNS, is the body's "fight-or-flight" system that is activated in moments of distress. When this system is activated, the following things occur in the body: Heart rate increases, blood pressure increases, saliva production increases, pupils become dilated (get bigger), and digestion slows down. The body moves into action.*

*The **parasympathetic nervous system**, or PNS, is the body's natural emotion regulation system. This is the opposite of the" fight-or-flight" system; it is the "rest-and-slow-down" system. When this system is activated, the following things occur in the body: Heart rate slows down, blood pressure decreases, saliva production decreases, pupils constrict (get smaller), and digestion increases.*

The goal of the TIP skills is to activate the PNS so that emotions can decrease quickly and allow for clear thinking about what other skills can be used. TIP skills will only activate the PNS for about 5–20 minutes.

Give the following example:

You and your friends are leaving the movie theater and are about to cross the street. All of a sudden, you realize there is a car driving down the street toward you. What happens in your body?

Allow students to answer. As necessary, say something like this:

You may feel shock and freeze if the car is really going fast and you think you will be hit. You may start yelling at the driver and dart out of the way. Internally, your SNS has been activated to get you out of the way. This is helpful. Now imagine that you have just walked out of the movie theater, and your best friend starts discussing the movie. You say how much you liked it, and she starts saying how bad a movie it was and you must be an idiot to think it was any good. How are you starting to feel?

Again, allow students to answer. As necessary, say something like this:

> You are likely to become very angry and have the urge to start yelling at your friend and saying or doing things that may cause more problems later for you, such as not getting a ride home or damaging the relationship. This is a time when it would be helpful to activate the PNS, so that you do not act on your intense emotional urge and cause more problems for yourself in the long run. Remember, this doesn't mean that your friend is right and that you should accept everything she says. This is just about ways to decrease emotions quickly to keep from making impulsive decisions.

Discussion: TIP Skills (23 minutes)

Review of Handout 8.1. Distress Tolerance: TIP Skills for Managing Extreme Emotions

Have students turn to Handout 8.1. Explain that TIP is another mnemonic (that is, a memory helper), and that it stands for <u>T</u>emperature, <u>I</u>ntense exercise, and <u>P</u>aced breathing.

<u>T</u>EMPERATURE (9 MINUTES)

> The first TIP skill is using <u>T</u>emperature.

Have a student read the points in the box corresponding to the T on Handout 8.1.
Explain:

> Cold water will calm you down fast by activating your PNS. This comes from the dive reflex, which is what happens when you dive into a body of cold water. What do you think happens to someone who falls off a boat into the cold ocean or a cold lake?

Responses you are looking for include these: The person might panic, start screaming, and start swimming really hard and fast. If this happens, the person is likely to get tired fast and then drown. Go on:

> The body has this automatic reaction to keep you alive. That's where the PNS comes in, so that arousal will decrease so that the person can stay afloat. Just as the dive reflex can save someone from drowning, we can use it to save us from acting impulsively in response to extreme emotions. We are going to use cold water to simulate falling into a cold body of water and activate our own dive reflex. The key components here are that we have to apply something cold and wet to the face, while bent over and holding your breath.

Emphasize that the following is very important:

> It is important to know before you try this skill whether you have a heart condition because cold water slows down the heart rate. So if you have a heart condition, you <u>do not</u> want to use this one particular skill.

Now continue:

> *What you want to do is hold your breath, put your face in a bowl of cold water for 10 seconds (or as long as you can hold it), lift your face, breathe, and then repeat this up to three times. If you are in a place where you can't get to a bowl of ice water, you can put an ice pack or a cold beverage can to your cheekbones just below your eyes, while bending over and holding your breath.*

CLASS EXERCISE: USING COLD TO TIP TEMPERATURE

Before the class begins, fill zipper-lock plastic bags with water and freeze them. Freeze a bag for each student. (Or use cold compresses.) Bring the bags and a roll of paper towels (or compresses) to class. Students will each think of someone or something that they dislike or feel some disgust toward. The goal will be to induce a *moderate* level of emotion in students during the exercise.

> *We are going to practice something similar to dunking our face in cold water in class now. Rather than bringing a lot of bowls of ice water to class today, I brought frozen ice packs [or cold compresses]. For the next minute, I want you to think of someone or something you dislike or feel some disgust toward, or something that makes you moderately anxious or sad. I want you to allow your emotion to grow inside of you. Do not choose something that you know will elicit extreme emotions in your during this practice. Notice any urges to act on the emotion, and without acting on it, continue to think about the situation that generates the emotion. After 1 minute, I will tell you to put the ice pack wrapped in a paper towel [or the cold compress] on your face and to bend over in your seat and hold your breath. Remember, you want to make sure it is at least touching your cheekbones just under your eyes. While you have the ice pack [or compress] on your face, notice any changes that occur within your body or any changes to the emotion. Hold the ice pack [or compress] on your face about 30 seconds or longer if you can.*

Pass out the ice packs and paper towels (or the cold compresses). Allow about 1 minute for emotion induction. After about 1 minute, instruct students to place the ice packs and paper towels (or compresses) on their faces and hold them there for 30 seconds or longer, while bending over in their seats and holding their breath for about 10 seconds at a time.

After this is done, have students discuss any impact they noticed from putting the ice packs (or cold compresses) on their faces. Explain:

> *Using an ice pack [or compress] will not have the same intensity of impact as putting your face in a bowl of ice water, but it is the next best option.*

If any students are still aroused, inform them that the class is going to learn two more skills and practice one in a few minutes. Coach them to focus their attention mindfully on the lesson, and to bring their attention gently back to the class if they get distracted.

INTENSE EXERCISE (5 MINUTES)

Have a student read the points in the box corresponding to the I on Handout 8.1. Explain:

> *When we learn the emotion regulation skills, one thing we will learn is that emotions communicate to us the need for action. Therefore, when we are experiencing intense emotions, one way to get in control of our behaviors is to engage in intense exercise rather than in the emotional urge behavior. For example, if you are angry, you often want to attack; if you are scared, you want to run and hide. So the goal here is to engage in 20 minutes of intense exercise. This could be going for a run, power walking, doing jumping jacks, jumping rope, or doing any other type of exercise as long as you do it intensely. What other types of intense exercise could someone engage in for 20 minutes?*

Possible examples/answers include (but are not limited to) rowing, using a punching bag, fast bicycling, mountain climbing, shooting basketball hoops, and swimming laps.

> *The key is that when the exercise stops, then your body will also slow down for about 20 minutes because the PNS becomes activated. This should be enough time to think about what other skills you can us to continue to stay in control of your behavior. In addition, this exercise needs to be done mindfully. If you are thinking about whatever it was that cued the intense emotion, it will be harder for the emotion to go down.*

Ask students:

> *Have you ever experienced this slowdown after you just finished a moment of intense exercise, like at the gym or at a sports event or just when playing something with your friends? If you have, what does that feel like? Do you think that this would be helpful if you were experiencing intense emotions and you needed to bring them down quickly? Again, this is the PNS at work.*

Add:

> *Since we do not have 20 minutes to do the intense exercise in class today, this will be part of your homework assignment this week.*

PACED BREATHING (9 MINUTES)

Have a student read the points in the box corresponding to the P on Handout 8.1. Explain:

> *Paced breathing is another method we can use to activate the PNS. This strategy can be used anywhere because we always have access to our breath, which may not be the case for cold water or intense exercise. Naturally, our heart rate increases when we inhale and slows down slightly when we exhale. So we are going to pace our breathing in order to increase the effects of our exhales and activate our PNS. The goal is to make our exhales longer than our inhales. We are going to inhale for 4 seconds and then exhale for 6–8 seconds. We could also inhale for 5 seconds and exhale for 7 seconds, as long as the exhale*

is longer than the inhale. Remember, our PNS is activated during the exhale. We need to breathe in deeply from our abdomens and not from our chests.

CLASS EXERCISE: PACED BREATHING

Students will practice paced breathing for 2 minutes. Instruct students:

Place one hand on your abdomen right around your belly button, and notice the rise and fall with each deep breath. This is the type of breathing you want to do, not shallow breaths that only go to your chest. We are going to practice paced breathing now. We are going to do the same thing we did for cold water. For the next minute, I want you to think of someone you dislike or feel some disgust toward, or something that makes you moderately anxious or sad. It can be the same situation or something else. I want you to allow your emotion to grow inside of you. Notice any urges to act on the emotion, and without acting on it, continue to think of the emotional situation. After about 1 minute, I will instruct you to begin the paced breathing. You can use the clock to count your breaths, or you can count in your head. Count to 4 on the inhale and up to 6 or 8 on the exhale. If you can, also track the total number of breath cycles (inhale plus exhale) you do in the minute. It is easiest to count the breath cycles by using your fingers.

Allow 1 minute for emotion induction. After 1 minute, instruct students to begin the paced breathing, counting to 4 on the inhale and 6 or 8 on the exhale. Have them do this for 2 minutes. Have students discuss any impact they noticed from the paced breathing, and describe any comparisons to the use of the ice packs.

Conclude by reminding students:

Remember, the TIP skills are going to help decrease the intensity of your emotions for only 5–20 minutes. During this time, you want to focus on what other skills you can use to help you tolerate or change the emotions.

Lesson Summary (3 minutes)

Review that there are times when emotions can be too high for us to practice skills, and to bring down the emotions quickly to get through the crisis, we can change our body chemistry by using TIP skills to activate the PNS. Ask for volunteers to review quickly what each letter stands for in TIP.

Homework Assignment (2 minutes)

Homework 8.2. Distress Tolerance: Using TIP Skills for Managing Extreme Emotions

Explain:

This sheet is your homework assignment. It is important to practice skills when not in a crisis, like practicing a sport before the big game. Therefore, you should practice each of the

TIP skills during the week when you are in any sort of situation, regardless of the intensity. It does not have to be a crisis. Since we weren't able to practice it in class today, you are to engage in 20 minutes of intense exercise this week and report on the impact when you stopped the exercise. Remember, it can be any type of intense exercise, as long as you do it mindfully for 20 minutes (and don't overdo it).

Review the different parts of the worksheet and ask whether there are any questions.

Diary Cards

Hand out new diary cards to the students. Highlight that they have now learned the TIP skills, and that when they practice these skills for their homework, they are to circle the days and rate the skill use for the week on the diary card (along with the other skills that they have been taught).

Finally, do some troubleshooting: Ask students whether they have any questions about the homework or any obstacles to completing it. If so, answer the questions and address the obstacles. Obstacles may include, but are not limited to, the following: Students have no intention of doing the assignment, have too much other homework this week, are likely to forget, or don't understand the assignment. Help students to identify their obstacles, and work with them to make a plan to overcome them. Examples include encouraging a student to write down the assignment and set a reminder in a cell phone or calendar to complete it; discussing why a student has no intention of doing the homework, and working on increasing his or her motivation and the relevance of the assignment (e.g., grades); or clarifying any other points. Troubleshooting should be done each week after the homework is assigned.

Distress Tolerance
Pros and Cons

SUMMARY

This lesson covers the final crisis survival skill: pros and cons. When people are trying to resist a powerful urge to engage in a problem behavior, using pros and cons helps them to think about the positive and negative aspects of tolerating their distress rather than acting on it. This process will help them have a stronger understanding of the decision they are making. For many people who struggle with impulsive decisions or with choices made in emotion mind, completing a pros-and-cons list at a time when not in crisis will help to decrease the likelihood of their acting on these behaviors in the future. Therefore, students will complete a pros-and-cons list for one of their primary target behaviors in class today.

MAIN POINTS

1. Pros and cons can be used to choose between two courses of action, and can be written out ahead of time to prepare for urges to engage in problem behaviors.
2. Unlike typical lists of pros and cons, the list used in DBT STEPS-A has four boxes, not two columns.

MATERIALS

1. Handouts for this lesson:
   - Handout 9.1. Distress Tolerance: Pros and Cons
   - Homework 9.2. Distress Tolerance: Practice with Pros and Cons (additional copies of this sheet should be provided; see the discussion of the homework assignment at the end of this lesson)
2. Extra student skills binders, with pens or pencils, for students who attend class without materials.
3. Dry-erase markers or chalk for writing on the board.

4. One small piece of chocolate for each student, for the mindfulness exercise.
5. Diary cards: Have new diary cards ready to distribute at the end of class. If possible, highlight the "Pros and cons" skill.

PREPARATION

1. Review the lesson plan as well as handouts in student skills binder.
2. Arrange desks in the classroom, if possible, so that students are able to see each other.

LESSON OVERVIEW AND TIMELINE

- Mindfulness exercise (5 minutes)
  - Observing and describing: Eating chocolate (3 minutes)
  - Describing observations of the exercise (2 minutes)
- Homework review (10 minutes)
  - Homework 8.2. Distress Tolerance: Using TIP Skills for Managing Extreme Emotions
  - Diary cards
- Introduction of main ideas (5 minutes)
  - Pros and cons compare advantages and disadvantages of behaviors.
- Discussion: Pros and cons (25 minutes)
  - Review of Handout 9.1. Distress Tolerance: Pros and Cons (5 minutes)
    - Pros and cons have four boxes.
    - Use wise mind to make a weighted decision.
  - Class exercise: Completing a pros-and-cons list (20 minutes)
    - Draw a pros-and-cons grid on the board.
    - Focus on both short-term and long-term goals.
    - Evaluate facts about and validity of each item.
- Lesson summary (3 minutes)
  - Review main points.
    - Pros and cons of engaging in a behavior *and* of not engaging in the behavior should be included in each list.
    - Identify both short- and long-term consequences.
    - Check the validity of each of our pros and cons.
- Homework assignment (2 minutes)
  - Homework 9.2. Distress Tolerance: Practice with Pros and Cons
    - Complete a pros and cons for at least one of your own target behaviors.
  - Diary cards

DETAILED LESSON PLAN

Mindfulness Exercise (5 minutes)

Observing and Describing: Eating Chocolate (3 minutes)

Welcome the class and introduce the exercise. For this exercise, you will need one small piece of chocolate for each student (e.g., Hershey's Kisses, miniatures). Say:

> *We are going to begin with another mindfulness practice that involves observing and describing. So often we eat food mindlessly and barely even taste it. Today we are going to eat chocolate mindfully. Who can remember what skill has us eating mindfully?*

Elicit (or give) this answer: self-soothe with taste. Pass out one piece of chocolate to each student. Explain:

> *Remember, we have more senses than just our eyes, but so often we rely on our sight for our observation. Today we are going to use our eyes, noses, and mouths to observe a piece of chocolate. The reason I say we are going to use all three is because when I tell you to begin, I don't want you just to open the chocolate and eat it. When I give the signal to begin, you will observe the chocolate in your hands: Observe the wrapper, the shape, anything and everything about it. When you are ready, you will open the wrapper. Notice the color, the texture, the shape, the way that the chocolate feels, the way that it smells. You can decide if you want to put the chocolate in your mouth or not. If you decide to eat the chocolate, put the chocolate in your mouth when you are ready, but don't start chewing or swallowing right away. Notice the sensations on your tongue, the urge to chew, the taste as part of it dissolves from the enzymes in your saliva. Simply observe the chocolate in your mouth without acting on it, and only allow swallowing to occur as a natural reflex.*

NOTE: You may have one or more students in your group who do not want to do this practice for various reasons (e.g., they have an allergy, they hate chocolate, or they have an eating disorder). Giving them the option not to eat the chocolate may alleviate this problem, but if it does not, you may decide to have other options available (such as a raisin or a cup of water). Ideally, you want to encourage the students to practice the observing part of the exercise and choose not to put the chocolate in their mouths. They can observe the wrapper, the smell, the patterns on the chocolate from the wrapper, and so on. Once you have explained this to students as necessary, continue:

> *When I say 1, that's the signal to sit in the mindful or wide-awake position we have often used before. As you know, this means keeping our feet flat on the floor, sitting up straight, and putting our hands in our laps. For this exercise, we will keep our eyes open.*
> *When I say 2, that's the signal to take a deep breath. When I say 3, that's the signal to begin the practice, and I will begin handing out the chocolate. As usual, I'll say, "Stop," to end the exercise.*

Now start the practice by counting to 3.

> *1: Get yourself into the mindful/wide-awake position.*
> *2: Take a deep breath.*
> *3: Begin the practice.*

Have students do the exercise for 1 minute. After 1 minute, say, "Stop," and instruct the students to eat the chocolate if they want to if it has not already melted in their mouths.

Describing Observations of the Exercise (2 minutes)

Go around the room and have students describe any observations they made during the practice. Follow up with questions comparing mindfully eating chocolate to their everyday experience of eating chocolate. Provide feedback about observations as needed, ensuring that each statement consists of something that a student can observe and describe nonjudgmentally (e.g., I noticed the thought that my object is rough, soft, I don't know what this is . . . , I noticed the urge to open my eyes and see the object, I noticed stopping with each pause, I noticed a thought about how this was different from last week. I noticed a thought . . . , I noticed the sensation . . . , I noticed my mind wandering to other thoughts. I had lots of thoughts about how this could be helpful to me, I noticed I liked last week's practice better, I noticed I was uncomfortable so had to move . . .).

Homework Review (10 minutes)

Homework 8.2. Distress Tolerance: Using TIP Skills for Managing Extreme Emotions

Ask:

> *Who practiced the Temperature skill with ice or cold water? Who practiced Intense exercise? Who practiced Paced breathing?*

Go through each skill with the class, and have a few students report on their experience of the skill. Ask specifically what they did, the differences they noticed before and after practicing the skill, whether there was any decrease in their distress ratings, and whether they were surprised by the outcome.

If there are skills that some students did not practice, encourage them to try practicing these this week, and troubleshoot with the students what got in the way of their completing their homework.

Diary Cards

As usual, ask all students to turn in their diary cards and homework sheets to be reviewed. If you are not able to review homework with each student each lesson, then be sure to get to each student over the course of several lessons.

Introduction of Main Ideas (5 minutes)

Say to students:

> *People can have powerful urges to engage in problematic behaviors, such as arguing with parents, skipping class or school, avoiding homework or studying, drinking, drugs, shoplifting, and so on. But there are usually better outcomes for tolerating distress.*
>   *So how do you decide whether or not to act on those urges?*

Allow students to answer. Then continue:

> *Most people often weigh the pros and cons of doing a behavior. For instance, they might ask themselves, "How much trouble will I get in versus how much fun will I have?" Pros and cons help a person to compare the advantages and disadvantages of different options when a decision needs to be made.*
>   *You make decisions every day when weighing your options; you just usually don't formally write these out. For example, you make a decision at night whether to do your homework or watch YouTube videos. You most likely think of the pros of how much more fun the videos would be, but then you think of the cons of getting in trouble or earning a bad grade. Let's hope that this outweighs the pros of watching the videos and you do your homework!*
>   *Today we are going to learn how to complete a list of pros and cons. However, this one will be a little different from simply looking at the advantages and disadvantages of acting on crisis urges.*

Discussion: Pros and Cons (25 minutes)

Review of Handout 9.1. Distress Tolerance: Pros and Cons (5 minutes)

Instruct students to turn to Handout 9.1. Say:

> *This version of pros and cons can be used when you are deciding between two courses of action, or trying to resist a powerful urge to engage in a destructive behavior. Either you can write this out when the situation comes up, or, if it is a problem behavior that you have been working on stopping, you can write out your pros and cons ahead of time and have the list handy to pull out the next time an urge hits to engage in the problem behavior. It can serve as a reminder for all of the reasons that you do not want to engage in it.*

Highlight that this version of a pros-and-cons list has four boxes.

> *Completing a pros-and-cons list is an example of dialectics: That is, there can be pros as well as cons to both of the courses of action you are considering. There are some pros to your problem behavior; otherwise you would not do it. The key here is that once we have listed all of the pros and cons of both acting on an urge and not acting on an urge we then go back and make a decision in wise mind. At times the pros of engaging in a behavior may have a longer list than the cons of not acting on it. When this occurs, it is important*

that we don't weigh each item with equal importance and that we understand whether each item is a short- or long-term consequence. Once we do this, wise mind will help us to make the decision.

CLASS EXERCISE: COMPLETING A PROS-AND-CONS LIST
(20 MINUTES)

Draw the pros-and-cons grid on the board. Figures L9.1 and L9.2 are two examples of pros-and-cons lists. One is for using drugs at a party; the second is for posting revealing pictures of oneself on social media. You may choose which example to use with your class. Tell students:

We are going to discuss the urge to [use drugs at a party] [post revealing pictures or sexually explicit pictures of yourself on social media] and create a list of pros and cons for this behavior.

Elicit responses from the class. Be sure to focus on both short-term and long-term goals. (These are designated in Figures L9.1 and L9.2 with the abbreviations ST and LT.) Explain:

The pros and cons can be either short-term or long-term consequences. Often the short-term consequences are more attractive or tempting than the long-term ones. However, the long-term ones are the goals we are striving toward—the exact reasons why we are learning to tolerate our distress. For example, having fun with your friends for one night is enjoyable in the short term, but not studying for tomorrow's test and failing it will have long-term repercussions on your ability to play in the next game or to pass the course.

Once the pros-and-cons list on the board is completed, discuss with students what a wise mind decision would be.

Finally, it is important for us to go back and to evaluate the facts about or validity of each of the pros and cons. Sometimes you may identify a consequence that is actually not true and may be emotion-based. For instance, if you are debating whether or not to sleep late instead of getting up early to exercise, you may think, "If I skip waking up early to exercise before school, I will have more energy to get through the day." The reality of this statement is that if one does exercise in the morning, it often increases one's energy throughout the day, and not exercising in the morning may decrease one's energy for the day. Let's look back at our list and see if we need to check the facts about any of our pros and cons.

You can use one of these examples, depending on whether you have used the sample list in Figure L9.1 or Figure L9.2:

Pros: "It's the only way to have fun." Check the facts: Have you ever had fun with friends before without using drugs?

Pros: "Only my friends will see the pictures, and I trust their feedback." Check the facts: You can't control what happens to a picture once it is posted or texted.

	Pros	Cons
Acting on crisis urges	Pros of using drugs 1. Fitting in (ST) 2. It's the only way to have fun (ST) 3. Decreased anxiety (ST)	Cons of using drugs 1. Getting sick (hangover, ER) (ST) 2. Getting in trouble (parents, law, school) (LT) 3. Drug and alcohol treatment (LT) 4. Acting foolishly (ST) 5. Acting against values (LT) 6. Losing trust of parents (LT) 7. Losing nonusing friends (LT) 8. Spending lots of money (ST, LT)
Resisting crisis urges	Pros of not using drugs 1. Self-respect (LT) 2. Maintaining trust (LT) 3. Being responsible 4. No consequences from parents (LT) 5. No worry of getting caught (LT) 6. Role modeling to younger siblings (LT) 7. Saving money (LT, ST) 8. Being able to study for tomorrow's test (ST)	Cons of not using drugs 1. Being boring (ST) 2. Others might have negative judgments (ST) 3. Guilty by association anyway (ST) 4. Friends might reject me or tease me (ST, LT)

FIGURE L9.1. Example of a pros-and-cons list for using drugs at a party. (ST, short-term consequence; LT, long-term consequence.)

	Pros	Cons
Acting on crisis urges	Pros of posting pictures 1. I get more attention, "likes" (ST) 2. It's fun (ST) 3. I feel good about myself (ST) 4. More people talk to me and want to hang out with me (ST) 5. Only my friends will see the pictures, and I trust their feedback	Cons of posting pictures 1. People might say mean things, call me names (ST) 2. Getting in trouble (parents, school) (LT) 3. Looking foolish (ST) 4. Losing trust of parents (LT) 5. Losing friends (LT) 6. People might try to use me (ST, LT) 7. Feeling worse about myself (LT) 8. I can't control who sees the pictures (ST, LT)
Resisting crisis urges	Pros of not posting pictures 1. Self-respect (LT) 2. Maintaining trust (LT) 3. Being responsible 4. No consequences from parents (LT) 5. No worry of getting caught (LT) 6. Role modeling to younger siblings (LT) 7. I won't have to wonder if someone is being my friend just because of my pictures (LT)	Cons of not posting pictures 1. My friends don't say nice things about me (ST) 2. Feeling alone (ST)

FIGURE L9.2. Example of a pros-and-cons list for posting pictures of oneself on social media. (ST, short-term consequence; LT, long-term consequence.)

Highlight:

> *Just because your pros-and-cons list may favor [not using drugs] [not posting pictures on social media], this does not mean that acting in wise mind will be easy. Once you have made your wise mind decision, you may need to employ other skills to help you tolerate not doing the behavior.*

If time allows, engage the class in another pros-and-cons exercise, using an example generated by one of the students. Have one to four students come up to the board and fill in one of the quadrants in the pros-and-cons grid, as the class generates pros and cons for the behavior.

Lesson Summary (3 minutes)

Congratulate the students for their hard work and coming up with such great examples and participating in class today. Ask for a volunteer to briefly review the main points of pros and cons. The review should include these points:

- Pros and cons of engaging in a behavior *and* of not engaging in the behavior should be included in each list.
- It is important to identify both short- and long-term consequences. Often short-term consequences are more powerful, but we want to keep our eye on long-term goals.
- It is also important to check the validity of each of our pros and cons.

Homework Assignment (2 minutes)

Homework 9.2. Distress Tolerance: Practice with Pros and Cons

Distribute extra copies of Homework 9.2. Tell students that their homework assignment will be to complete at least one copy of Homework 9.2 for one of their own target behaviors. Remind them that they should use a behavior that they are committed to stopping, and that they should keep in mind both their long-term and short-term goals. Add these instructions:

> *If the behavior that you want to change is one of the behaviors that we talked about on the first day that we don't discuss in class, then complete the pros-and-cons sheet for that behavior because that is important. On one of the extra worksheets provided, complete a different set of pros and cons for a behavior that would be appropriate to share in class.*
>
> *Remember that when you create your own pros-and-cons sheet for a problem behavior ahead of time, it can then be used to resist the problem behavior or urge when you are in emotion mind. Just like your list of the ACCEPTS skills, you want to have this pros-and-cons list handy for when the urge hits.*

Review the homework sheet and ask if there are any questions.

Diary Cards

Hand out new diary cards to the students. Highlight that they have now learned pros and cons, and that when they practice this skill for homework, they are to circle the days and rate the skill use for the week on the diary card (along with the other skills that they have been taught).

Finally, do some troubleshooting: Ask students whether they have any questions about the homework or any obstacles to completing it. If so, answer the questions and address the obstacles. Obstacles may include, but are not limited to, the following: Students have no intention of doing the assignment, have too much other homework this week, are likely to forget, or don't understand the assignment. Help students to identify their obstacles, and work with them to make a plan to overcome them. Examples include encouraging a student to write down the assignment and set a reminder in a cell phone or calendar to complete it; discussing why a student has no intention of doing the homework, and working on increasing his or her motivation and the relevance of the assignment (e.g., grades); or clarifying any other points. Troubleshooting should be done each week after the homework is assigned.

Distress Tolerance

Introduction to Reality Acceptance Skills, and Radical Acceptance

SUMMARY

Today's lesson begins the second part of the Distress Tolerance module: the skills for accepting reality. Whereas the crisis survival skills focus on tolerating distress in the short term for problems that cannot be solved right now, the reality acceptance skills focus on tolerating distress for problems that cannot be solved in the long term—either because they occurred in the past and cannot be changed or because they are off in the future and cannot be solved right now. The focus is on helping individuals to accept the world and themselves as they are. Suffering comes from nonacceptance of reality, so using the specific skill of radical acceptance is the way out of suffering. In today's lesson, students will identify something that they need to practice radical acceptance of in their life.

MAIN POINTS

1. Pain is inevitable, but suffering is optional.
2. Accepting reality through radical acceptance—complete and total acceptance with the mind, body, and heart—can alleviate suffering.
3. Accepting reality also requires a willingness to accept; turning the mind in the direction of acceptance, sometimes over and over again; and mindfulness of current thoughts.
4. Acceptance does not mean approval or passivity.

MATERIALS

1. Handouts for this lesson:
   - Handout 10.1. Distress Tolerance: Overview of Reality Acceptance Skills
   - Handout 10.2. Distress Tolerance: Accepting Reality

- Handout 10.3. Distress Tolerance: Radical Acceptance, Step by Step
- Homework 10.4. Distress Tolerance: Choosing Things for Radical Acceptance Practice
2. Extra student skills binders, with pens or pencils, for students who attend class without materials.
3. Dry-erase markers or chalk for writing on the board.
4. Diary cards: Have new diary cards ready to be distributed at the end of class. If possible, highlight the "Radical acceptance" skill.

PREPARATION

1. Review the lesson plan as well as handouts in student skills binder.
2. Arrange desks in the classroom, if possible, so that students are able to see each other.

LESSON OVERVIEW AND TIMELINE

- Mindfulness exercise (5 minutes)
  - Participating: Standing on one leg (3 minutes)
  - Describing observations of the exercise (2 minutes)
- Homework review (10 minutes)
  - Homework 9.2. Distress Tolerance: Practice with Pros and Cons
    - Sharing with class
    - Sharing with partners
  - Diary cards
- Introduction of main ideas (5 minutes)
  - Review of Handout 10.1. Distress Tolerance: Overview of Reality Acceptance Skills
  - What is the difference between crisis survival and reality acceptance skills?
  - Generate an example of something you need to radically accept.
- Discussion: Reality acceptance skills and radical acceptance (25 minutes)
  - Review of Handout 10.2. Distress Tolerance: Accepting Reality (8 minutes)
    - Brief review of four solutions to any problem.
    - Suffering = pain + nonacceptance.
    - Accepting facts of the past and present moments, but not the future.
    - Awareness, acceptance, action.
  - Class exercise: Practicing Radical Acceptance 10.4 (7 minutes)
    - Use Homework 10.4. Distress Tolerance: Choosing Things for Radical Acceptance Practice.
    - Identify items you need to radically accept.
  - Class exercise: Small-group discussion of Handout 10.3 (10 minutes)
    - Discuss 10 steps of practicing radical acceptance.
    - Determine two steps to use over the next week.
- Lesson summary (3 minutes)
  - Radical acceptance is for problems that cannot be solved in the long term.
  - Nonacceptance of reality turns pain into suffering.

- Homework assignment (2 minutes)
  - Homework 10.4. Distress Tolerance: Choosing Things for Radical Acceptance Practice
    - Practice at least two steps in radical acceptance.
  - Diary cards

DETAILED LESSON PLAN

Mindfulness Exercise (5 minutes)

Participating: Standing on One Leg (3 minutes)

Welcome the class and introduce the exercise. Explain:

Today we are going to begin with a mindfulness activity that involves the skill of participation. We are going to practice mindfully standing on one leg. You will need to pay attention to your balance and throw yourself fully into standing on one leg. Find a place on the floor about 5–6 inches in front of you where you can gently hold your gaze during the practice. Practice being aware of the position of your body, the sensations in your leg, and any urges that you might have, while focusing on your balancing. If you notice your mind starting to drift to other thoughts, or if you start to have judgments, gently bring yourself back to standing on one leg. If you feel like you are going to fall, go ahead and put your hand on your desk to steady yourself. If you do fall, put a hand down, or put a leg down, just notice it without judgment, and return to standing on one leg when you are able.

Continue:

When I say 1, that's the signal to stand in a mindful position, the way I just described. When I say 2, that's the signal to take a deep breath. When I say 3, that's the signal to begin the practice by lifting one leg. As usual, I'll say, "Stop," to end.

Now start the practice by counting to 3.

1: Stand in the mindful position. 2: Take a deep breath. 3: Lift one leg and begin the practice.

Have the students do the exercise for 1 minute, and then say, "Stop," to end the practice.

Describing Observations of the Exercise (2 minutes)

Highlight:

You had to be very mindful while maintaining your balance. If your mind were to drift to other thoughts or judgments, you would be out of the present moment of standing on one leg and could potentially lose your balance and fall. That is a key to mindfulness: maintaining your stance in the present moment.

Have students share their observations of the mindfulness exercise. Provide feedback about observations as needed, ensuring that each statement consists of something that a student can observe and describe nonjudgmentally (e.g., I noticed starting to fall when my thoughts were not focused on my body, I noticed stopping with each pause, I noticed a thought about how this was different from last week, I noticed a thought . . . , I noticed the sensation . . . , I noticed my mind wandering to other thoughts. I had lots of thoughts about how this could be helpful to me, I noticed I liked last week's practice better, I noticed I was uncomfortable so had to move . . .).

Homework Review (10 minutes)

Homework 9.2. Distress Tolerance: Practice with Pros and Cons

SHARING WITH THE CLASS

Begin by briefly reviewing one Homework 9.2 example of completing a pros-and-cons list with the entire class. As you review the list, be sure to highlight the use of all four quadrants, short- and long-term consequences, and checking the facts or validity of the items. Invite the entire class to add further pros and cons to the list.

SHARING WITH PARTNERS

Divide the students into pairs. Instruct each student in each pair to read to the other what the problem behavior is and then share the pros-and-cons list. (Remind the students that they should be discussing their class-appropriate pros-and-cons lists.) In addition, have the partners briefly discuss with each other any other skills they used that week that they may need help with.

Walk around listening as the dyads talk about their lists. Make sure that each list was filled out correctly, as well as that the pros for resisting crisis urges and the cons for acting on crisis urges are greater than the cons for resisting crisis urges and the pros for acting on them. Encourage students to discuss the difference between short- and long-term consequences, as well as to challenge any items that may not be valid. Check with students to ask whether they used their pros-and-cons lists, and, if so, whether they were effective.

Encourage students to keep their lists in an easily accessible place, especially if they have written pros and cons for avoiding problem behaviors they typically engage in. Some troubleshooting may be necessary to make sure that the students will in fact keep their lists in their designated places.

Follow up on any students who did not complete the homework, and briefly problem-solve what interfered with the homework completion.

Diary Cards

As usual, ask all students to turn in their diary cards and homework sheets to be reviewed. If you are not able to review homework with each student each lesson, then be sure to get to each student over the course of several lessons.

Introduction of Main Ideas (5 minutes)

Review of Handout 10.1. Distress Tolerance: Overview of Reality Acceptance Skills

Begin by pointing out that Handout 10.1 simply lists the skills the class will learn in the next few weeks and that you will not be teaching all of the skills here and now. Then say:

> We have now completed the crisis survival skills in the Distress Tolerance module, and we are moving into the reality acceptance skills. Who can remind us what the difference is between crisis survival and reality acceptance skills?

Elicit (or give) this answer: Crisis survival skills are used to tolerate short-term problems that can't be solved right now. Reality acceptance skills are used to tolerate long-term problems—ones that either occurred in the past or are in the future and cannot be solved. Then go on:

> These are the skills for recognizing and accepting reality when problems occur that we cannot solve, and these problems cause pain. These skills are designed to help you work with your life/reality instead of against it. Although you can use these skills in a crisis, they are mainly skills to help with problems you cannot solve in the long term.

Refer to Handout 10.1:

> There are four reality acceptance skills: radical acceptance, turning the mind, willingness, and mindfulness of current thoughts. Today we are going to focus on learning the skill of radical acceptance.

Ask students to start thinking about things in their own lives that they think are unfair or painful, but that they must accept. Provide examples such as these:

- *Your GPA falls below 2.0, and now you cannot play in the next game.*
- *Your ex-boyfriend/ex-girlfriend is dating someone else.*

Give the students about 1 minute to identify and write down something they need to radically accept in their lives. Then tell the class:

> As we go through and learn the skills of accepting reality, I want you to keep your example in mind to see if it fits our definition of acceptance or how you might need to change it.

Discussion: Reality Acceptance Skills and Radical Acceptance (25 minutes)

Review of Handout 10.2. Distress Tolerance: Accepting Reality (8 minutes)

Write on the board the four solutions to any problem:

- Solve the problem.
- Change how you feel.

- Accept it.
- Stay miserable (or possibly make things worse).

Then say:

During the first lesson, we discussed these four solutions to any problem. Today we are going to focus on accepting the problem or accepting reality by using radical acceptance. When we get to the emotion regulation skills, we will focus on solving the problem and changing how we feel about the problem.

Continue:

Reality is "what is." Everything is caused, and pain is inevitable in our lives. Cause and effect are the rules of the universe; everything should be as it is, because everything is caused. If we want to change an effect, we have to change the cause. We have to accept what we cannot change in this moment.

Ask students to read the points in Handout 10.2 under "Radical Acceptance." Then discuss the following examples.

First, let's say you are at track practice before a big meet and you twist your ankle. You refuse to accept that you are injured and you keep practicing, but the more you run, the more your ankle hurts. Radical acceptance is fully and completely accepting the reality that you have a hurt ankle and are going to need to rest it and that you will not be able to run in tomorrow's meet. Nonacceptance or rejecting reality is likely to be experienced through anger and blaming someone (including possibly yourself) or something for causing you to hurt your ankle. You may be also judging yourself or others by calling yourself stupid or an idiot for not watching where you were going. Nonacceptance is saying things like "This shouldn't have happened. I should be able to run." How do you think you would feel if you were saying these things to yourself?

Allow students to answer. Then go on:

In this example, radical acceptance is completely and totally accepting the facts of the reality that regardless of what caused you to hurt your ankle, your ankle is hurt; it hurts even to walk; and you will not be able to compete in tomorrow's meet. It is likely that sadness or other painful emotions may arise once you reach acceptance. But when those emotions do arise, you can validate your emotions and allow yourself to feel them and then let them go. Acceptance turns suffering you can't cope with into pain you can cope with; it can help you to acknowledge, recognize, and endure. If you don't reach acceptance, the emotions will keep growing and growing and make things more difficult for you, and you begin to suffer.

On the board, write this equation: "Suffering = Pain + Nonacceptance." Say:

Another way to think about this equation is through this statement: "Pain is inevitable, but suffering is optional." The way to stop suffering is through acceptance of the pain or reality.

Let's look at another example of radical acceptance: having to accept the fact of a breakup when the person you liked has moved on to someone else. Nonacceptance of the fact—writing letters, stalking the person on social media, or otherwise acting from emotion mind to get the person back—only leads to suffering. Once you accept the breakup, the pain will still be there, but it will just be pain—pain without suffering.

Continue:

Radical acceptance is acknowledging real life rather than rejecting it. It is accepting the things that we cannot change in life. With acceptance, we can turn suffering into pain you can manage. Once we get to the emotion regulation skills, you will learn how to experience painful emotions or change them if you want.

Radical acceptance is completely and fully accepting the facts of the present moment and the past; it is also knowing that the future does not yet exist, and is therefore not a fact we have to accept. For instance, you don't have to accept that you will never have a boyfriend or girlfriend or never get into college; those are thoughts, not facts. You may need to accept in the present moment that you don't have a boyfriend or girlfriend, or accept facts about the past, such as that you failed biology last year, and this may hurt your chances of getting into a top-ranked college. This allows you to acknowledge your current pain and endure it until you are able to let it go.

Write "Awareness, Acceptance, and Action" on the board as steps to change. Then go on:

Refusing to accept reality does not make things simply go away. First you must be Aware of the problem; then you Accept the reality of the problem; and that must occur before Actions, such as problem solving or grieving, can occur. If you continue to reject reality, it will continue to cause suffering and haunt you. Think of this as the triple-A model: Awareness, Acceptance, Action.

Further, radical acceptance is not approval. Accepting something does not mean that you like it or that you are giving in. It is also not passivity, helplessness, or weakness; accepting something does not mean that you do not try to change it. Remember, pain is inevitable, but suffering is optional. We will all have pain in our lives. It is how we manage the pain that is important.

CLASS EXERCISE: PRACTICING RADICAL ACCEPTANCE
(7 MINUTES)

Have students take out Homework 10.4. Distress Tolerance: Choosing Things for Radical Acceptance Practice. They will continue to complete this sheet for homework as well. Ask:

Think about the example you came up with at the beginning of class. How does what you thought you needed to accept now fit with our definition of radical acceptance?

Then explain:

We are going to use this worksheet both now and as part of your homework to determine two very important things and two less important things you need to practice radically accepting. Determine now whether the thing you wrote down at the beginning of class is a very important thing or a less important thing, and write it down in the section for either the first or second step.

Next, have everyone start Step 1 on Homework 10.4 (identifying two very important things to accept right now, and then rating current acceptance of these things on the 0–5 scale in the handout). Then have everyone start Step 2 (identifying two less important things to accept this week, and again rating current acceptance of those things on the 0–5 scale). Ask for a student or two to share a class-appropriate example.

Finally, have students start Step 3 (going back and checking the facts of their problems, as well as checking that they are not judgments and represent reality). Again, ask a few students to share examples with the class and provide feedback regarding judgments and reality.

Students will complete Steps 4–6 of Homework 10.4 as their homework for practicing radical acceptance. Step 5 lists several ways in which students can practice radical acceptance of something. (Note that the skill of opposite action will be taught during the Emotion Regulation module. Many of the other points focus on mindfully observing.)

CLASS EXERCISE: SMALL-GROUP DISCUSSION OF HANDOUT 10.3 (10 MINUTES)

Have students break into small groups (two to four students each), and read through Handout 10.3. Distress Tolerance: Radical Acceptance, Step by Step. Explain:

Handout 10.3 describes a step-by-step plan of how to practice radical acceptance. These same 10 steps are listed on Homework 10.4 that we just looked at. Part of your homework will be to practice using some or all of these steps in order to increase your level of acceptance for step 4. In groups, I want you to discuss each of the different ways to practice radical acceptance, and determine at least two ways in which you can practice radical acceptance over the next week for one of your very important items and one of the less important items.

Lesson Summary (2 minutes)

Congratulate the students for their hard work on thinking through such a big topic.

Review, and ask students to describe, radical acceptance. The following points should be covered:

- Radical acceptance is for problems that cannot be solved in the long term.
- Denying reality will not change reality. Changing reality requires first accepting the facts of reality.
- Pain is a part of reality that cannot always be prevented.
- Nonacceptance of reality turns pain into suffering.

Ask the students whether they have any questions.

Homework Assignment(3 minutes)

Homework 10.4. Distress Tolerance: Choosing Things for Radical Acceptance Practice

Some of this homework sheet will already have been completed in class. The primary homework is for students to practice radically accepting the two things identified earlier and completing the worksheet. Read through the entire sheet to ensure clarity, and ask whether there are any questions.

Diary Cards

Hand out new diary cards to the students. Highlight that they have now learned radical acceptance, and that when they practice this skill for their homework, they are to circle the days and rate the skill use for the week on the diary card (along with the other skills that they have been taught).

Finally, do some troubleshooting: Ask students whether they have any questions about the homework or any obstacles to completing it. If so, answer the questions and address the obstacles. Obstacles may include, but are not limited to, the following: Students have no intention of doing the assignment, have too much other homework this week, are likely to forget, or don't understand the assignment. Help students to identify their obstacles, and work with them to make a plan to overcome them. Examples include encouraging a student to write down the assignment and set a reminder in a cell phone or calendar to complete it; discussing why a student has no intention of doing the homework, and working on increasing his or her motivation and the relevance of the assignment (e.g., grades); or clarifying any other points. Troubleshooting should be done each week after the homework is assigned.

Distress Tolerance
Turning the Mind and Willingness

SUMMARY

Today's lesson focuses on the reality acceptance skills of turning the mind and willingness. Turning the mind is based on the awareness that radical acceptance is a choice that we sometimes must make over and over again. Just because we have radically accepted something one time, this does not mean that we will have accepted it forever. The skill of willingness is similar to the practice of effectiveness from the mindfulness "how" skills. Making a choice to approach something with willingness over willfulness can be a difficult skill at times. Willingness includes choosing to be active and effective when responding to the reality of our lives. Willfulness is the opposite: It is choosing to sit on our hands or dig in our heels to be right rather than effective. Students will also engage in a class exercise where they develop short skits to demonstrate the use of these skills.

MAIN POINTS

1. Accepting reality requires choosing to accept and turning the mind in the direction of acceptance (sometimes over and over again).
2. Accepting reality through willingness is playing the cards we are dealt and doing what works, rather than sitting on our hands or trying to fix the situation.

MATERIALS

1. Handouts for this lesson:
   - Handout 11.1. Distress Tolerance: Turning the Mind
   - Handout 11.2. Distress Tolerance: Willingness
   - Homework 11.3. Distress Tolerance: Practice with Turning the Mind and Willingness
2. Extra student skills binders, with pens or pencils, for students who attend class without materials.

3. Dry-erase markers or chalk for writing on the board.
4. Bowl and jellybeans for mindfulness.
5. Diary cards: Have new diary cards ready to distribute at the end of class. If possible, highlight the "Turning the mind" and "Willingness" skills.

PREPARATION

1. Review the lesson plan as well as handouts in student skills binder.
2. Arrange desks in the classroom, if possible, so that students are able to see each other.

LESSON OVERVIEW AND TIMELINE

- Mindfulness exercise (5 minutes)
  - Observing: Bowl of jellybeans (3 minutes)
  - Describing observations of the exercise (2 minutes)
- Homework review (10 minutes)
  - Homework 10.4. Distress Tolerance: Choosing Things for Radical Acceptance Practice
    - Sharing with class
  - Diary cards
- Introduction of main ideas (2 minutes)
  - Acceptance does not occur just one time, but involves turning the mind back to acceptance when you find yourself in nonacceptance again.
  - Willingness is doing what is needed to be effective.
- Discussion: Turning the mind (13 minutes)
  - Review of Handout 11.1. Distress Tolerance: Turning the Mind
    - Three steps to turning the mind
    - Small-group discussions
    - Full-class discussion
- Discussion: Willingness (15 minutes)
  - Review of Handout 11.2. Distress Tolerance: Willingness (5 minutes)
    - Class exercise: Small-group skits of willfulness versus willingness (10 minutes)
- Lesson summary (2 minutes)
  - Briefly review turning the mind and willingness.
- Homework assignment (3 minutes)
  - Homework 11.3. Distress Tolerance: Practice with Turning the Mind and Willingness
    - Identify a situation when you were experiencing non-acceptance and practiced turning the mind.
    - Identify a situation when you may have been willful and used willingness to increase your acceptance of reality.
  - Diary cards

DETAILED LESSON PLAN

Mindfulness Exercise (5 minutes)

Observing: Bowl of Jellybeans (3 minutes)

Welcome the class and state that today's mindfulness exercise will involve observing. Place in the center of your desk or table, or in a place where all students can see it, a bowl full of jellybeans. Depending on the classroom setup, you may need to use more than one bowl of jellybeans and to move students around the bowls. Explain:

> *Today we are going to practice observing our thoughts, urges, and possible judgments. I am not going to count to 3 as I usually do to start our exercise. Today I will give you a set of instructions as we go through the exercise. Throughout the exercise, I want you to observe or notice the thoughts that you have, any urges you have, and any judgments you may have.*
>
> *First, get into our usual mindful/wide-awake position, and be sure you can see the bowl of jellybeans from where you are.*
>
> *Now I want you to start observing the jellybeans. Notice the colors, the shapes, and the sizes. Imagine what each different color tastes like. Now think about your favorite color. Look at a jellybean in your favorite color, and imagine what it tastes like.*

Allow this for 30 seconds.

> *Now go ahead and pick out your two favorite jellybeans from the bowl. If someone else takes your jellybean before you do, or if you get the jellybean you wanted, notice the emotions, sensations, or thoughts that arise, and then let them go. Notice them and then bring your attention back to the jellybeans in your hand.*
>
> *Observe the jellybeans in your hand. Notice any urges that you may have to eat the jellybeans without acting on that urge.*

Allow students 30–45 seconds to observe their jellybeans.

> *Now pass your jellybeans to the person to your right.*

After students have passed their jellybeans, continue by saying:

> *Now observe the jellybeans that were just passed to you, and notice any other thoughts, urges, sensations, or emotions that occur.*

Have students observe the new jellybeans for another 45–60 seconds. Then instruct the students to stop.

Describing Observations of the Exercise (2 minutes)

Ask a few students to share their observations in the moment. In particular, ask whether any students had difficulty letting go of their original two jellybeans.

> *What emotions, urges, thoughts, or sensations did you notice arising within you? Did anyone have difficulty accepting that they had to let go of their original jellybeans?*

Then state:

> *Reality acceptance doesn't always have to be about big, huge deals in your life. It can be necessary to radically accept something as simple as the fact that you had to pass your candy that you were excited to eat to the person next to you, and maybe you ended up with colors that you really don't like. Smaller things like this are also part of accepting reality.*

Provide feedback about observations as needed, ensuring that each statement consists of something that a student can observe and describe nonjudgmentally (.e.g., I noticed the urge and thought that I could quickly eat my jellybeans before passing them, I noticed stopping with each pause, I noticed a thought about how this was different from last week, I noticed a thought . . . , I noticed the sensation . . . , I noticed my mind wandering to other thoughts. I had lots of thoughts about how this could be helpful to me, I noticed I liked last week's practice better, I noticed I was uncomfortable so had to move . . .).

Homework Review (10 minutes)

Homework 10.4. Distress Tolerance: Choosing Things for Radical Acceptance Practice

SHARING WITH CLASS

Have the students take out their completed copies of Homework 10.4. Explain:

> *Radical acceptance can be a difficult concept to learn, and we are going to deepen our understanding by hearing how you did on practicing this skill over the last week.*

Have students share with the class which of the methods in Step 5 of this sheet they used to practice radical acceptance, and how much, if at all, their level of acceptance changed during the week.

Validate and reinforce each student, as appropriate:

> *Thank you for sharing. It sounds like you tried really hard.*

Troubleshoot by eliciting more information from the students to deepen their understanding by asking whether they noticed a difference after practicing radical acceptance; whether it was difficult; and, if so, what they did to get past the difficulty. If appropriate, ask for things that they might do differently if they were to try this activity again.

Diary Cards

As usual, ask all students to turn in their diary cards and homework sheets to be reviewed. If you are not able to review homework with each student each lesson, then be sure to get to each student over the course of several lessons.

Introduction of Main Ideas (2 minutes)

Congratulate the class for almost finishing the Distress Tolerance module. Then say:

> *Today we will learn two more skills for accepting reality, and next week will be our final week in the Distress Tolerance module. The first skill is called turning the mind, and the second skill is called using willingness over willfulness.*

Ask:

> *Do you think that if you radically accept something, then you have accepted it forever?*

Allow students to respond, and then continue.

> *Sometimes we have to keep radically accepting the same thing over and over again. Turning the mind will teach us how to do that. Often acceptance can come and go, and when we find ourselves in a place of nonacceptance, we must turn our minds back to acceptance. We may recognize when we have gone back to nonacceptance—when anger or willfulness appear and we are rejecting reality again. Turning the mind is about choosing to turn back to accepting reality; it's like making a decision when we come to a fork in the road. Turning the mind may need to occur once a year, once a month, once a week, once an hour, or 30 times a minute. We must practice being mindful to notice when nonacceptance or rejecting reality occurs.*
>
> *Using willingness over willfulness is similar to practicing being effective from the mindfulness "how" skills. Sometimes it is hard to be willing to do what is needed and effective. So we have to actively practice ungluing our feet from our position or being willful in order to be effective. Willingness is doing just what is needed to get through the situation.*

Discussion: Turning the Mind (13 minutes)

Review of Handout 11.1. Distress Tolerance: Turning the Mind

Have students turn to Handout 11.1. Say:

> *Radical acceptance is a choice that is made, and turning the mind is the act of making that choice. It is turning your mind toward acceptance and away from rejecting reality. It is like coming to a fork in the road, where you have the choice between acceptance and nonacceptance—the acceptance road and the rejecting-reality road. It is your choice which fork to choose. The choice itself is not yet acceptance; it just turns you toward the path.*

SMALL-GROUP DISCUSSIONS

Have students break into small groups of two to four to discuss the steps in Handout 11.1. Say:

> We are going to read the bullet points under "Turning the Mind" in Handout 11.1. These can be thought of as a step-by-step guide in how to turn the mind.

Ask a student to read one step (one bullet point) at a time. After each step, have the small groups discuss the points. Instruct the students:

> Step 1: Step 1 is about being mindful and observing or noticing when you may not be accepting reality. Typical signs of nonacceptance are anger, bitterness, being judgmental of yourself or a situation, or using lots of "shoulds," as in "Things should be different then they are."
>
> Step 2: Step 2 is to make an inner commitment or a wise mind decision to choose to accept reality completely—to turn your mind toward reality when you are at the fork in the road. It's like sitting on a swivel chair and having to actively turn your mind and body toward acceptance. How do you access your wise mind? Do you use one of the practices from the mindfulness lessons? Share an example of a time when you came to a fork in the road.
>
> Step 3: Step 3 is about recognizing that acceptance doesn't occur just one time and then you are home free. Choosing to radically accept something may need to be done over and over again, from once a month to 30 times a minute. Also, think about what your cues or signs are for nonacceptance. How do you know when you are not accepting something? Make a plan to be on the lookout for those cues in the future. And how might you remind yourself to turn back to acceptance?

Have the students discuss in small groups as well:

> Are there other times when you can recall that you were not accepting reality? Did you know it in the moment? Now that you are learning these skills, what could you have done differently?

FULL-CLASS DISCUSSION

Discuss the students' answers to the previous questions. Check in to see whether any students realized that they might have been choosing to be in nonacceptance. How might they turn to acceptance in the future?

Discussion: Willingness (15 minutes)

Review of Handout 11.2. Distress Tolerance: Willingness (5 minutes)

Have students turn to Handout 11.2. Explain:

> Denying that things are happening in your life, refusing to be part of these things, or ignoring problems do not make them go away. This is being willful. Imagine yourself standing in front of a pitching machine in order to stop it from throwing balls at you. Refusing to hit

the balls doesn't stop the machine from having them shoot out at you. You have to swing. If you don't swing, you will get a strike; if you stand in front of the machine and tell it to stop, the machine will pitch the next ball anyway, and you will get hit by the ball.

Have one student read the bullet points under "Willfulness." Then ask:

Can you give some examples of willful behavior, personal or general? Has anyone in this class ever been willful?

Elicit students' examples, or give these:

- *Digging your feet into the ground and not moving.*
- *Not being willing to listen to a friend explain his or her side of the story.*
- *Washing your parents' car, but doing it grudgingly the whole time.*

Then ask the class:

If this is willfulness, what would willingness look like?

Gather examples, and then ask one student to read the bullet points under "Replace Willfulness with Willingness." After this reading, continue:

Willingness is wisely responding to what happens in life voluntarily, without complaint and bitterness. It is accepting "what is" and participating in it completely. Willingness is responding from wise mind, whereas willfulness is responding from emotion mind or reasonable mind. Willfulness is focused on "me" and saying "no" or "yes, but" to life's situations.

We've all had times in life where we want to fight reality. Think about the first day back at school after your last break this year. I bet that when the alarm clock went off and you realized that your vacation was over, you put the pillow over your head and went back to sleep. That was willfulness—saying no to the reality of life. Willingness, on the other hand, would be getting up, accepting that the vacation was over, and being ready to experience what school had to bring.

Willingness is accepting what is and responding appropriately and effectively. It is doing just what is needed in the current situation or moment. It is complete openness to the moment. It doesn't mean you have to like it.

Discuss ways of being able to tell willfulness from willingness. Include body differences and posture. Then have students fill out the questions at the bottom of Handout 11.2, and ask for a few volunteers to share what they wrote.

CLASS EXERCISE: SMALL-GROUP SKITS OF WILLFULNESS VERSUS WILLINGNESS (10 MINUTES)

Divide the class into groups of four or five. Instruct the students that each group is to come up with two 30-second skits involving the same scenario. The first skit is to demonstrate willfulness, and the second, willingness. The students are to come up with their own appropriate scenarios. They can use examples similar to the ones already discussed. Remind them that class is almost over, so everyone has to come up with their skits in 3–4 minutes.

After 3–4 minutes, have the groups each act out their two skits without stating which one is willingness and which is willfullness. Ask students to identify which skit is which. Provide feedback as needed about what they did well and what corrections (if any) might be needed.

Encourage students to continue actively practicing the skills of turning the mind and willingness and to be mindful of when they are engaging in willful behavior. As the teacher, you may now also identify and ask about when you suspect willful behavior on the part of the students (e.g., "Is it possible that you are being willful right now?").

Lesson Summary (2 minutes)

Congratulate the students for their hard work in thinking through some tough topics, both today and over the course of this module. Then ask for volunteers to review briefly what turning the mind and willingness mean.

- Turning the mind: Making the choice of acceptance when we come to a fork in the road.
- Willingness: Choosing to be effective and do what is needed; the opposite of willfulness.

Ask the students whether they have any questions.

Homework Assignment (3 minutes)

Homework 11.3. Distress Tolerance: Practice with Turning the Mind and Willingness

Review this homework sheet with the students, making sure that it is clear to them. Explain:

You are to identify a time over the coming week when you are experiencing nonacceptance and use the steps to practice turning your mind toward acceptance. You will also identify and describe a time when you practice willingness over the week.

Remind the students that next week they will finish the Distress Tolerance module (and that the module test also will be next week, if the test is given). As preparation for the test, they should review all of their handouts and notes for the Mindfulness and Distress Tolerance modules since the test also includes a few questions on the core mindfulness skills.

Diary Cards

Hand out new diary cards to the students. Highlight that they have now learned turning the mind and willingness, and that when they practice these skills for homework, they are to circle the days and rate the skill use for the week on the diary card (along with the other skills that they have been taught).

Finally, do some troubleshooting: Ask students whether they have any questions about the homework or any obstacles to completing it. If so, answer the questions and address the obstacles. Obstacles may include, but are not limited to, the following: Students have no intention of doing the assignment, have too much other homework this week, are likely to forget, or don't understand the assignment. Help students to identify their obstacles, and work with them to make a plan to overcome them. Examples include encouraging a student to write down the assignment and set a reminder in a cell phone or calendar to complete it; discussing why a student has no intention of doing the homework, and working on increasing his or her motivation and the relevance of the assignment (e.g., grades); or clarifying any other points. Troubleshooting should be done each week after the homework is assigned.

Distress Tolerance
Mindfulness of Current Thoughts
(and Distress Tolerance Test)

SUMMARY

The final skill of the Distress Tolerance module is mindfulness of current thoughts. This skill is the method by which we can act and feel separately from our thoughts. Mindfulness of current thoughts is the opposite of trying to change thoughts; it is about allowing thoughts to come in and go out without holding on to them. Mindfulness of current thoughts includes the practice of observing, as well as the skill of labeling a thought as just a thought (which may be a fact or may not be). Through observing our thoughts, we gain distance from them and can watch them come and go, without holding on to them or believing that they must be true. The module test can be given during the second half of today's class. If you choose not to give the test within this lesson, then there are additional teaching points and exercises to strengthen this skill.

The test allows students to demonstrate what they have learned in the Distress Tolerance module, and enables you to assess for any areas of weakness that may need further review.

MAIN POINTS

1. Through mindfulness of current thoughts, we can allow our thoughts to be just thoughts, rather than holding on to them or suppressing them and treating all thoughts as facts.
2. The test is used to examine students' knowledge and understanding of the different distress tolerance skills (as well as the core mindfulness skills).

MATERIALS

1. Handouts for this lesson:
   • Handout 12.1. Distress Tolerance: Mindfulness of Current Thoughts, Step by Step

- Handout 12.2. Distress Tolerance: Ways to Practice Mindfulness of Current Thoughts
- Homework 12.3. Distress Tolerance: Practicing Mindfulness of Current Thoughts

2. Distress Tolerance Test, if the test is being administered within this lesson (make enough copies for the whole class).
3. Extra student skills binders, with pens or pencils, for students who attend class without materials.
4. Dry-erase markers or chalk for writing on the board.
5. Diary cards: Have new diary cards ready to distribute at the end of class. If possible, highlight the "Mindfulness of current thoughts" skill.

PREPARATION

1. Review the lesson plan as well as handouts in student skills binder.
2. If you are not giving the Distress Tolerance Test today, arrange desks, if possible, so that students are able to see each other.
3. If you are giving the test today, arrange desks as usual for taking exams.

LESSON OVERVIEW AND TIMELINE

- Mindfulness exercise (5 minutes)
  - Observing: Counting one breath (3 minutes)
  - Describing observations of the exercise (2 minutes)
- Homework review (10 minutes; 6 minutes if administering test today)
  - Homework 11.3. Distress Tolerance: Practice with Turning the Mind and Willingness
    - Sharing with class
    - Diary cards
- Introduction of main ideas (3 minutes)
  - Boat on a river metaphor
- Discussion: Mindfulness of current thoughts (10 minutes)
  - Review of Handout 12.1. Distress Tolerance: Mindfulness of Current Thoughts, Step by Step
    - Observe your thoughts.
    - Adopt a curious mind.
    - Remember: You are not your thoughts.
    - Don't block or suppress thoughts.
- (If not giving the test today:)
  - Review of Handout 12.2. Distress Tolerance: Ways to Practice Mindfulness of Current Thoughts (15 minutes)
  - Module and test review (5 minutes)
  - Homework assignment (2 minutes)
    - Homework 12.3. Distress Tolerance: Practicing Mindfulness of Current Thoughts
      - Practice observing and describing thoughts each day.
    - Diary cards

- (If giving the test today:)
  - Homework assignment (1 minute)
    - Homework 12.3. Distress Tolerance: Practicing Mindfulness of Current Thoughts
      - Practice observing and describing thoughts each day.
    - Diary cards
  - Module and test review (5 minutes)
  - Administration of test (20 minutes)

DETAILED LESSON PLAN

Mindfulness Exercise (5 minutes)

Observing: Counting One Breath (3 minutes)

Welcome the class and introduce the mindfulness exercise. Explain:

> Today we are going to practice observing and practicing our breath again. In past exercises, we have simply observed our breath, or we have observed our breath and counted to 10 repeatedly. Today we are going to focus on noticing just one breath at a time and letting each breath go, just as we practice letting each moment go. We are going to count our breath because focusing on our bodily sensations helps anchor us in the present moment. Remember, since we always have our breath with us, it is something we can always use as a focusing point.

Continue:

> For this practice, we are going to observe our inhale and count to 1 on the exhale. On the next breath, we will observe the inhale again, and then count to 1 on the exhale. We are only focusing on counting to 1, for just this one breath, just this one moment. If you notice that all of a sudden you are at 2, 5, or 9, just notice it, let it go, and return to 1. If you notice that your mind is drifting away from your breathing, notice it, and gently bring your attention back to your breath and counting. If you find yourself having judgmental thoughts, notice them, let them go, and return to your breath. If you notice any urges to move other than blinking or swallowing, notice each urge without acting on it, and return your focus to your breath.

Go on:

> When I say 1, that's the signal to sit in the mindful/wide-awake position we have often used before. This means keeping our feet flat on the floor, sitting up straight, and putting our hands in our laps. For this exercise, we will keep our eyes open, but with a soft gaze, which means looking forward and down but at nothing in particular. We don't always want to practice mindfulness with our eyes closed because we don't live our lives with our eyes always closed. When I say 2, that's the signal to take a deep breath. When I say 3, that's the signal to begin the practice. I'll say, "Stop," to end the practice.

Now start the practice by counting to 3.

1: Get yourself into the mindful/wide-awake position. 2: Take a deep breath. 3: Begin the practice.

Have students do the exercise for 2 minutes, and then say, "Stop."

Describing Observations of the Exercise (2 minutes)

Ask some students to share one observation of their experience of the exercise. (Depending on the number of students in class, you may not be able to call on each student every time.) Ask whether any students lost track of their counting; if so, how often? Provide feedback about observations as needed, ensuring that each statement consists of something a student can observe and describe nonjudgmentally (e.g., I noticed the urge and thought to count past 1, I noticed stopping with each pause, I noticed a thought about how this was different from last week, I noticed a thought . . . , I noticed the sensation . . . , I noticed my mind wandering to other thoughts. I had lots of thoughts about how this could be helpful to me, I noticed I liked last week's practice better, I noticed I was uncomfortable so had to move . . .).

Finally, for this exercise, emphasize the importance of catching distractions:

Remember, it is just as important for us to notice when we are distracted as it is to stay focused on counting our breath. By noticing when we are distracted and bringing our attention back to our breath, we are strengthening our "observing muscles." This is important because when we are in emotion mind, we need to notice this in order to get back to wise mind. When we are daydreaming in class and not paying attention to the lecture, we want to recognize or observe that we are daydreaming, so we can bring our attention back to the present moment. Over time and with a lot of practice, these skills will get stronger.

Homework Review (6 minutes if administering test; 10 minutes if not administering test)

Homework 11.3. Distress Tolerance: Practice with Turning the Mind and Willingness

SHARING WITH THE CLASS

Have the students take out their completed copies of Homework 11.3. Ask some students to describe how they practiced turning the mind and using willingness over willfulness. Did they all notice a time during the week when they had to make a choice between acceptance and nonacceptance?

Diary Cards

As usual, ask all students to turn in their diary cards and homework sheets to be reviewed. If you are not able to review homework with each student each lesson, then be sure to get to each student over the course of several lessons.

Introduction of Main Ideas (3 minutes)

Explain:

> *Today is the last day we will be working on the distress tolerance skills. Nice work!*
>
> *Today's skill is called mindfulness of current thoughts. This skill will help us to notice and react to our thoughts as just thoughts. Do you ever notice that sometimes you can get caught up in your thoughts, and then your thoughts start spiraling into bigger thoughts and may even begin to start causing the intensity of your emotions to increase? We are going to work on stopping that.*

Introduce this metaphor:

> *Imagine you are sitting on a large and beautiful riverbank. Coming down the river is a boat. And on that boat are all of your thoughts, emotions, sensations, and urges. You have two choices: You can jump in the water, swim out to the boat, climb aboard, and go down the river with all of your thoughts, emotions, sensations, and urges. Or you can simply remain on the riverbank and watch the boat go down the river until it is out of sight. Which choice would you make?*

Allow students to discuss this question for 2 minutes. Then say:

> *Through mindfulness of current thoughts, you are allowing your thoughts to come and go rather than suppressing them or holding on to them.*

Discussion: Mindfulness of Current Thoughts (10 minutes)

Review of Handout 12.1. Distress Tolerance:
Mindfulness of Current Thoughts, Step by Step

Have the students turn to Handout 12.1. Explain:

> *Mindfulness of current thoughts can also be thought of as "allowing the mind." By this, we mean allowing the mind to do what it does—generate thoughts from continuous firings of our brain cells. Have you ever tried <u>not</u> to think about something, such as flying pink elephants? What probably happens is that you keep thinking about flying pink elephants. As another one of our reality acceptance skills, we are going to practice being mindful of our current thoughts by simply letting them come in and go out, without holding on to them and without pushing them away.*
>
> *This skill is different from the emotion regulation skill of checking the facts, which we will learn later. This skill is about building a new relationship with our thoughts, rather than reacting to every thought we have or trying to stop or suppress our thoughts; we are going to practice allowing our thoughts just to come and go as they please. In some ways, we can think of it as taking away the power of our thoughts, and acknowledging them as just words or images passing over a screen in our minds.*

> *As we discussed during the Mindfulness module, you are not your thoughts. Thoughts are just thoughts, and often thoughts are not even the facts of the situation. A good way to think about this is with the sentence "Just because I think it, this doesn't mean that it's true."*

Write this sentence on the board: "Just because I think it, this doesn't mean that it's true." Students can also change this statement into "Just because someone said it, this doesn't mean that it's true." This is effective for countering the judgments that they make of themselves, or that they think others are making of them. Both sentences may help students to detach themselves from their thoughts if they learn that a thought is simply a thought and not all thoughts are facts.

The boxes in Handout 12.1 present four steps to practicing mindfulness of current thoughts. Go around the room and have a different student read each box.

OBSERVE YOUR THOUGHTS

Explain:

> *This is the same observing skill we learned during the Mindfulness module—noticing the thought and allowing it to move on.*

Ask:

> *Why would we want to detach or push away our thoughts?*

Allow students to generate answers. Then say:

> *Because our thoughts can take control of our minds. We will all have painful and distressing thoughts; the goal is not to let those thoughts cause us to suffer or lose control. The goal of observing a thought is not to change the thought; it is simply to change our reaction to the thought. By acknowledging the presence of the thought, we can choose to validate that it is there, without validating the content of the thought. Imagine sitting at the edge of the ocean and just allowing your thoughts to wash over you and wash away, just like a wave coming and going.*

ADOPT A CURIOUS MIND

Explain:

> *Rather than completely believing every thought that comes into your mind, assess where the thought comes from and where it goes. Track the path of your thoughts. Notice how one thought can lead to another and then another. Become an objective bystander watching your thoughts as if they are going across an electronic billboard—wondering what will come next, and noticing how quickly the last one is gone. Practice being nonjudgmental of your thoughts.*

REMEMBER: YOU ARE NOT YOUR THOUGHTS

A thought is only a thought, a firing of the brain cells. You do not have to act on every thought your brain produces. Imagine what that would be like if you did. Have you ever had a thought that you just noticed and then let go? Some thoughts are harder than others to do this with, but with practice it will become easier.

DON'T BLOCK OR SUPPRESS THOUGHTS

Just like trying not to think about flying pink elephants, it is really hard to suppress or block our thoughts from coming into our minds. Practice playing with your thoughts. Sing them to the tune of "The Star-Spangled Banner," "Happy Birthday to You," "Twinkle, Twinkle, Little Star," or any other favorite song. When we see words as just words or thoughts as simply firings of the brain cells, they can become meaningless and create only the impact we allow them to.

This skill is truly about building a new relationship with your thoughts—allowing them to come and go. This is a way to decease the suffering that may come with holding on to our thoughts and stewing over them.

Now have students turn to Handout 12.2. Distress Tolerance: Ways to Practice Mindfulness of Current Thoughts. Tell students they can use this handout for ideas about practicing mindfulness of current thoughts. For homework, they should read through this handout and then complete Homework 12.3. Distress Tolerance: Practicing Mindfulness of Current Thoughts.

If you are giving the Distress Tolerance Test today to students, assign the homework now, and then move to module review and the test for the remainder of the class. If you are not giving the test today, you may choose to spend more time on reviewing and practicing mindfulness of current thoughts, as described below (and reviewing the entire module, if time permits). If you are giving the test today, skip to page 170 at the end of this lesson. If you are not giving the test, continue:

Review of Handout 12.2. Distress Tolerance: Ways to Practice Mindfulness of Current Thoughts (15 minutes)

Explain:

There are multiple ways to practice allowing your thoughts to come and go or to stop reacting to our thoughts. Handout 12.2 describes many of these.

Ask one student to read the first section of the handout (about practicing by using words and voice tone). Say:

We often have emotional responses to our thoughts. Our goal is to change how we react to those thoughts by seeing them as just thoughts or images. One way to do this is by saying the word over and over again until it is just a sound.

CLASS EXERCISE

Tell students:

> *We are going to start practicing this by saying the word "fat." This word has a lot of judgments attached to it in our society, and when we think it, we often start down a long path of other judgments about ourselves or others.*
>
> *When I tell you to begin, we are simply going to start saying the word "fat" over and over again for about 1 minute. You can't stop until I say to stop. Feel free to change the speed in which you say it or your voice tone as you go along. Ready, begin: "FAT FAT FAT FAT FAT FAT FAT . . . "*

Stop after 1 minute. Ask:

> *What did you notice during that exercise?*

Elicit responses. Then say:

> *Eventually it just becomes a sound. Another way is to sing the thought/phrase out loud to the tune of a song, such as "Twinkle, Twinkle, Little Star" or "The Star-Spangled Banner."*

Have another student read through the second section of Handout 12.2 (about practicing with opposite action). Then have students think about what thoughts get in the way of their doing things, such as "I can't wear that type of shirt because I will look funny in it," or "I am stupid, so I cannot answer questions in class." Have them write down those thoughts on the handout (under item 4), and imagine what it would be like if they didn't believe those thoughts. Allow 2–3 minutes for this exercise, and then ask students to share their thoughts and what they imagined would be different if they didn't believe all of their thoughts.

Now explain:

> *The final two sections of Handout 12.2 are examples of mindfulness practices: observing thoughts and describing thoughts through imagery.*

Have another student read through the third section of the handout (about practicing by observing thoughts). Then say:

> *Rather than judging our thoughts or letting them take control of where our mind goes, you can practice commenting on your thoughts as they come into your awareness.*

CLASS EXERCISE

Tell students:

> *For the next minute, we are going to simply practice saying to ourselves each time we have a thought, regardless of what the thought is about, "A thought came into my mind," or "Another thought just came into my mind." The goal here is simply to describe each*

thought as a thought, rather than react to its content. When I say, "Begin," start doing this for 1 minute.

Say, "Begin," and stop the class after 1 minute. Ask for observations from students.

Have another student read through the final section of Handout 12.2 (about practicing by imagining). Say:

This way of practicing is similar to the story I told at the beginning of this lesson about sitting on the riverbank. Our goal is to simply allow our mind to watch our thoughts non-judgmentally.

The ultimate goal with mindfulness of current thoughts is to remember that you are not your thoughts and that your thoughts can come and go like the wind. We want to practice letting them go rather than trying to push them away or hold on to them.

Homework Assignment (1 minute if administering test; 2 minutes if not administering test)

Congratulate the students for their hard work in thinking through some tough topics over both today's lesson and the course of this module. Students should read through the rest of Handout 12.2 if it has not been covered in class.

Homework 12.3. Distress Tolerance: Practicing Mindfulness of Current Thoughts

Tell students:

This week you are to practice observing your thoughts throughout the week at least one time per day, and check off which exercises you did, in order to change your relationship with your thoughts versus changing the thoughts themselves. In addition, you will describe three thoughts that you were mindful of during the week, the strategies you used, and how effective they were.

Diary Cards

Hand out new diary cards to the students. Highlight that they have now learned mindfulness of current thoughts, and that when they practice these skills for homework, they are to circle the days and rate the skill use for the week on the diary card (along with the other skills that they have been taught). Remind them that they have now learned all of the mindfulness and distress tolerance skills.

Finally, do some troubleshooting: Ask students whether they have any questions about the homework or any obstacles to completing it. If so, answer the questions and address the obstacles. Obstacles may include, but are not limited to, the following: Students have no intention of doing the assignment, have too much other homework this week, are likely to forget, or don't understand the assignment. Help students to identify their obstacles, and work with them to make a plan to overcome them. Examples include encouraging a student to write down the assignment and set a reminder in a cell phone or calendar to complete it; discussing why a student has no intention of doing the homework, and working on increasing his or her motivation and the relevance of the assignment (e.g., grades); or clarifying any other points. Troubleshooting should be done each week after the homework is assigned.

Note: If you are giving the Distress Tolerance Test today, proceed as follows.

Module and (Test) Review (5 minutes)

Answer students' questions about the skills presented in the Mindfulness and Distress Tolerance modules. Remind them that the next two lessons return to reviewing the core mindfulness skills.

Administration of Test (20 minutes)

Administer the Distress Tolerance Test.

Mindfulness
Wise Mind

SUMMARY

Today's class focuses mostly on reviewing and practicing the concepts of mindfulness and wise mind. Jon Kabat-Zinn (1994) describes mindfulness as paying attention in a particular way, on purpose, and in the present moment. Students will engage in an activity about generating solutions based on the different states of mind: reasonable mind, emotion mind, and wise mind. The purpose of this exercise is to help students practice finding wise mind solutions to different dilemmas. Students will be able to work together and provide feedback and suggestions to each other. It is another example of how one person's wise mind solution may be different from someone else's wise mind solution.

MAIN POINTS

1. Mindfulness is learning to be in control of your own mind.
2. There are three states of mind: reasonable mind, emotion mind, and wise mind.
3. Mindfulness skills require practice.

MATERIALS

1. Handouts for this lesson:
   - Handout 3.1 Mindfulness: Taking Hold of Your Mind
   - Handout 3.3. Mindfulness: Three States of Mind
   - Homework 13.1. Mindfulness: Solutions Using Three States of Mind
2. Extra student skills binders, with pens or pencils, for students who attend class without materials.
3. Dry-erase markers or chalk for writing on the board.
4. Diary cards: Have new diary cards ready to distribute at the end of class.

PREPARATION

1. Review the lesson plan as well as handouts in student skills binder.
2. Review Lesson 3 for complete teaching points.
3. Arrange desks, if possible, so that students are able to see each other.

LESSON OVERVIEW AND TIMELINE

- Mindfulness exercise (5 minutes)
    - Participating: The Hokey Pokey (3 minutes)
    - Describing observations of the exercise (2 minutes)
- Homework review (10 minutes; 5 minutes if time is needed for test review)
    - Homework 12.3. Distress Tolerance: Practicing Mindfulness of Current Thoughts
        - Sharing with class
    - Diary cards
- Test review (if applicable; 5 minutes)
- Introduction of main ideas (5 minutes)
    - Review of Handout 3.1. Mindfulness: Taking Hold of Your Mind
        - Goals of mindfulness
        - Mindfulness versus mindlessness
- Discussion: Wise mind (25 minutes)
    - Review of Handout 3.3. Mindfulness: Three States of Mind (10 minutes)
        - Reasonable mind
        - Emotion mind
        - Wise mind
    - Class exercise: Practice in using different states of mind (15 minutes)
        - Groups of three students each
        - Students will develop different solutions for multiple scenarios based on assigned state of mind.
- Lesson summary (2 minutes)
    - Wise mind is the balanced middle path.
    - The goal is not to eliminate all reason or emotions. The key is to not let one guide all of your decisions at the expense of the other.
- Homework assignment (3 minutes)
    - Homework 13.1. Mindfulness: Solutions Using Three States of Mind
        - Develop reasonable mind, emotion mind, and wise mind solutions for two different situations.
    - Diary cards

DETAILED LESSON PLAN

Mindfulness Exercise (5 minutes)

Participating: The Hokey Pokey (3 minutes)

Welcome the class and state that today's mindfulness activity will involve participating. Explain:

> Today we are going to sing and dance for our mindfulness practice. We are going to practice throwing ourselves completely into an activity, and being nonjudgmental of others and ourselves, while doing the Hokey Pokey. To do the Hokey Pokey, we will use our right and left arms, our right and left legs, and our whole bodies.

For students who may not know the Hokey Pokey song, read the lyrics (or write them on the board before class):

> You put your [right hand] in,
> You put your [right hand] out,
> You put your [right hand] in,
> And you shake it all about.
> You do the Hokey Pokey,
> And you turn yourself around.
> That's what it's all about!
> [Repeat with left hand, right leg, left leg, and whole body]

Continue:

> When I say 1, that's the signal to stand in a mindful position. Make sure there is enough space around you to do the Hokey Pokey. When I say 2, that's the signal to take a deep breath. When I say 3, that's the signal to begin the practice by starting to sing. We will stop and sit down after we sing the final verse with "whole body."

Now start the practice by counting to 3.

> 1: Stand up and get in a mindful position where there is space around you to dance. 2: Take a deep breath. 3: Begin singing.

End the exercise after the last verse is finished.

Describing Observations of the Exercise (2 minutes)

Ask:

> What did you observe while doing the practice? Did you notice any judgments of yourself or others? Did those judgments stop you from throwing yourself completely into the song and dance?

Have students share their observations of the mindfulness exercise. Provide feedback about observations as needed, ensuring that each statement consists of something a student can observe and describe nonjudgmentally(e.g., I noticed judgmental thoughts of 'I am a terrible singer,' I noticed joy in my body, I noticed a smile on my face, I noticed a thought about how this was different from last week, I noticed a thought . . . , I noticed the sensation . . . , I noticed my mind wandering to other thoughts. I had lots of thoughts about how this could be helpful to me, I noticed I liked last week's practice better, I noticed I was uncomfortable so had to move . . .).

Homework Review (10 minutes; only 5 minutes if reviewing test)

Homework 12.3. Distress Tolerance: Practicing Mindfulness of Current Thoughts

SHARING WITH CLASS

Have the students take out their completed copies of Homework 12.3. Ask:

> *Please share one thought you were mindful of over the week, and describe which strategies you used to gain distance from the thought, or simply to allow the thought without trying to push it away or hold on to it. Also, share your rating of how effective the strategy was.*

Reinforce all efforts made, and thank the students for sharing with the class. Remind the class:

> *This is a very difficult skill and will take practice. As with all the skills, none of these will become automatic until we practice them on a regular basis.*

Diary Cards

As usual, ask all students to turn in their diary cards and homework sheets to be reviewed. If you are not able to review homework with each student each lesson, then be sure to get to each student over the course of several lessons.

Test Review (if Applicable; 5 minutes)

If you administered the Distress Tolerance Test in Lesson 12, return the tests to students. Review any questions the students may have about the test. If you have found that any items were answered incorrectly by a large number of students, you may choose to review those items in more detail with the class.

Introduction of Main Ideas (5 minutes)

Review of Handout 3.1. Mindfulness: Taking Hold of Your Mind

Have students turn back to Handout 3.1 in their binders. Ask:

> *Who can tell us why we are going through the mindfulness skills again?*

Elicit answers, and then give this one, if necessary:

The mindfulness skills are the core skills for all the other skills we use. We need to be mindful in order to be able to use all of our skills.

Mindfulness is learning to be in control of our own minds, instead of our minds' being in control of us. It is about putting our minds where we want them to be.

Now ask:

What is mindfulness?

The goal is to generate answers such as these: being present in the moment; paying attention on purpose; controlling where we focus our minds; being aware of what we are experiencing right now.

Next, have a few students share examples of when and how they have practiced mindfulness over the last 12 weeks (since Lesson 1). In each case, ask:

How has that been different from how you were doing things in the past?

Discussion: Wise Mind (25 minutes)

Review of Handout 3.3. Mindfulness: Three States of Mind (10 minutes)

Have students turn to Handout 3.3. Then ask three students to come up to the board. Have each one write one of the states of mind on the board, allowing for space to write underneath each. Ask the entire class:

How do we describe the different states of mind?

Have the students at the board write descriptions under each respective heading. The following are examples:

Emotion mind:

   Scared, excited, happy, joy, sad, angry . . . [or other emotions]
   Emotions are leading your behaviors
   Not thinking about short- and long-term consequences of behavior
   Not in the present moment
   Ignoring logic and reason

Reasonable mind:

   Mechanic, air traffic controller, pilot, completing a chemistry lab . . . [occupations or
      situations in which reasonable mind is needed]
   Reason and logic are leading your behaviors
   Not taking your emotions into consideration

Wise mind:

> Intuitive—a balance of emotion and reason
> Everyone has a wise mind
> It is the wisest part of you
> But even sometimes when you know what wise mind tells you to do, it can still be hard to overcome emotion mind

Now ask:

If we are not sure whether we are making a decision in wise mind or in emotion mind, how can we figure it out?

Elicit answers, or give this one:

If we sit with the decision, time will tell us. If we still reach the same decision 1–2 days later, then it is a wise mind decision. If it changes, then the first decision was probably made in emotion mind. In the Emotion Regulation module, we will learn that emotions only last 60–90 seconds unless they are fired again. Therefore, if our decision changes over time, it was probably an emotion-based decision to start with.

CLASS EXERCISE: PRACTICE IN USING DIFFERENT STATES OF MIND (15 MINUTES)

Explain:

We are going to practice using our different states of mind.

Divide students into groups of three. Continue:

For this activity, we will go through a variety of situations for which we need to make decisions. Each group will generate a solution for reasonable mind, emotion mind, and wise mind. Once the groups have their solutions, each group will present its solutions to the rest of the class in front of the room.

Instruct students to stand in front of the board as they present each solution. In the presentation, one student will represent reasonable mind, one will represent emotion mind, and one will represent wise mind. Have the student representing each state of mind stand in front of where that state has been written on the board earlier in the lesson.

After the students in each group present their solutions, allow the rest of the class to provide feedback or generate other possible solutions for the different states of mind. Highlight that one student's wise mind solution may be different from someone else's.

You may also ask students to volunteer other scenarios that they have experienced or are currently experiencing and for which they are trying to determine wise mind solutions. Write each of the different situations on a sheet of paper and hand one out to each group. You may also generate your own examples, or assign one of the following examples to two groups, depending on the size of the class.

- There is a substitute teacher in math class today, and some of your friends are skipping class and asked you to join them.
- The new group of friends you are hanging out with are having a party this weekend, and you are invited, but it's your mom's birthday.
- Your friend Sofia asked you to share your math homework with her to copy because she did not do it.
- You have been arguing a lot with the person you have been dating for 3 months. You are thinking about breaking up with this person, but you really like him or her when you are not arguing.
- You just broke up with your boyfriend or girlfriend before third period. You are really sad and angry, and you want to ditch school for the rest of the day.
- You just heard that a kid in your grade was busted for smoking marijuana and arrested. You want to post the information on Facebook, Instagram, or Twitter.
- You are dating someone in the grade above you, and you really like him or her. This person tells you, "I love you and want to have sex with you" (i.e., oral sex or intercourse). You do not think you want to, but you are afraid that the person will break up with you if you do not. (You can change this example as needed based on age appropriateness (6th graders compared to 12th graders) for the class.
- You are spending the night at your friend Josh's house. You told your parents who will be there and said that you will be staying in all night. Josh gets a call from some other friends, and they want to pick you both up and go hang out in the park. Josh wants to sneak out and go, since his parents are already asleep.

Lesson Summary (2 minutes)

Review the three states of mind, and emphasize that the ultimate goal is to be in wise mind. Explain:

What we just did was a way to practice generating solutions based on your different states of mind. Remember that wise mind is not simply a compromise between emotion mind and reasonable mind; it is honoring both your reasonable and emotion mind at the same time. In other words, it's a dialectic! The goal is not to eliminate the experience of emotions or logic; the key is not to allow either one to guide all of your decisions at the expense of the other.

Homework Assignment (3 minutes)

Homework 13.1. Mindfulness: Solutions Using Three States of Mind

Explain:

For homework, you will use Homework 13.1 to continue doing what we did in class today: You will generate reasonable mind, emotion mind, and wise mind solutions for two different situations you are experiencing. Remember that, at least for the homework, you are to write down examples of situations you are willing to share in class.

Review the homework sheet with the class, and ask if there are any questions about the assignment.

Diary Cards

Hand out new diary cards to the students. Highlight that they now know all of the mindfulness skills and the distress tolerance skills. Remind them to circle the days and rate their skill use for the week on the diary card for each of the skills.

Finally, do some troubleshooting: Ask students whether they have any questions about the homework or any obstacles to completing it. If so, answer the questions and address the obstacles. Obstacles may include, but are not limited to, the following: Students have no intention of doing the assignment, have too much other homework this week, are likely to forget, or don't understand the assignment. Help students to identify their obstacles, and work with them to make a plan to overcome them. Examples include encouraging a student to write down the assignment and set a reminder in a cell phone or calendar to complete it; discussing why a student has no intention of doing the homework, and working on increasing his or her motivation and the relevance of the assignment (e.g., grades); or clarifying any other points. Troubleshooting should be done each week after the homework is assigned.

Mindfulness
"What" and "How" Skills

SUMMARY

Today's lesson focuses on reviewing and strengthening the mindfulness "what" and "how" skills. Students will have the opportunity to generate teaching points and lead the class through practice exercises for each of the six skills.

MAIN POINTS

1. Mindfulness skills are divided into the "what" and "how" skills.
2. The "what" skills are observe, describe, and participate.
3. The "how" skills are nonjudgmentally, one-mindfully, and effectively.

MATERIALS

1. Handouts for this lesson:
   - Handout 4.1. Mindfulness: "What" Skills
   - Handout 5.1. Mindfulness: "How" Skills
   - Homework 14.1. Mindfulness: Practicing "What" and "How" Skills
2. Extra student skills binders, with pens or pencils, for students who attend class without materials.
3. Dry-erase markers or chalk for writing on the board.
4. Diary cards: Have new diary cards ready to distribute at the end of class.

PREPARATION

1. Review Lessons 4 and 5 for complete teaching points, as well as student handouts.
2. Arrange the desks in the classroom, if possible, in order for students to be able to see each other.

LESSON OVERVIEW AND TIMELINE

- Mindfulness exercise (5 minutes)
  - Observing: Observing your partner (3 minutes)
  - Describing observations of the exercise (2 minutes)
- Homework review (10 minutes)
  - Homework 13.1. Mindfulness: Solutions Using Three States of Mind
    - Sharing with partners
    - Sharing with class
  - Diary cards
- Introduction of main ideas (2 minutes)
  - What skills: observe, describe, participate
  - How skills: nonjudgmentally, one-mindfully, and effectively
  - Why return to mindfulness between each module?
- Discussion: "What" and "how" skills (29 minutes)
  - Review of Handout 4.1. Mindfulness: "What" Skills, and Handout 5.1. Mindfulness: "How" Skills (2 minutes)
  - Class exercise: Demonstrations of "what" and "how" skills (27 minutes)
- Lesson summary (2 minutes)
  - Provide feedback about student demonstrations.
- Homework assignment (2 minutes)
  - Homework 14.1. Mindfulness: Practicing "What" and "How" Skills
    - Practice at least one "what" and "how" skill.
  - Diary cards

DETAILED LESSON PLAN

Mindfulness Exercise (5 minutes)

Observing: Observing Your Partner (3 minutes)

Welcome the class and state that today's mindfulness activity will involve observing. Have students pair off with partners. Explain:

> *You are going to observe your partner mindfully for 1 minute. When 1 minute has passed, I will let you know, and you and your partner will turn your backs to each other. You are then to change three things about yourself; for example, put your watch on your other wrist, take off your glasses, or change your hair. You will then face each other again, and you and your partner will see whether you can notice what was changed.*

Continue:

> *When I say 1, that's the signal to turn toward your partner and sit in our usual mindful/wide-awake position. As we know by now, this means keeping our feet flat on the floor, sitting up straight, and putting our hands in our laps. Eyes stay open for this exercise, of course. If you notice any urges to move, other than blinking or swallowing, notice each urge without*

acting on it, and return to your breath. When I say 2, that's the signal to take a deep breath. When I say 3, that's the signal to begin the practice by observing your partner.

I'll say, "Turn around," when it is time for you to turn around and change three things. Once you have quickly changed the three things, turn back around and face your partner. Continue to observe your partner and notice any differences. I'll say, "Stop," to end the practice.

Now start the practice by counting to 3.

1: Get yourself into the mindful/wide-awake position and face your partner. 2: Take a deep breath. 3: Begin the practice.

After 1 minute, say, "Turn around and change." After another minute, say, "Stop."

Describing Observations of the Exercise (2 minutes)

Allow students to share briefly with their partners what they noticed that was changed.

Then call on two or three students to share their observations of the exercise. Provide feedback about observations as needed, ensuring that each statement consists of something a student can observe and describe nonjudgmentally (.e.g., I noticed his watch was on his left wrist and the comparison thought that this was different from before, I noticed stopping with each pause, I noticed a thought about how this was different from last week, I noticed a thought . . . , I noticed the sensation . . . , I noticed my mind wandering to other thoughts. I had lots of thoughts about how this could be helpful to me, I noticed I liked last week's practice better, I noticed I was uncomfortable so had to move . . .).

Homework Review (10 minutes)

Homework 13.1. Mindfulness: Solutions Using Three States of Mind

SHARING WITH PARTNERS

Have the students take out their completed copies of Homework 13.1. Divide students into pairs. Have the partners in each pair share with each other the two situations and the different reasonable, emotion, and wise mind solutions they generated. Students can provide feedback to each other on the different solutions. (Ask students to put their diary cards out so you can collect them while the students are reviewing homework.)

SHARING WITH THE CLASS

Have one student from each dyad share examples of the different solutions the dyad generated based on the three states of mind. Ask:

Did anyone have difficulty determining or following through with the wise mind decision?

If any students report that they did have trouble, coach these students through the skill with the help of the class to determine what was in the way of determining or following through on the wise mind decision. Model and reinforce for all students that figuring out and following wise mind can be difficult at times. In addition, remind students that one person's wise mind may be different from another's.

Diary Cards

As noted above, collect diary cards while students are working in pairs. Briefly review the level of skills use over the past week for students. Comment on the amount of skills practice students are reporting. Explain:

> *We have now gone through the entire first module and are reviewing mindfulness. We want to see continued practice of all these skills.*

If you notice that any students are not recording regular practice of skills on their diary cards, use this time to troubleshoot with the class as a whole any obstacles that may be getting in the way of practicing or using the skills.

Introduction of Main Ideas (2 minutes)

Review that there are seven mindfulness skills.

- Wise mind: Synthesis of emotion mind and reasonable mind.
- Three "what" skills: What to do.
- Three "how" skills: How to do the "what" skills.

Call on students who remember what the different skills are, and have them name the seven skills. Then ask students:

> *Why do we review the core mindfulness skills at the beginning of each new module?*

Elicit answers, or give this one: Because mindfulness skills are at the core or base of all the other skills. In order to use the other skills well, we need to be mindful of the need for skills use and then mindfully use them.

Discussion: "What" and "How" Skills (29 minutes)

Review of Handout 4.1. Mindfulness: What Skills, and Handout 5.1. Mindfulness: How Skills (2 minutes)

Have students turn to Handouts 4.1 and 5.1, which outline the mindfulness "what" and "how" skills, respectively, and any additional notes they have about the skills. Let them look briefly over these handouts and notes, and then explain:

> *For the remainder of class today we will review and practice the "what" and "how" skills.*

CLASS EXERCISE: DEMONSTRATIONS OF "WHAT" AND "HOW" SKILLS (27 MINUTES)

Divide the students up into six groups. Explain:

Each group will be assigned one of the "what" or "how" skills. Each group is to generate a description or teaching points about the skill and one exercise to demonstrate the skill.

Make the group assignments, and allow about 4 minutes for students to generate teaching points for the exercise.

After all six groups have come up with their teaching points and exercises, each group will have about 3 minutes to teach the class and 1 minute for feedback. The goal here is to help the class generate multiple methods of practicing each mindfulness skill. As each group presents the skill, ask for other students' feedback, and clarify any key points from Lessons 4 and 5 and from Handouts 4.1 and 5.1 that may have been missed.

One extra minute has been built into this exercise to allow for general feedback as needed. You may also use the time allotted for the lesson summary to provide additional feedback as needed.

Lesson Summary (2 minutes)

Provide feedback to students about their class demonstrations. Review and clarify any points as needed.

Homework Assignment (2 minutes)

Homework 14.1. Mindfulness: Practicing "What" and "How" Skills

Explain:

> *For homework this week, you are to practice at least one "what" skill and one "how" skill. Use Homework 14.1 to describe how you practiced the skill and how it affected your thoughts, feelings, or behaviors.*

Diary Cards

Hand out new diary cards to the students. Highlight that they now know all of the mindfulness and distress tolerance skills. Although they are only assigned to practice the "what" and "how" skills this week, they should be using all the skills regularly. They should rate their use of each skill over the course of the week as they practice every day.

Finally, do some troubleshooting: Ask students whether they have any questions about the homework or any obstacles to completing it. If so, answer the questions and address the obstacles. Obstacles may include, but are not limited to, the following: Students have no intention of doing the assignment, have too much other homework this week, are likely to forget, or don't understand the assignment. Help students to identify their obstacles, and work with them to make a plan to overcome them. Examples include encouraging a student to write down the assignment and set a reminder in a cell phone or calendar to complete it; discussing why a student has no intention of doing the homework, and working on increasing his or her motivation and the relevance of the assignment (e.g., grades); or clarifying any other points. Troubleshooting should be done each week after the homework is assigned.

Emotion Regulation

Goals of Emotion Regulation and Functions of Emotions

SUMMARY

This lesson begins the Emotion Regulation module. Overall, this module teaches students how to label, identify, and regulate emotions through decreasing their vulnerability factors and changing their behaviors. Students will also learn how to be mindful of their emotions and how to tolerate their emotions, therefore eliminating the need to change them. Today's lesson focuses on introducing this module by reviewing its goals, followed by discussing the overall purposes of having emotions.

MAIN POINTS

1. The goals of emotion regulation skills are to understand the emotions we experience, decrease unwanted emotions, decrease our emotional vulnerability, and decrease our emotional suffering.
2. Emotions are good for motivating and organizing action, communicating and influencing others, and communicating to ourselves.
3. People often have myths about emotions that interfere with their abilities to manage their emotions effectively.

MATERIALS

1. Handouts for this lesson:
   - Handout 15.1. Emotion Regulation: Goals of Emotion Regulation
   - Handout 15.2. Emotion Regulation: Short List of Emotions
   - Handout 15.3. Emotion Regulation: What Good Are Emotions?

- Homework 15.4. Emotion Regulation: Myths about Emotions
- Homework 15.5. Emotion Regulation: Emotion Diary

2. Extra student skills binders, with pens or pencils, for students who attend class without materials.
3. Dry-erase markers or chalk for writing on the board.
4. Diary cards: Students will not be learning a new skill today; rather, they will learn the purpose of emotions and how to identify and challenge their own myths about emotions. Therefore, no skills need to be highlighted on the diary cards this week.

PREPARATION

1. Review the lesson plan as well as handouts in student skills binder.
2. Arrange desks in the classroom, if possible, in order for students to be able to see each other.

LESSON OVERVIEW AND TIMELINE

- Mindfulness exercise (5 minutes)
  - Participating: Snap, crackle, pop (3 minutes)
  - Describing observations of the exercise (2 minutes)
- Homework review (10 minutes)
  - Homework 14.1. Mindfulness: Practicing "What" and "How" Skills
    - Sharing with class
  - Diary cards
- Introduction of main ideas (5 minutes)
  - Emotion regulation is the process of influencing which emotions you have, when you have them, and how you will express them.
  - Generate a list of emotions with the class.
- Discussion: Goals of emotion regulation (13 minutes)
  - Review of Handout 15.1. Emotion Regulation: Goals of Emotion Regulation (10 minutes)
    - Understand the emotions you experience.
    - Reduce emotional vulnerability.
    - Decrease the frequency of unwanted emotions and decrease emotional suffering.
  - Review of Handout 15.2. Emotion Regulation: Short List of Emotions (3 minutes)
    - Identify "families of emotions."
- Discussion: What good are emotions? (10 minutes)
  - Review of Handout 15.3. Emotion Regulation: What Good Are Emotions?
    - Emotions give us information.
    - Emotions communicate to and influence others.
    - Emotions motivate and prepare us for action.
- Lesson summary (2 minutes)
  - Review goals of emotion regulation and function of emotions.
- Homework assignment (5 minutes)
  - Homework 15.4. Emotion Regulation: Myths about Emotions
    - Write a challenge to each myth.

- Homework 15.5. Emotion Regulation: Emotion Diary
  - Analyze the function of three emotions during the week.
- Diary cards

DETAILED LESSON PLAN

Mindfulness Exercise (5 minutes)

Participating: Snap, Crackle, Pop (3 minutes)

Welcome the class and state that today's mindfulness activity will involve participating. Explain:

> *Today we are going to practice mindfully participating by playing a game called Snap, Crackle, Pop. This game has three sets of instructions, one for each word. First, when I say to, we will stand up and get into a large circle.*

Smaller circles of five or six students can also be made, as necessary.

> *What we will do is this:*
> *One person points over his or her head with the right arm to the person on the left, or points over his or her head with the left arm to the person on the right, and says, "Snap."*
> *The person who just received the "snap" (the person to either the left or right of the first person) will use the left arm to point across his or her chest to the person on the right, or the right arm to point across his or her chest to the person on the left, and says, "Crackle."*
> *The person who received the "crackle" will then point to anyone in the circle, even across the circle, and say "Pop." The person who received the "pop" will begin again with "snap" to the person on his left or right. The practice continues in this way. We want to go fast and spontaneously. If someone makes a mistake, then we just notice it, and anyone else can just start again with "snap."*
> *Because this is an exercise in participating, remember that we want to throw ourselves into the activity fully, without judgment. If you notice yourself having a judgmental thought, just notice it, and then let it go and bring yourself back to the exercise. If you notice yourself anticipating what you will do when it is your turn, then you are not participating in the moment. Notice that and jump back into the moment. Again, if anyone makes a mistake, simply notice it and let it go, and the group can begin again.*

Continue:

> *When I say 1, that's the signal to stand up and mindfully and quietly create a large circle [or smaller circles, depending on class size]. I will let you take your positions before I say 2. When I say 2, that's the signal to take a deep breath. When I say 3, that's the signal for the group to begin playing the Snap, Crackle, Pop game.*

Now start the practice by counting to 3.

1: Stand and mindfully create a circle. 2: Take a deep breath. 3: Begin playing Snap, Crackle, Pop.

After 3 minutes, say, "Stop," to end the exercise.

Describing Observations of the Exercise (2 minutes)

Highlight:

> *It can be difficult not to judge ourselves or others when a mistake was made, or to mindfully wait rather than think about when it is going to be your turn. Our goal is, first, to be nonjudgmental, and second, if we are judgmental, to notice it and quickly let it go and throw ourselves back into the exercise.*

Have students share their observations of the mindfulness exercise. Provide feedback about observations as needed, ensuring that each statement consists of something a student can observe and describe nonjudgmentally (e.g., I noticed having judgmental thoughts about the exercise, I noticed that I repeatedly forgot which hand motion was next, I noticed stopping with each pause, I noticed a thought about how this was different from last week, I noticed a thought . . . , I noticed the sensation . . . , I noticed my mind wandering to other thoughts. I had lots of thoughts about how this could be helpful to me, I noticed I liked last week's practice better, I noticed I was uncomfortable so had to move . . .).

Homework Review (10 minutes)

Homework 14.1. Mindfulness: Practicing "What" and "How" Skills

SHARING WITH CLASS

Have the students take out their completed copies of Homework 14.1. Ask which students completed their homework, and reinforce these students by having some of them share an example of how they practiced their "what" and "how" skills and how doing this affected their thoughts, emotions, and behaviors. You may review several students' homework at once by asking whether any other students practiced the same skill as the student describing that skill. Ask for similarities or differences in experiences. Then ask who practiced a different "what" or "how" skill. Continue in a similar fashion with as many students as possible.

If any students had difficulty practicing, troubleshoot what happened, and provide coaching for future practice. Ask classmates for suggestions as well.

Diary Cards

Ask all students to turn in their diary cards and homework sheets to be reviewed. If you are not able to review homework with each student each lesson, then be sure to get to each student over the course of several lessons.

Introduction of Main Ideas (5 minutes)

Explain:

> *We all have emotions, and sometimes these emotions can be intense, like giant waves. Sometimes these intense emotions can lead to self-destructive or other problematic behaviors. However, we can learn skills to ride the waves, or to decrease the size of the waves, and therefore avoid those problematic behaviors.*
>
> *We will be learning how to be skillful with our emotions, not how to get rid of them. Emotions themselves are neither good nor bad; they just are. Some are pleasurable, and some are painful. As we learned in the Distress Tolerance module, our emotions are inevitable, so we need to learn how to regulate them because we can't simply get rid of them.*
>
> *"Emotion regulation" is the process of influencing which emotions you have, when you have them, and how you will express them.*

Generate a list of emotions: Invite two students up to the board. Ask the class to name as many emotions as possible, and have the two students at the board write these down.

Discussion: Goals of Emotion Regulation (13 minutes)

Review of Handout 15.1. Emotion Regulation: Goals of Emotion Regulation (10 minutes)

Have students turn to Handout 15.1. This handout is an overview of the general goals for the skills students will learn in this module.

UNDERSTAND EMOTIONS YOU EXPERIENCE

> *The first goal is to understand the emotions you experience. This relates to the mindfulness skills of observing and describing emotions and the functions of emotions. Emotions can be reactions to events around you or to your own thoughts and feelings.*
>
> *Ask a student to read the bullet points under the first goal on Handout 15.1. Explain: Every emotion has a biological function.*

Write the following four emotions on the board if they have not already been written there, or circle them if they have been: fear, anger, sadness, and guilt. Ask:

> *Let's see if we can figure out what the functions of these four emotions would be. What is the purpose of fear?*

Elicit responses from students. (Answer: Alerting us to danger.)

> *What is the purpose of anger?*

Elicit responses. (Answer: Alerting us when goals are being blocked.)

> *What is the purpose of sadness?*

Elicit responses. (Answer: Alerting us that something has been lost.)

> *What is the purpose of guilt?*

Elicit responses. (Answer: Alerting us to when we have acted against our own values.) Then say:

> *Something we all need to learn is how to know when our emotions fit the situation, whether our emotions are being effective and helping us, or whether they are making things more difficult for us in the moment.*

REDUCE EMOTIONAL VULNERABILITY

Ask a student to read the bullet points under the second goal on Handout 15.1, or say:

> *The second goal is to reduce our emotional vulnerability by stopping unwanted emotions from starting in the first place. This can be done through skills that will decrease our vulnerability to emotion mind and increase our pleasurable activities.*

DECREASE THE FREQUENCY OF UNWANTED EMOTIONS, AND DECREASE EMOTIONAL SUFFERING

Continue:

> *The last two goals are to decrease the frequency of unwanted emotions and to decrease our suffering from unwanted emotions once they start. In this module, we will learn a variety of skills that will teach us how to change what we are feeling or how to experience the emotions we have by using mindfulness.*

> Finally, ask:

> *In the Distress Tolerance module, we learned how to distract ourselves from our emotions. Do you think it is effective to distract from our emotions all of the time?*

Elicit a "No," and add:

> *In this module, we will learn how to sit with and experience an emotion without becoming overwhelmed by it and ending up in emotion mind.*

Review of Handout 15.2. Emotion Regulation: Short List of Emotions (3 minutes)

Have students turn to Handout 15.2. Ask:

> *Are there any emotions on the list that are not on the board?*

If so, have a student add them to the board. Then ask:

> *Are there any emotions on the board that are not on the short list?*

If so, have students add them to the short list on the handout. Continue:

> *As you can all see, there are a lot of emotions. Some represent differing intensities of an emotion, such as frustration, anger, and rage. Can you identify other "families of emotions" based on their intensity levels?*

Elicit responses. Finally, say:

> *For the remainder of this module, we are going to be learning how to identify, label, and regulate our emotions. I am glad we are able to start off with you all knowing so many of the different emotions already.*

Discussion: What Good Are Emotions? (10 minutes)

Review of Handout 15.3. Emotion Regulation: What Good Are Emotions?

Have students turn to Handout 15.3. Remind the students that the purpose of this module is to regulate emotions, not to get rid of them. Ask:

> *Can any of you think of a time in your lives when emotions have been useful?*

> *Allow one or two students to share how emotions have been helpful. Then have a student read the bullet points under "Emotions give us information" in Handout 15.3. Highlight: Emotions can be like an internal alarm clock, alerting you to something important. If you get a gut feeling about something, don't treat it as a fact, just a message—but you might not want to ignore it. It is important to check the facts when you get a "gut feeling."*

Encourage students to share experiences when they listened to their "gut feeling" in a situation and it proved to be correct. Note that this may have also been a wise mind experience. But add:

> *Treating our emotions as facts can bring about problems. If we only listened to our fear emotions about dentists and interpreted those as facts that dentists are harmful, many of us would have mouths full of rotten teeth! Similarly, feeling guilty that you are a bad person does not make it true that you are a bad person.*

Now have a student read the bullet points under "Emotions communicate to and influence others" on Handout 15.3. Discuss the importance of being able to communicate emotions through facial expressions, and note how that can be lifesaving in a dangerous situation where there is no opportunity for words. Say:

> *Our faces are hard-wired to show emotions, and our brains are hard-wired to recognize the emotion on the faces of others. Sadness communicates to others the message "I need help," and anger communicates to others the message "Stop!" For example, at the time of the 2004 Indian Ocean tsunami, people saw the expressions on the faces of others, and these immediately organized them to move.*
>
> *Studies have found that despite cultural differences, people can still recognize the emotional facial expressions of others. These expressions are universal. Since expressions are similar to a "universal language," if people's words don't match their expressions of an emotion in their faces, posture, or tone of voice, other people may believe the nonverbal expression of the emotion over what is being said. Sometimes, when people are reading your nonverbal expressions and not listening to your words, this can create problems. For instance, if a classmate is joking around at your expense, then you may laugh to save face, and tell the classmate to stop. The classmate sees you laughing, pays attention to that and not your words, and misinterprets that you are fine with the joke.*

Ask the students for examples of their experiences with a mismatch between verbal and nonverbal expressions of emotion. Have the students ever paid attention to someone's nonverbal expressions over their words, as in the example above?

Now call on a student to read the bullet points under "Emotions motivate and prepare us for action" in Handout 15.3. Say:

> *As we discussed earlier, every emotion has a function that motivates us for action. Fear organizes the body to run or freeze. This helps us avoid danger. Anger organizes the body to fight or attack. This helps us defend ourselves or gain control. Emotions make us act quickly in a situation, and this can save important time in an emergency. Or think of the last time you were anxious about a test: Test anxiety motivates the action of studying.*

Draw on the board a Yerkes–Dodson curve (see Figure L15.1). Explain:

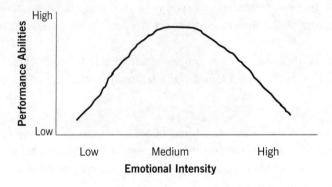

FIGURE L15.1. A Yerkes–Dodson curve.

People have a zone of peak performance—a state of mind where they are challenged but not overloaded. This occurs when emotional intensity is not too high or too low, but medium for that individual. If your test anxiety were low, you might not study, but if it were too high, you would be too distressed to learn anything or even sit down with your book.

Lesson Summary (2 minutes)

Acknowledge the students for their hard work at beginning a new module and learning a lot of information in one class. Review the goals of emotion regulation and the functions of emotions.

Homework Assignment (5 minutes)

Homework 15.4. Emotion Regulation: Myths about Emotions

Explain:

> *Before we start looking at different emotions next week, we will discuss some of the myths that people hold regarding emotions. Why do you think it is important that we discuss myths about emotions?*

Allow students to answer. Then discuss:

> *Some people have beliefs about emotions that sometimes get in the way of how they feel. For example, I have heard people say things like "I don't let myself ever feel sad," or "Only weak people get scared." What do you think about those statements? Do you have any beliefs like that about emotions?*
>
> *Homework 15.4 has a list of myths about emotions. Each myth also has a challenge provided for it. For homework, you are going to write down another challenge, and I want you to personalize the challenge so that it is meaningful to you. Let's go through item 1 on this homework sheet together.*

Ask a student to read item 1: "There is a right way to feel in every situation." Ask the class:

> *Is that true? Does anyone believe there is a right way to feel in every situation?*

Elicit responses. Then ask a student to read the challenge for number 1. Ask the class:

> *How can you personalize this challenge or restate it in a way that is meaningful to you?*

Examples of responses:

- *I may feel different than other people do in a situation, and that is OK. Everyone is different.*
- *It's OK that different people have different emotional reactions.*
- *My emotions are just as valid as yours.*

As the first part of their homework, students will complete Homework 15.4. The worksheet lists several myths about emotions and one possible challenge to each myth. Students will generate their own challenge for each myth.

Homework 15.5. Emotion Regulation: Emotion Diary

Explain:

> *Today we learned the functions our emotions serve. To further strengthen your understanding of these functions, your second assignment is to use Homework 15.5 to keep a diary of your emotions this week. It can be really effective in helping you to start understanding the impact your emotions have on yourself and others. I want you to record at least three emotions you feel this week—either the strongest emotion of the day or the longest-lasting one—and describe whether it motivated you into action, what it communicated to others, and what it communicated to you. Again, do this at least three times.*

Diary Cards

Hand out new diary cards to the students. This week they are assigned to practice all of the mindfulness and distress tolerance skills. Students should circle the days and rate their skill use for the week on the diary card.

Finally, do some troubleshooting: Ask students whether they have any questions about the homework or any obstacles to completing it. If so, answer the questions and address the obstacles. Obstacles may include, but are not limited to, the following: Students have no intention of doing the assignment, have too much other homework this week, are likely to forget, or don't understand the assignment. Help students to identify their obstacles, and work with them to make a plan to overcome them. Examples include encouraging a student to write down the assignment and set a reminder in a cell phone or calendar to complete it; discussing why a student has no intention of doing the homework, and working on increasing his or her motivation and the relevance of the assignment (e.g., grades); or clarifying any other points. Troubleshooting should be done each week after the homework is assigned.

Emotion Regulation
Describing Emotions

SUMMARY

There are many types of emotions and several words to describe each type. Today's lesson focuses on teaching students what an emotion is: a complex, full-system response that is primarily biologically hard-wired and made up of multiple components, including the prompting events, interpretations, biological changes, expressions, and aftereffects. This lesson uses a model of emotions to help students understand the different components. The lesson ends with a small-group activity in which each group is assigned an emotion to discuss and explain, using the model of emotions.

MAIN POINTS

1. An emotion is a full-system response that last approximately 60–90 seconds. Emotions that seem to last longer are due to repeated refiring of the neurons in the brain.
2. Emotions are complex and can be best understood through examining the prompting event, the interpretation, the biological changes, the expressions, and the aftereffects experienced by the body.

MATERIALS

1. Handouts for this lesson:
   - Handout 16.1. Emotion Regulation: Model of Emotions
   - Handout 16.2a–h. Emotion Regulation: Ways to Describe Emotions
   - Homework 16.3. Emotion Regulation: Practice with the Model of Emotions (2 copies)
2. Extra student skills binders, with pens or pencils, for students who attend class without materials.

3. Ten sheets of light-colored construction paper and markers for the homework review activity.

4. Dry-erase markers or chalk for writing on the board.

5. Diary cards: Have new diary cards ready to distribute at the end of class. If possible, highlight the "Describing emotions" skill.

PREPARATION

1. Review the lesson plan as well as handouts in student skills binder.

2. Arrange the desks in the classroom, if possible, in order for students to be able to see each other.

LESSON OVERVIEW AND TIMELINE

- Mindfulness exercise (5 minutes)
  - Observing/wise mind: Breathing in "Wise," breathing out "Mind" (3 minutes)
  - Describing observations of the exercise (2 minutes)
- Homework review (10 minutes)
  - Homework 15.4. Emotion Regulation: Myths about Emotions
  - Homework 15.5. Emotion Regulation: Emotion Diary
    - Sharing in small groups
  - Diary cards
- Introduction of main ideas (2 minutes)
  - Emotions are a full-system response made up of multiple components.
  - Emotions last 60–90 seconds.
- Discussion: Model of emotions (28 minutes)
  - Review of Handout 16.1. Emotion Regulation: Model of Emotions (15 minutes)
    - Class exercise: Walking though the model with an example
    - Prompting event 1
    - Vulnerability factors
    - Thoughts about the event
    - Internal experience: Inside the body effects
    - External experience: Outside the body effects
    - Emotion name
    - Consequences of Actions
    - Prompting event 2
  - Review of Handout 16.2a–h. Emotion Regulation: Ways to Describe Emotions (5 minutes)
    - Review anger
  - Class exercise: Small-group activity with Homework 16.3 (8 minutes)
- Lesson summary (2 minutes)
- Homework assignment (3 minutes)
  - Homework 16.3. Emotion Regulation: Practice with the Model of Emotions
  - Diary cards

DETAILED LESSON PLAN

Mindfulness Exercise (5 minutes)

Observing/Wise Mind: Breathing in "Wise," Breathing out "Mind"
(3 minutes)

Welcome the class and introduce the mindfulness exercise.

> *Today we are going to practice observing our breath and accessing wise mind. Sometimes, in order to access our wise mind, we need to deliberately slow ourselves down and quiet our minds. For today's practice, we will focus on our breath. To ourselves, we will say the word "Wise" on the in-breath, and say the word "Mind" on the out-breath. In other words, we will inhale "Wise" and exhale "Mind." So we are going to practice accessing wise mind while focusing all of our attention on only our breath. You may remember that we did this exercise during Lesson 3.*
>
> *When I say 1, that's the signal to sit in the mindful/wide-awake position we know pretty well by now. This means keeping our feet flat on the floor, sitting up straight, and putting our hands in our laps. For this exercise, we will keep our eyes open, finding a place 4–6 inches in front of you to rest your gaze. If you notice any urges to move, other than blinking or swallowing, notice each urge without acting on it, and return to your breath. When I say 2, that's the signal to take a deep breath. When I say 3, that's the signal to begin the practice. I'll say, "Stop," to end.*

Now start the practice by counting to 3.

> *1: Get yourself into the mindful/wide-awake position. 2: Take a deep breath. 3: Begin the practice.*

Have students do the practice for 2 minutes, and then say, "Stop."

Describing Observations of the Exercise (2 minutes)

Ask:

> *What did you observe while doing the practice? Did you notice any judgments or difficulties in accessing wise mind?*

Have students share their observations of the mindfulness exercise. (Depending on the number of students in class, you may not be able to call on each student every time.) Provide feedback about observations as needed, ensuring that each statement consists of something a student can observe and describe nonjudgmentally (.e.g., I noticed judgmental thoughts, I noticed the urge to move, I noticed sadness arise within me, I noticed a smile on my face, I noticed a thought about how this was different from last week, I noticed a thought . . . , I noticed the sensation . . . , I noticed my mind wandering to other thoughts. I had lots of thoughts about how this could be helpful to me, I noticed I liked last week's practice better, I noticed I was uncomfortable so had to move . . .).

Homework Review (10 minutes)

Homework 15.4. Emotion Regulation: Myths about Emotions
Homework 15.5. Emotion Regulation: Emotion Diary

SHARING IN SMALL GROUPS

Have the students take out their completed copies of Homework 15.4 and Homework 15.5. Say:

> *Generating challenges to myths and describing the functions of your emotions can be difficult tasks. Did anyone have difficulty with the homework assignment this week?*

Answer any general questions students have about their difficulties. Then have students break into groups of three to four. Evenly split up the eight myths among the different groups, and explain:

> *Share the challenges you developed this week with your group for the myth you were assigned. We will also make some signs with those challenges on them to help decorate the room. I will hand out the paper when it is time for that. Once you have discussed some of your challenges, especially any that you had difficulty coming up with, make any necessary changes to challenges that may still support the myth. Once you have completed the myths, turn to your Emotion Diary in Homework 15.5. Discuss the emotions you experienced during the week that you feel comfortable sharing, and describe what the emotions motivated you to do, communicated to others, and communicated to yourself.*

After 5 minutes, pass out the construction paper and markers. Instruct the students that they have the next 5 minutes to write up their favorite of the challenges in an artistic way, to be put up on the classroom wall. When everyone is done, bring the class back together, and have the students share their challenges and the functions of their emotions.

If any students had difficulty practicing, troubleshoot what happened and provide coaching for future practice. Ask classmates for suggestions as well.

Diary Cards

Ask all students to turn in their diary cards and homework sheets to be reviewed by. If you are not able to review homework with each student each lesson, then be sure to get to each student over the course of several lessons.

Introduction of Main Ideas (2 minutes)

Review with students:

> *What are the three purposes of an emotion?*

Elicit:

- To motivate us into action.
- To communicate to ourselves.
- To communicate to others.

Now ask:

How long does an emotion last?

Allow multiple students to answer this question, in order to get a variety of lengths. Then go on:

An emotion actually only lasts about 60–90 seconds. However, sometimes an emotion feels as if it can last for hours or days because we are continually refiring the neurons (or brain cells) that cause the emotion in our bodies. Today we are going to learn about the different components of an emotion, so that throughout the rest of this module we can identify different places to intervene in order to regulate our emotions, because changing one component can have an impact on the entire emotion response. Sometimes it seems like emotions last a really long time because they can be self-perpetuating: Once an emotion starts, its impact can then be the trigger for another emotion's prompting event.

Discussion: Model of Emotions (28 minutes)

Review of Handout 16.1. Emotion Regulation: Model of Emotions (15 minutes)

Explain:

It is important that before we learn how to regulate our emotions, we learn how to identify and label them. How many of you have been asked before, "How are you feeling?" How many of you have responded with, "I'm upset"?

Allow students to explain what "I'm upset" means. Then ask:

OK, so what emotion is "upset"? "Upset" is usually a shorthand term we use for any negative emotion, such as scared, sad, worried, angry, or frustrated. So our focus for today will be on learning to identify and label our specific emotions, because once we can identify what we are feeling, we can then begin working on how to regulate the emotions. It is important to be able to name your emotions in order to be able to communicate to yourself and to other people how you feel and to be able to guide yourself to change an emotion when you need to.

CLASS EXERCISE: WALKING THROUGH THE MODEL WITH AN EXAMPLE

Continue:

> We are going to walk through this model of emotions, one component at a time, so that we can identify and understand each of the different components. After we go through the entire model with an example, we will break into small groups and go through the model for each of the different emotions.
>
> So first, when someone says, "I am scared," what does this mean?

Elicit answers from the class. Then say:

> An emotion is a full-system response that includes our thoughts, the sensations in our bodies, and our actions. Today we are going to go over all of the different components that make up an emotion.

Draw each component on the board as you go through the model, so that you end with a full picture. Begin with the box in Handout 16.1 for the **first prompting event** Say:

> The first prompting event is the event that sets off the entire emotion process. It can occur internally, like a thought or sensation; however, typically it is something that has happened around you, such as something you saw or heard, or something someone else said or did. External prompting events are things that happen around you—somebody saying something to you, getting back a test, seeing a fight. Internal prompting events are things that happen inside of you—a memory or a thought. What might be a prompting event for "scared"?

Write the examples on the board.

Now draw in the **vulnerability factors** that lead into the prompting event. Ask:

> Have you ever noticed that some days you are more emotionally sensitive or reactive than others?

Allow students to answer and provide some examples of when this may have occurred. Then go on:

> Emotions can be made stronger by certain vulnerabilities, like not getting enough sleep, or not having eaten, or being sick. You are more likely to have a reaction to the prompting event of somebody not saying hello to you if you are tired, hungry, and/or sick than you would be if you were feeling like your usual well-fed, well-rested, healthy self. Things that happened in the past can be also vulnerabilities, such as the anniversary of your grandmother's death or your anniversary with your ex-boyfriend or ex-girlfriend. These factors may not be the prompting events themselves, but they make us more vulnerable to our emotions when a prompting event does occur. In addition to being tired, hungry, and/or sick, can anyone think of any other vulnerability factors?

Write examples on the board.

Now draw in **thoughts about the event**. Say:

Thoughts are your interpretations about the prompting event. A person not saying hello to you is an external prompting event. Then this could lead to many different interpretations. You might think, "Sydney just didn't see me," or "Jackson is mad at me." Or you might think that the person is really depressed and doesn't want to talk. When something happens, we have thoughts about the event; we interpret the event in our minds and give it some kind of meaning. Now, are our thoughts about an event always accurate? Sometimes they are not. However, how we think about an event can have a big impact on what we feel. What are some thoughts we might have about the prompting events for "scared" that we generated?

Write the examples on the board. Highlight that the same prompting event can have multiple interpretations, which may lead to different emotional responses. For example, a snake for one person may prompt thoughts "it will hurt me" and prompt fear, and another person may think "it's so cool" and prompt curiosity or excitement.

Then draw in and discuss what happens **inside the body.**

Each emotion affects the body differently because of things that happen internally that cannot be seen by others. The things that cannot be seen are things like neurons firing in the brain or physiological changes, such as heart beating faster, temperature going up, and muscles tensing. We also internally experience our action urges. An action urge is the urge to do a behavior that we all have just before we engage in the actual behavior. Sometimes the action urge is so fast we don't even notice it, but now that we have our mindfulness skills, we are going to become more aware of noticing our urges to act before we actually do. How many of you have noticed the urge to pack up your backpack or tote bag before the bell rings, without actually packing up your bag? The urge to fight or attack associated with the anger is an example of this that most people are familiar with, since it is usually unacceptable in society to punch people with whom you are angry. The important thing is that the urge to act on a behavior is different from the actual behavior. We want to be able to observe and describe our urges. It is important to notice and strengthen our ability to observe an urge without acting on it as a way to decrease our impulsive behaviors. What are some of the physical sensations and action urges we might experience in response to our prompting event for scared and our interpretations about the event?

Write the examples on the board.

Next, draw and discuss what happens **outside the body**.

So if we know what happens inside the body, what occurs on the outside? What types of things can other people observe?

Allow students to answer. Then continue:

The things that can be seen—that are observable on the outside of the body—are facial expressions, posture, the words we say, and the behaviors we engage in. The clearest way to express emotions is with words. What are some of the external body reactions and actions we might experience in response to our "scared" prompting events and thoughts?

Write those examples on the board, and add:

It is important to note that expressing an emotion differently is not the same as suppressing an emotion. Suppressing an emotion can lead to more extreme emotions. Expressing an emotion differently means that you are expressing it in a more effective way. (Remember that being effective is one of the mindfulness "how" skills.)

Next, draw the **consequences of actions** box on the board, and say:

Consequences are the events that occur after our actions and/or body reactions. We can also call these the "aftereffects" of the emotion. Have you ever noticed that after you are really sad and crying, you become really tired or cannot think clearly? This is an aftereffect or consequence. Sometimes a consequence can then become a new prompting event for another emotion or even the same emotion. This is how the emotion gets refired in the brain over and over again. What are some of the consequences of being scared?

Write the examples on the board.
Finally, draw the **Prompting Event 2** box on the board.

Sometimes, the consequences can lead to a second prompting event that sets off another emotion path. It can continue the current emotion or prompt a second one. For example, if I am feeling scared and I screamed, followed by someone laughing at me. Someone laughing at me can be the second prompting event that may lead to experiencing embarrassment. What are some examples of other prompting events that could occur in our model of feeling scared?

Write the examples on the board.
Explain the solid and dotted lines in the model. Say:

Notice that there are both solid and dotted lines that lead to some of the different components. Why do you think that is?

Allow students to answer, then add as necessary:

The solid lines represent the paths that could occur in the full system response of one emotion. Notice that the first prompting event can lead to thoughts about the event or go directly to the internal experience. Why do you think that is?

Allow students to answer, then continue.

Sometimes we don't think about something that happens, we just automatically have a response. This can be our body's natural alert system to danger. If you are riding your bike or driving a car down the road and something runs out in front of it, you likely don't have enough time to think about the potential danger; your body reacts quickly. Your heartbeat increases, your blood pressure rises, and you slam on the brakes or swerve out of the way. The dotted lines are possible paths that might occur that refire the next emotion. The consequences of one emotion do not always set off another prompting event or other emotions.

Take questions from the students about this whole process. Then say:

Now let's go back and think again about that friend who didn't say hi to you. You might have different sensations, depending on how you interpreted the event. If you thought that the person was ignoring you on purpose, what might be the internal and external experiences you have?

Allow students to answer. Add, as necessary:

You might have your heart rate increase, the sensation of feeling like you are going to explode, or the urge to yell at the person. Your body language might be that your fists are clenched, your face is turning red, and maybe you do yell; that would be the action. This would be the emotion of anger.

If you interpreted the event as meaning that your friend no longer likes you, what internal and external experiences might you have?

Again, allow students to answer. Add, as necessary:

You might have the physical sensation of your throat closing or the urge to cry, and your body language might be that you are withdrawing. This would be sadness. Thinking then about that friend who stopped talking to you could restart the whole cycle of emotions for sadness. Or it might bring up a fear reaction—worries that you will never have any friends.

Review of Handout 16.2. Emotion Regulation: Ways to Describe Emotions (5 minutes)

Have students turn to Handout 16.2a. Refer back to the diagram of emotions on the board for each section of the emotion description. Explain:

Learning to observe and describe your emotions helps you to be able to understand and regulate your emotions. The next handout is multiple pages long, and each page is dedicated to a different emotion and each of the components of that emotion. We are going to start with anger, in Handout 16.2a. As you can see, each section on the page that we discuss will fit into one of the parts of the diagram. One benefit of the various parts of Handout 16.2 is that, if you are not sure what emotion you are feeling, you can identify the other components, such as your thoughts or action urges, and then look through the handout to see which emotion these experiences fit. The rest of Handout 16.2 (parts b–h) describes other emotions for you to read about.

Highlight to the students the different words for anger. Then discuss the different prompting events for feeling anger; the thoughts about the events that prompt feelings of anger; the "inside the body" reactions (body changes and sensations); and then the "outside the body" components (expressions and actions).

Class Exercise: Small-Group Activity with Homework 16.3 (8 minutes)

Divide students into small groups (depending on the number of students, there should be one group for each of the remaining seven emotions). Have students turn to Homework 16.3. Emotion Regulation: Practice with the Model of Emotions. Assign an emotion to each of the groups, and instruct the students that they are to read about their group's emotion and then fill in the appropriate parts of the diagram with the corresponding information for that emotion, based on one personal example that the group agrees upon. It is up to the group members to choose one prompting event that guides their emotional response. If groups have time after they finish their first example, the students should go through the process a second time, using the same prompting event. However, they should identify different interpretations, which may lead to different internal and external experiences, resulting in a different emotion.

When time is up, allow students to ask questions for clarification or make comments about the process.

Lesson Summary (2 minutes)

Congratulate the class for learning the model of emotions and for describing some emotions. Ask students to review the different components of the emotions briefly. Then say:

Now that we know the different components of an emotion, in the next lesson we will start learning the different skills to use to change each area. Remember, by changing one component, we can have an impact on the entire system.

Homework Assignment (3 minutes)

Homework 16.3. Emotion Regulation: Practice with the Model of Emotions

Explain:

For homework, you are going to do just what was done in class today for an emotion that you experience sometime over the course of the week. You are to identify a prompting event and then fill in each area of the homework sheet based on the components that occurred after the prompting event and the vulnerability factors that may have been present.

Ask whether there are any questions.

Diary Cards

Hand out new diary cards to the students. Highlight that they have now learned the skill of describing emotions, and that when they practice observing the different components of the emotions, they are to circle the days and rate the skill use for the week on the diary card (along with the other skills that they have been taught).

Finally, do some troubleshooting: Ask students whether they have any questions about the homework or any obstacles to completing it. If so, answer the questions and address the obstacles. Obstacles may include, but are not limited to, the following: Students have no intention of doing the assignment, have too much other homework this week, are likely to forget, or don't understand the assignment. Help students to identify their obstacles, and work with them to make a plan to overcome them. Examples include encouraging a student to write down the assignment and set a reminder in a cell phone or calendar to complete it; discussing why a student has no intention of doing the homework, and working on increasing his or her motivation and the relevance of the assignment (e.g., grades); or clarifying any other points. Troubleshooting should be done each week after the homework is assigned.

Emotion Regulation
Check the Facts and Opposite Action

SUMMARY

In Lesson 16, students have learned to identify and label emotions, with all of their different components. Today's lesson teaches two skills that students can use to change their emotional responses. As Lesson 16 has made clear, changing one component in the model of emotions can have an impact on the entire emotional response. First, students will learn to check the facts of a situation as a method of modifying their thoughts and beliefs about the event. Second, they will learn the skill of opposite action: Students will learn to change their emotions by changing their behaviors. Every emotion is linked with the urge to engage in some type of behavior. For example, if we are scared, we have the urge to avoid; if we are angry, we may have the urge to attack. Therefore, one strategy to change or regulate an emotion is to change our behavior by acting in a way that opposes or is inconsistent with the action urge associated with the emotion.

MAIN POINTS

1. Through checking the facts, we can change our beliefs or interpretations of an event, which can change our emotions.
2. Determining whether our emotions fit the facts (i.e., are justified by the facts) or don't fit the facts (i.e., are unjustified by the facts) will allow us to determine whether to use problem solving or opposite action to change the emotion. (Problem solving is covered in Lesson 18.)
3. Every emotion has a behavior or action urge associated with it. Reversing the expressive and action components of emotional responses can effectively change emotions.

MATERIALS

1. Handouts for this lesson:
   - Handout 17.1. Emotion Regulation: Overview of Skills for Changing Emotional Responses
   - Handout 17.2. Emotion Regulation: Check the Facts
   - Handout 17.3. Emotion Regulation: Examples of Emotions That Fit the Facts
   - Handout 17.4. Emotion Regulation: Opposite Action to Change Emotions
   - Homework 17.5. Emotion Regulation: Practice with Check the Facts
   - Homework 17.6. Emotion Regulation: Practice with Changing Emotion by Opposite Action
2. Extra student skills binders, with pens or pencils, for students who attend class without materials.
3. Dry-erase markers or chalk for writing on the board.
4. Diary cards: Have new diary cards ready to distribute at the end of class. If possible, highlight "Check the facts" and "Opposite action."

PREPARATION

1. Review the lesson plan as well as handouts in student skills binder.
2. Arrange the desks in the classroom, if possible, in order for students to be able to see each other.

LESSON OVERVIEW AND TIMELINE

- Mindfulness exercise (5 minutes)
  - Participating: Zen counting (3 minutes)
  - Describing observations of the exercise (2 minutes)
- Homework review (10 minutes)
  - Homework 16.3. Emotion Regulation: Practice with the Model of Emotions
    - Sharing with class
  - Diary cards
- Introduction of main ideas (2 minutes)
  - Review of Handout 17.1. Emotion Regulation: Overview of Skills for Changing Emotional Responses
    - Check the facts
    - Opposite action
    - Problem solving
- Discussion: Check the facts (13 minutes)
  - Review of Handout 17.2. Emotion Regulation: Check the Facts (8 minutes)
    - Thoughts can affect emotions.
    - Emotions can affect thoughts.
    - Three steps to check the facts

- Review of Handout 17.3. Emotion Regulation: Examples of Emotions That Fit the Facts (5 minutes)
  - Cheat sheet for determining if the emotion fits the facts
  - Class exercise: Small-group activity with Handout 17.3
- Discussion: Opposite action (15 minutes)
  - Review of Handout 17.4. Emotion Regulation: Opposite Action to Change Emotions
    - Emotions impact behaviors and behaviors impact emotions.
    - Opposite action works best when emotion does not fit the facts or behavior is not effective.
    - Opposite action must be done all the way.
    - Seven steps to opposite action
- Lesson summary (3 minutes)
  - Three steps to check the facts
  - Seven steps to opposite action
- Homework assignment (2 minutes)
  - Homework 17.5. Emotion Regulation: Practice with Check the Facts
    - Identify if your thoughts and interpretations fit the facts.
  - Homework 17.6. Emotion Regulation: Practice with Changing Emotion by Opposite Action
    - Practice opposite action by going through each step when you want to change your emotion.
  - Diary cards

DETAILED LESSON PLAN

Mindfulness Exercise (5 minutes)

Participating: Zen Counting (3 minutes)

Welcome the class and introduce the mindfulness activity. Explain:

> *Today we are going to practice another mindfulness exercise that involves participating. As we've learned, this means that everyone in the class participates fully by doing just one thing in the moment. We are going to do what is called "Zen counting."*
>
> *This is how it works: We will start counting one person at a time, with random people calling out the numbers in order. If we reach 20, then we will start back at 1. One person calls out 1, then another 2, then another 3, and so on. If two people say the same number at the same time, then we have to start back at 1, and the same person cannot say two consecutive numbers. Furthermore, we cannot communicate to each other in any way.*
>
> *This is an important example of letting go of judgments. If everyone were to be worried about calling out a number at the same time as someone else or worried about what others will think of them, then nobody would call out a number. The key is to throw yourself into the activity. If you should call out a number at the same time as someone else, let go of any judgments or worries that you might be feeling, and get back into the counting.*

For classes with more than 15 students, you may break the class up into two groups. Depending on the students, this exercise may go quickly, or it may take a full 3 minutes. If students make it to 20 right away, do it again with counting to 20, or substitute the alphabet.

Continue:

When I say 1, that's the signal to stand up and mindfully create a circle [or two circles, depending on class size]. I will let you take your positions before I say 2. When I say 2, that's the signal to take a deep breath. When I say 3, that's the signal for the group to begin Zen counting to 20.

Now start the practice by counting to 3.

1: Stand and mindfully create a circle. 2: Take a deep breath. 3: Begin Zen counting to 20.

After 3 minutes, say, "Stop," to end the exercise.

Describing Observations of the Exercise (2 minutes)

Highlight:

We had to be very mindful while counting. It can be difficult not to judge ourselves or others when multiple people said a number. Our first goal is to be nonjudgmental; our second goal, if we are judgmental, is to notice it, quickly let it go, and throw ourselves back into the exercise.

Have students share their observations of the mindfulness exercise. Provide feedback about observations as needed, ensuring that each statement consists of something a student can observe and describe nonjudgmentally(e.g., I noticed the urge to say a number and then being anxious about saying it, I noticed a judgmental thought about myself for saying the same number as [another student], I noticed stopping with each pause, I noticed a thought about how this was different from last week, I noticed a thought . . . , I noticed the sensation . . . , I noticed my mind wandering to other thoughts. I had lots of thoughts about how this could be helpful to me, I noticed I liked last week's practice better, I noticed I was uncomfortable so had to move . . .).

Homework Review (10 minutes)

Homework 16.3. Emotion Regulation: Practice with the Model of Emotions

SHARING WITH THE CLASS

Have the students take out their completed copies of Homework 16.3. Explain:

This can be a difficult concept to learn, and we are going to deepen our understanding by hearing how you did on practicing this skill over the last week.

Ask for any volunteers who would like to share their diagrams with the class. Go through one or two complete examples of the homework model with the class. As you are reviewing the model of emotions, ask students to generate other possible interpretations of a prompting event that could have occurred, and check to see whether this event might have had a different emotion-based response.

Also, ask whether any students had any difficulties with observing and describing an emotion that they had over the week. Follow up on any students who did not complete the homework, and briefly problem-solve what interfered with the homework completion.

Diary Cards

Ask all students to turn in their diary cards and homework sheets to be reviewed. If you are not able to review homework with each student each lesson, then be sure to get to each student over the course of several lessons.

Introduction of Main Ideas (2 minutes)

*Review of Handout 17.1. Emotion Regulation: Overview of Skills
for Changing Emotional Responses*

Have the class turn to Handout 17.1. This is an overview handout for the next three skills that will be taught. Explain:

> *In Lesson 16, we learned about all of the different components of an emotion, and we learned that by changing one component we can change the response of the entire system. Today we are going to focus on learning how to change two of the components: interpretations and actions. We will learn about checking the facts of a situation, and we will learn how changing our behavior can also change our emotional responses.*

Call on three students to read through each of the descriptions in the handout, or summarize them as follows:

- *Check the facts: Do our interpretations match the reality of the situation?*
- *Opposite action: Changing our behavior can change our emotions.*
- *Problem solving: When our thoughts do fit the facts, we need to solve the problem. (This skill will be taught in the next lesson.)*

Discussion: Check the Facts (13 minutes)

Review of Handout 17.2. Emotion Regulation: Check the Facts (8 minutes)

Have students turn to Handout 17.2. Ask a student to read the first statement in the handout: "Many emotions and actions are set off by our thoughts and interpretations of events, not by the events themselves." Explain:

> *As we learned in the lesson on describing emotions, our thoughts and interpretations of an event can affect the way that we respond to that event. Sometimes, though, what we are reacting to are not the actual facts of the situation, but our interpretations of the event. For example, being mad at a person who ignored you as you walked down the hall wouldn't fit the facts of the situation if the person did not see you.*

Ask the class to generate some examples of when someone might be responding to an interpretation of the event rather than the facts, or provide one or more of the following examples. Once each example has been provided, have other students generate other possible interpretations. Then ask students what different emotions they might experience, based on the different interpretations.

> *Example 1: Your friend Antonio walked past you in the hall and did not say hi (fact). This must mean he was mad at you (interpretation 1; emotions: anger, feeling rejected). Or he was feeling sick and going to the nurse's office (interpretation 2; emotion: worry). When you see Antonio later, you ask him why he didn't say hi, and he says he did not see you because he was focusing on preparing for a test he was about to take next period (fact; emotion: minimal or no emotional response).*
>
> *Example 2: Your mother tells you to wait a minute while she is talking to your brother before you can share some great news with her, and then she doesn't come back to talk to you (fact). Therefore, she doesn't really care about how you are doing and what's important to you (interpretation 1; emotions: anger, feeling rejected, envy). Or there must be something wrong with your brother that she had to attend to (interpretation 2; emotion: worry, fear). You find out later that your mother ran into the kitchen because she remembered she had water boiling on the stove (fact; emotion: disappointment, no other emotional response).*

Continue:

Faulty beliefs can also affect our emotions. If we have a belief that everyone should be our friend or a belief that our best friend should only hang out with us, this belief can cause emotional suffering. Another type of faulty belief that people sometimes have is all-or-nothing thinking. Examples of this kind of thinking (sometimes also called black-and-white thinking) are "If I don't get straight A's in all of my classes, then I am a failure," and "If I don't win every game, then I am a terrible athlete." These absolutes are extreme, and can lead to extreme negative emotions.

Now ask a student to read the second point in Handout 17.2: "Our emotions can also have a big effect on our thoughts about events." Explain:

Our emotions also affect how we think about things. When we are sad, happy people may seem really annoying; or when we are angry, it may seem like everyone is walking too slow or getting in our way. Our emotions influence how we interpret events. And if we are angry, those slow-moving people may just cause us to be angrier, perpetuating the cycle of angry emotions. Knowing the facts is important for problem solving.

Ask the students whether they have any questions so far.

Read through the rest of Handout 17.2 with the students. First, call on volunteers to read the "Three Steps to Check the Facts," and discuss each step in turn.

Step 1: In regard to "What is the emotion I want to change?", highlight:

In order to change how we are feeling, we need to know what emotion we are feeling. How can we know whether we want to change our emotion if we don't know what we are feeling?

Step 2: In regard to "What is the event prompting my emotion?", highlight:

> *It is important to just pay attention to describing the facts of the situation—the who, the what, and the where. Notice if you are engaging in any extreme thinking.*

Step 3: In regard to "Am I interpreting the situation correctly?", highlight:

> *Many of the negative emotions we feel occur because of how we thought about or interpreted an event. We may have a tendency to think about the worst possible outcome. A friend may eat lunch at a different table one day and that is the fact, but our interpretation that the person doesn't want to be our friend any more is what leads to feeling sad. Checking the facts helps us see the situation more clearly.*

Now continue the discussion with the "Additional Questions . . . ":

> *The next three questions may or may not apply to each situation. These are additional questions to ask yourself as you analyze your thoughts.*

In regard to "a": "Am I thinking in extremes . . . ?", encourage students to ask themselves:

> *"Is this really a catastrophe? Is this the end of the world? If the catastrophe did occur, how could I cope with it effectively?" Sometimes it helps to ask ourselves what the worst thing is that can happen, and then really examine that situation and remind ourselves that even then, there still would be other alternatives. Catastrophizing just focuses on the most hopeless aspects and doesn't do any good. People sometimes react to failing a test as if they are flunking out of school, or react to being grounded as if they will never get to hang out with their friends again, when this isn't the case. Checking the facts is important.*

In regard to "b": "What is the likelihood of the worst thing happening?", encourage students to ask themselves:

> *"What's the likelihood that the worst thing possible will occur? What's the likelihood that if I don't get to play in tomorrow's game, my life will be ruined? What's the likelihood that if I can't go to the party this weekend, I will lose all of my friends?"*

In regard to "c": "Even if the worst were to happen, can I imagine coping well with it?", say:

> *Can you imagine yourself coping effectively with the worst possible outcome? In an upcoming lesson, we will learn the skill of coping ahead. This skill focuses on preparing yourself for any possible outcome by imagining yourself coping effectively with it.*

Review of Handout 17.3. Emotion Regulation: Examples of Emotions That Fit the Facts (5 minutes)

Have students turn to Handout 17.3. Explain:

> *How do we know when our emotions don't fit the facts? Handout 17.3 is a "cheat sheet" we can use to understand when our emotions fit the facts or are justified by the facts.*

This part of the lesson is similar to the earlier lesson about the function of emotions. Going through this handout will be the introduction for the skill of opposite action. Because of this, you will revisit many of these facts, so do not spend too much time here now and move quickly into the class exercise.

CLASS EXERCISE: SMALL-GROUP ACTIVITY WITH HANDOUT 17.3

Have students break up into small groups of two or three students apiece. Assign each group one of the seven emotions. Students are to read through the examples of emotions that fit the facts on Handout 17.3, and then identify a situation for the identified emotion that fits the facts for the emotions. Students should also read the three questions at the bottom of the handout to determine whether the intensity and duration of their emotion fit the facts. Below are some key points listed about each of the emotions that you may review prior to the activity.

- *Fear: This emotion fits the facts when an actual threat is present. A perceived threat may not fit the facts: "I think I will be teased if I go to the party."*
- *Anger: This emotion fits the facts when a goal is blocked or when someone you care about is being attacked or hurt. However, just because your anger fits the facts, it does not mean that you can always act on your anger.*
- *Jealousy: This emotion fits the facts when someone or something is threatening to take something important away from you. It may be hard to know for sure when a relationship is being threatened, and then the more important question to ask is whether acting jealous is effective.*
- *Love: This emotion fits the facts when a person, animal, or object improves quality of life for you or for those you care about, and has qualities you value. Many abusive relationships do not fit these facts.*
- *Sadness: This emotion fits the facts when you have lost something or someone very important to you.*
- *Shame: This emotion fits the facts when your behaviors lead to public rejection by others.*
- *Guilt: This emotion fits the facts when your behavior goes against your own values or moral code.*

Allow students to ask questions and share examples of their situations that fit the facts.

Discussion: Opposite Action (15 minutes)

Handout 17.4. Emotion Regulation: Opposite Action to Change Emotions

Have students turn to Handout 17.4. Explain:

> *Every emotion has an action urge, and by changing our behaviors, we can also change our emotions.*

Draw only the top set of circles in Figure L17.1 on the board. Explain:

> *Typically, emotions lead to behavior: We have an emotion, and we behave a certain way. When we are angry, our action urge is to attack. When scared, our action urge is to avoid.*

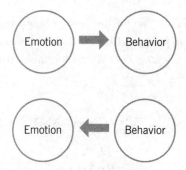

FIGURE L17.1. Diagram of how emotion leads to behavior (top two circles) and how behavior leads to emotion (bottom two circles).

> *When sad, our action urge is to withdraw. When feeling shame or guilt, our action urge is to hide.*

Ask a student to read aloud the action urges for jealousy and love from Handout 17.4. Then ask:

> *Who can share examples of when they had one of these emotions and the accompanying action urge?*

Allow a couple of students to share, and then say:

> *We know that if our emotion has an impact on our behavior, then the reverse also may be true: Our behavior can have an impact on our emotion.*

Now draw the second set of circles in Figure L17.1, with the arrows going in the opposite direction, on the board. Explain:

> *This means you can change your emotion by changing your behavior. For instance, when we attack, we may feel angry. Have you ever started yelling at someone, and the more you yelled at that person, the angrier you became? This is an example of how our behaviors can escalate our emotions. In the same way, when we avoid, we may feel scared or anxious. When we withdraw, we may feel sad. When we hide, we may feel shame or guilt.*
> *Now, is our goal to change our behaviors to cause more painful emotions? No. So the skill we are going to engage in to decrease or change our painful emotions is called "opposite action." We are going to focus on acting opposite to the action urge we are experiencing in response to our emotion.*

Go through each emotion listed under "Emotion → Opposite Action" on Handout 17.4. Begin by asking:

> *What would be the opposite behavior of running or avoiding if you are scared or afraid?*

Allow students to answer, then continue.

The answer is to approach the thing that makes you scared. Do the thing you are scared of over and over again, until you are no longer scared. For example, if someone is afraid of nonpoisonous snakes because he or she thinks they are dangerous, making the fear unjustified because it doesn't fit the fact that these snakes actually are not dangerous, then the way to decrease that fear is to have the person go toward snakes repeatedly until the fear goes down. For some people, the fear may be so high at first that this has to be done slowly and gradually—maybe starting with just showing these persons a picture of a snake, and working up to them holding the snake. The key is that if the fear is unjustified, meaning that it doesn't fit the facts, then we want to do the opposite action of approaching the situation over and over again.

Next, ask:

What would be the opposite behavior of attacking when you are angry?

Allow students to answer, then continue.

There are three things you can do. First, gently avoid the person rather than attacking. This means not stomping out and slamming the door. Second, take time out, and breathe in and out deeply and slowly. This will help reduce your action urge of attacking. Third, do something kind for the person, such as making the person's favorite meal or sending him or her a kind and encouraging note. Put yourself in the other person's shoes, and imagine having sympathy or empathy for the person.

Continue:

What would be the opposite behavior of withdrawing when you are sad?

Allow students to answer, then continue.

The answer is to get active with other behaviors and do things you enjoy or make you feel confident. Have you ever noticed that when you are sad, you don't want to do much of anything? You may even think, "I am going to wait until I feel better to do something." Well, it is likely that we will be waiting a very long time if we wait for our emotion to change on its own.

Go on:

What is the opposite of hiding when you feel shame or guilt and the emotion is unjustified, meaning that it does not fit the facts?

Allow students to answer, then continue.

The answer is to repeat the behavior over and over again until you no longer feel guilt or shame about it. Remember, this is for only when the behavior is <u>not</u> justified. For example, if you don't raise your hand in class to ask questions because you think the teacher will *kick you out for not understanding and you feel shame, you are likely to find once you check the facts that the shame does not fit the facts. Therefore, we want you to ask a lot of questions until you no longer feel shame about asking questions. However, in a situation where the shame or guilt is justified, meaning that it fits the facts and you violated your own values or the group's values, then in order to get the emotion to change, you must "face the music" and repair what you did wrong.*

Instruct students to read the descriptions of Face the Music and Go Public for both shame and guilt. Then say:

As you can see with shame and guilt, you must first figure out whether the emotion fits the facts to determine if opposite action will work. Opposite action works best when the emotion does not fit the facts (is not justified) or when acting on your emotions is not effective for the situation (remember that effectiveness is a mindfulness skill).

Now read through the sections of Handout 17.4 on jealousy and love with the class.

What is the opposite of trying to control someone, or making verbal accusations of someone, when you are jealous and the emotions don't fit the facts? In order to actively work on decreasing your jealousy, you will have to stop trying to control the other person and give him or her more freedom. For instance, don't spy or stalk the person on social media sites.

What if love is the emotion you want to change because it does not fit the facts? What would be the opposite action for love? Typically, when you love someone, you want to be around that person and think about him or her all day. However, if love for this person does not fit the facts—either because the relationship is truly over, or because it never was as strong as you thought it was, or because it is an abusive relationship—then you have to practice acting opposite by avoiding the person, reminding yourself about the cons of the relationship, and avoiding things that remind you of the person. For example, don't sleep with your ex-partner's t-shirt at night, or listen to "your" song over and over again.

We can determine whether an emotion fits the facts by referring back to Handout 17.3.

Now go on to the "Opposite Action Works Best When:" section of Handout 17.4. Have a student read point 1 in this section, or say:

Opposite action works the best when the emotion does not fit the facts. For example, if you came to class today and there was a tiger in the room, you would be afraid, and that fear would fit the facts because there would be an actual threat to your life. Now let's suppose that before the next class, the tiger gets taken out of the room, but you come to class tomorrow and are still afraid. This time your fear does not fit the facts because there is no actual threat to your life. Your fear is understandable, but not justified.

In addition, if an emotion is justified by the facts but not effective for the situation, you can use opposite action to change the emotion. Or you can use problem solving (which we will learn later on) as the other option.

Ask:

> *Who can provide an example of when an emotion might be justified by the facts <u>and</u> not effective?*

Elicit responses, or say:

> *Anger is an example of this. Although the anger may be justified by the facts, physically or verbally attacking another person is often not the effective solution. Therefore, using opposite action to decrease your anger is important even when the emotion is justified.*

Now have a student read point 2 under "Opposite Action Works Best When:", or say:

> *Opposite action has to be done all the way for it to work—with action, thinking, facial expressions, and tone of voice. This means that if you go to a party, opposite action doesn't just mean showing up at the party. You could show up at the party and stand in the corner, but that isn't really going to the party. Doing opposite action all the way would mean going to the party and making an effort to talk to people.*

Finally go through the seven required steps for opposite action. Have a student read these from the end of Handout 17.4, or say:

> *There are seven main steps to opposite action. First, identify and label the emotion you are feeling. Second, identify the action urges associated with your emotion. Third, check the facts: Does the emotion fit the facts? Is expressing or acting on this emotion effective? Fourth, ask yourself: "Do I want to change my emotion?" This is a key question because if you don't want to change the emotion, then this is not the time to use opposite action. There will be times when you want to be able to sit with your emotion and experience it. We will learn that in a future lesson.*
>
> *Fifth, if the answer from the fourth step is yes, then determine the opposite action to your emotion action urge. Sixth, do this opposite action <u>all the way</u>. This includes thoughts, appearance (eye contact, smiling), and behaviors. Seventh, repeat acting opposite until the emotion goes down enough for you to notice it.*

Lesson Summary (3 minutes)

Praise the class for doing a great job thinking of so many examples today. Briefly review the three key steps for checking the facts, and the seven key steps for taking opposite action. Then say:

> *In the next lesson, we will learn about problem solving in a situation when the emotion does fit the facts (is justified). For now, we are focusing on understanding how to determine whether our interpretations fit the facts and how to change our emotions by changing our behaviors.*

Homework Assignment (2 minutes)

Homework 17.5. Emotion Regulation: Practice with Check the Facts

Explain to students that because checking the facts is so important for opposite action, the first part of their homework assignment is to get more practice at it. Students should complete Homework 17.5 for an emotion experienced over the course of the coming week. Explain:

> For this homework sheet, you will ask yourself the same questions we asked during the class examples. Your goal is to identify whether your thoughts and interpretations fit the facts of the situation. Notice whether your emotion changes if you change your interpretations to fit the actual facts of the situation.

Homework 17.6. Emotion Regulation: Practice with Changing Emotions by Opposite Action

Explain that the second part of the homework assignment is to practice opposite action for an emotion that students experience during the week and to complete Homework 17.6. Say:

> You will walk through the steps of opposite action by identifying the emotion, identifying the action urge, deciding whether it fits the facts or not, identifying the opposite action, and then doing it all the way. Finally, comment on your emotion after you engaged in opposite action all the way.

Remind students that the homework is assigned to help them learn skills, that practice is the best way to learn, and that the worksheets are an aid to learning.

Diary Cards

Pass out new diary cards. Highlight that the students have now learned checking the facts and opposite action, and that when they practice these skills for their homework, they are to circle the days and rate the skill use for the week on the diary card (along with the other skills that they have been taught).

Finally, do some troubleshooting: Ask students whether they have any questions about the homework or any obstacles to completing it. If so, answer the questions and address the obstacles. Obstacles may include, but are not limited to, the following: Students have no intention of doing the assignment, have too much other homework this week, are likely to forget, or don't understand the assignment. Help students to identify their obstacles, and work with them to make a plan to overcome them. Examples include encouraging a student to write down the assignment and set a reminder in a cell phone or calendar to complete it; discussing why a student has no intention of doing the homework, and working on increasing his or her motivation and the relevance of the assignment (e.g., grades); or clarifying any other points. Troubleshooting should be done each week after the homework is assigned.

Emotion Regulation
Problem Solving

SUMMARY

Lesson 17 has focused on teaching the skills of check the facts and opposite action to change emotions. We use check the facts to verify whether an emotion fits the facts (i.e., whether it's justified). When the emotion does not fit the facts, we use opposite action to decrease or change the emotion. When the emotion does fit the facts, it is time to use the skill of problem solving. Today's lesson focuses on problem solving.

MAIN POINTS

1. Problem solving is a skill that identifies effective solutions for emotions that fit the facts.
2. It is important to determine what the actual problem is to be solved.
3. How do we problem-solve when an emotion is unwanted, yet fits the facts?

MATERIALS

1. Handouts for this lesson
   - Handout 18.1. Emotion Regulation: Problem Solving
   - Handout 18.2. Emotion Regulation: Putting Opposite Action and Problem Solving Together
   - Homework 18.3. Emotion Regulation: Practice with Problem Solving to Change Emotions
2. Extra student skills binders, with pens or pencils, for students who attend class without materials.
3. Dry-erase markers or chalk for writing on the board.
4. Diary cards: Have new diary cards ready to distribute at the end of class. If possible, highlight the "Problem solving" skill. Music player device (e.g., CD player, iPod, smartphone), with music that is older or novel, is to be played during the mindfulness exercise.

PREPARATION

1. Review the lesson plan as well as handouts in student skills binder.
2. Arrange the desks in the classroom, if possible, in order for students to be able to see each other.

LESSON OVERVIEW AND TIMELINE

- Mindfulness exercise (5 minutes)
  - Observing: Listening to novel music (3 minutes)
  - Describing observations of the exercise (2 minutes)
- Homework review (10 minutes)
  - Homework 17.5. Emotion Regulation: Practice with Check the Facts
  - Homework 17.6. Emotion Regulation: Practice with Changing Emotions by Opposite Action
    - Sharing with class
  - Diary cards
- Introduction of main ideas (3 minutes)
  - Four solutions to any problem
  - When the emotion does fit the facts, use problem solving.
- Discussion: Problem solving (17 minutes)
  - Review of Handout 18.1. Emotion Regulation: Problem Solving (7 minutes)
    - Describe the problem situation.
    - Check the facts.
    - Identify your goal(s).
    - Brainstorm lots of solutions.
    - Choose at least one solution that is likely to work.
    - Put solution(s) into action.
    - Evaluate each outcome.
  - Class exercise: Small-group activity with Homework 18.3 (10 minutes)
    - Small groups work through individual examples of problem-solving steps.
- Discussion: Putting it all together to change emotions (10 minutes)
  - Review of Handout 18.2. Emotion Regulation: Putting Opposite Action and Problem Solving Together
    - Summary of opposite action and problem solving for seven emotions
    - Students generate examples for emotions when emotions fit the facts and when they don't fit the facts.
- Lesson summary (3 minutes)
  - What questions guide you when checking the facts?
  - List the steps of problem solving.
- Homework assignment (2 minutes)
  - Homework 18.3. Emotion Regulation: Practice with Problem Solving to Change Emotions
    - Practice the steps of problem solving.
    - If students generated possible solutions to a problem in class, take the next step of putting one solution into action and evaluating outcomes.
  - Diary cards

DETAILED LESSON PLAN

Mindfulness Exercise (5 minutes)

Observe: Listening to Novel Music (3 minutes)

Prepare the music you are going to play for this mindfulness activity ahead of time, so you can start it easily. This should be music that is not popular with your students, so that it represents a genuinely novel experience to most of them. It can be music such as instrumental music, soundtracks from older films, "soft" jazz, or something similar. Welcome the class and state that today's mindfulness activity will involve a new type of observing. Explain:

> *Today we will mindfully listen to and observe music. This is most likely not music that you would typically listen to or buy. The purpose of this exercise is to let go of judgments and listen to the music, noticing pitch, rhythm, melody, volume changes, instrumental arrangement, and lyrics, or anything else that you may observe while listening. If you notice your mind wandering from the music, gently bring it back. If you find yourself having judgments (either positive or negative) about the music, just notice each thought as a judgment, let it go, and bring your attention back to the music.*

Continue:

> *When I say 1, that's the signal to sit in the mindful/wide-awake position we have often used before. Again, this means keeping our feet flat on the floor, sitting up straight, and putting our hands in our laps. For this exercise, we will keep our eyes open with a soft gaze, looking forward and down, but at nothing in particular. If you notice any urges to move, other than blinking or swallowing, notice each urge without acting on it, and return to your breath. When I say 2, that's the signal to take a deep breath. When I say 3, that's the signal to begin the practice. I'll say, "Stop," to end the practice.*

Now start the practice by counting to 3.

> *1: Get yourself into the mindful/wide-awake position. 2: Take a deep breath. 3: Begin the practice.*

Play the music for 2 minutes; then turn it off and say, "Stop."

Describing Observations of the Exercise (2 minutes)

Have a couple of students share observations of the exercise in the moment. Provide feedback about observations as needed, ensuring that each statement consists of something a student can observe and describe nonjudgmentally (e.g. I noticed the urge to move my body to the music, I noticed a thought about how this was different from last week, I noticed a thought . . . , I noticed the sensation . . . , I noticed my mind wandering to other thoughts. I had lots of thoughts about how this could be helpful to me, I noticed I liked last week's practice better, I noticed I was uncomfortable so had to move . . .).

Homework Review (10 minutes)

Homework 17.5. Emotion Regulation: Practice with Check the Facts
*Homework 17.6. Emotion Regulation: Practice with Changing Emotions
by Opposite Action*

SHARING WITH THE CLASS

Have the students take out their completed copies of Homework 17.5, and ask whether any students had difficulty with checking the facts. Review one to three students' homework, and review concepts as needed. Have other students generate additional possible interpretations for these students' examples.

Then move to Homework 17.6, and ask whether anyone had any difficulty with opposite action. Again, review one to three students' homework with the class.

Ask whether there are any additional questions about these two skills, and reinforce students for completing their assignments. If any students did not complete the homework, troubleshoot what may have been in their way, and ask them how they will complete the homework this week.

Diary Cards

Ask all students to turn in their diary cards and homework sheets to be reviewed. If you are not able to review homework with each student each lesson, then be sure to get to each student over the course of several lessons.

Introduction of Main Ideas (3 minutes)

Ask:

> Who can remember the four solutions to any problem?

Write the solutions on the board as students generate the answers:

1. Figure out how to solve the problem.
2. Change how you feel about the problem.
3. Accept the problem.
4. Stay miserable (or make things even worse).

Explain:

> What we learned in Lesson 17 and just reviewed were the skills of check the facts and opposite action. Opposite action is the skill to use when your emotion does not fit the facts or when it is not effective for the situation. But what do you do when you have an emotion that is justified—when the emotion does fit the facts of the situation, and it is not an emotion that you want to keep? When this occurs, you want to use the skill of problem solving, which is what we will learn today. The great thing about problem solving is that it is really effective in helping us to change an emotion when it fits the facts—and, in general, it is a really useful skill in all parts of our lives when we are faced with any problem for which we

need to find a solution. For today's lesson, we are going to focus on using the problem-solving skill to change our emotions, but I also want you to think about how you could apply the same steps we are going to learn today to any problem you have. In addition, remember that what may be a problem for you may not be a problem for your friends; these situations and emotions depend on the person.

Discussion: Problem Solving (17 minutes)

Review of Handout 18.1. Emotion Regulation: Problem Solving (7 minutes)

Have students turn to Handout 18.1. Explain:

> *Today we are going to focus on figuring out how to solve the problem. Sometimes it is the problem itself that is causing us to have unwanted emotions. And sometimes our emotions can keep us from seeing how we can solve a situation. In addition, sometimes we need to step back to figure out what the actual problem is that we are experiencing.*
>
> *For instance, you might identify a problem as "not doing your homework." And we can figure out all the ways to get you to do your homework. However, if not doing your homework is actually your solution to the problem and not the problem itself, then we might be trying to solve the wrong issue. It might be that your problem is that you get really anxious every time you think about doing your homework because you don't understand it. And when you avoid your homework, your anxiety goes away. If that is the case, then we need to do some problem solving to figure out how to help you understand the material and tolerate some anxiety.*

Continue:

> *There are seven steps to problem solving. We are going to read through each of them one by one, and then we will go back and go through several examples together.*

Read through the seven problem-solving steps on Handout 18.1, or have a student do so. Then go through the example below with the students.

> *Let's look at this example. Suppose you want to spend the weekend at a friend's house, but because you haven't been doing your chores and your last progress report had you failing two classes because of incomplete assignments, your parents have said no. They have told you that you are going to spend the weekend at home doing chores and completing your assignments. You experience the emotion of anger, which fits the facts because an important goal and activity are being blocked. However, attacking your parents would probably not be an effective plan. So you might use opposite action to get your anger down when you interact with them. Since anger fits the facts because your goal has been blocked, it also would be the time to use problem solving to figure out what you can do to overcome the obstacle to your goal of hanging out at your friend's house over the weekend. Overcoming this obstacle would also decrease your anger.*
>
> *First, ask yourself: Can this problem be solved? Do your parents have a history of changing their minds if you complete the tasks they are requesting? If no, use radical acceptance. If yes, use problem solving.*

Let's say that today is Monday and that your parents do have a history of changing their minds if you complete their goals.

Now go through each of the problem-solving steps with the students, asking for ideas and feedback at each step.

1. DESCRIBE THE PROBLEM SITUATION

The first step is to describe the problem situation. You want to go to a friend's house for the weekend. Your parents have said no. They have said no because you have failed two classes due to missing assignments and because you have not been doing your chores. You feel angry and sad, because you are going to miss out on what you think will be a fun weekend. Remember that when we describe a problem situation, we want just the facts, but that the facts also include the description of our emotional response. The core of the problem is that you think you will miss out on a lot of fun with your friends and will be lost next week when everyone is talking about it.

2. CHECK THE FACTS

The second step is to check the facts. Remember from Lesson 17 that there are several questions to ask ourselves when we check the facts. Our goal is to determine whether our interpretation of the situation fits the facts. The questions we are about to read are brief reminders of the steps to use when we check the facts.

Have students read each point, and then discuss each one.

Am I interpreting the situation correctly?

Your parents said you can't spend the weekend at your friend's house because of your grades and because you have not been doing your chores.

Am I thinking in extremes (all-or-nothing thoughts, catastrophic thinking)?

You are thinking, "I am going to miss out on everything this weekend. I won't know what anyone is talking about next weekend. Everyone will think I am a loser for not being around." The first two thoughts are all-or-nothing thoughts: Not everything is going to happen this weekend at your friend's house, and not everyone will be talking about it. The third thought is catastrophic thinking: When other friends have missed something over the weekend, you didn't dismiss them as "losers."

What is the probability of the worst thing happening?

It seems pretty unlikely that everyone will think you are a loser. But if you don't get your assignments completed, your grades improved, and your chores done this week, it is pretty unlikely that your parents will let you go.

Even if the worst thing happened, could you imagine coping well?

You can say to yourself, "I can keep in touch with my friends through texting and social media over the weekend. I can get my assignments completed so I don't have to miss out on the following weekend too."

Now continue:

If you are still faced with the problem and you still want to get your emotion down, start the steps below. It is likely that, although you understand why your parents are saying no to you, you still want to go. So let's go through the next step.

3. IDENTIFY YOUR GOAL(S)

The third step is to identify your goal or goals in solving the situation. In this example, what is your goal? Your goal is to get to your friend's house for the weekend.

4. BRAINSTORM LOTS OF SOLUTIONS

The fourth step is to brainstorm lots of solutions. "Brainstorming" is the process of generating as many possible solutions as you can think of, without judging any of the solutions. If you are having a difficult time coming up with possible solutions, ask for suggestions from people you trust—people you know will help you to be effective. For example, don't ask a friend who is likely to get you into more trouble. What does it mean not to judge any of the solutions?

Allow students to answer. Then continue:

In brainstorming, the trick is to write down anything and everything that comes to mind, not judging or throwing away any ideas.

Work with the class to generate solutions. As the teacher, you can model by suggesting extreme possibilities if the students are not doing so (e.g., running away, hiring a maid to clean the house, bribing your teacher to change your grades), and noting that during brainstorming we don't evaluate until all possible solutions are generated. Other examples of possible solutions might include these: Go to your friend's house anyway, do housework every day, talk to your teacher about extra credit, complete the missing assignments before Friday, run away, do a lot of homework during the week. Write all of the suggestions on the board, or have a student do so.

5. CHOOSE AT LEAST ONE SOLUTION THAT IS LIKELY TO WORK

The fifth step is to pick at least one solution that you think is likely to work. Now that we have generated an exhaustive list of possibilities, we can go through and evaluate them to identify solutions that might work. With the class, go through all of the possible solutions and evaluate them as (1) "Yes, this could work" (put a check mark by each of these items); (2) "No, this won't work" (put an X by each of these items); or (3) "This is in between yes and no" (put a dash by each of these items). For illustrative purposes here, let's assume that the class settles on "Do housework every day" and "Complete the missing assignments before Friday." (It will need to be determined whether it is possible to complete the missing assignments before Friday; for this example, however, let's assume it can be done.)

Now draw a four-cell list of pros and cons on the board for the possible solutions (see Figure L18.1), and elicit the pros and cons from the students.

> *Again, pros and cons can be an aid in making a decision. For example, completing all of the missing assignments during the week may mean that you will have to miss some after-school activities this week in order to get everything completed.*

Have the students weigh the pros and cons to arrive at a decision. For illustrative purposes here, let's assume that the decision is to complete the missing assignments before Friday.

6. PUT THE SOLUTION(S) INTO ACTION

> *The sixth step is to put the solution or solutions you have chosen into action. What steps would need to be taken for "Complete the missing assignments before Friday"? These may include making a plan for what assignments are going to be completed daily. With this example, it may also include presenting the plan to your parents to see whether they will accept the plan and change their minds if all requirements are completed.*

7. EVALUATE EACH OUTCOME

> *The seventh and last step is to evaluate each outcome. Of course, you will have to wait until the end of the week to evaluate your outcomes. Did your solution solve the problem? Were you able to meet your goals?*
>
> *If it worked, reward yourself. If not, validate yourself for working so hard, and evaluate why the solution may not have worked. In this example, it may have been that complet-*

	Pros	Cons
Using this solution		
Not using this solution		

FIGURE L18.1. Four-cell pros-and-cons list for problem solving.

ing all of the missing assignments in 4 days was not possible, since each assignment took longer than you expected. Choose another solution, or move back to radical acceptance if the problem can't be solved.

CLASS EXERCISE: SMALL-GROUP ACTIVITY WITH HOMEWORK 18.3 (10 MINUTES)

Instruct students to break into groups of three or four, and to turn to Homework 18.3. Emotion Regulation: Practice with Problem Solving to Change Emotions. Explain:

In your small groups, you are going to spend the next 10 minutes practicing with using problem solving. First, each of you should identify a problem that you are having that is causing unwanted emotions. Choose one person's problem to work on, and go through the homework sheet together. I especially want you to practice brainstorming solutions without evaluating. If you finish with the first person's problem, go on to the next person's.

While students are working on this, be sure to walk around and listen to the conversations, and provide feedback to students on how they are working through the steps. After 7 minutes, ask students to share any observations they made or to ask questions about the process.

Discussion: Putting It All Together to Change Emotions (10 minutes)

Review of Handout 18.2. Emotion Regulation: Putting Opposite Action and Problem Solving Together

Have students turn to Handout 18.2. Explain:

Handout 18.2 lists seven emotions, along with the events that would make each emotion justified or fit the facts. If the emotion does not fit the facts, different opposite actions are listed. If the emotion does fit the facts, different approaches toward problem solving are listed. This handout is an excellent summary of what we have been talking about today and in Lesson 17. The decision to engage in opposite action or problem solving will depend on the facts of the situation.

Read through a few of the emotions with the students, allowing opportunities for questions to be asked. As you read through the examples, ask students to generate brief examples of situations where the emotion would fit the facts and would be justified, and then examples of situations where the emotion would not fit the facts and would be unjustified. If students are not able to generate examples, then you should provide examples.

Depending on class time, after a few examples are reviewed, inform students that reading through this handout will be part of their homework. In any case, they should use it as guidance for completing Homework 18.3.

Lesson Summary (3 minutes)

Today we reviewed the skill of checking the facts and learned how to use problem solving. What are some of the questions you can ask to help you check the facts?

Allow students to generate the questions to guide them in checking the facts. For guidance, use Handout 17.2. Emotion Regulation: Check the Facts.

> Am I interpreting the situation correctly? Are there other possible interpretations?
>
> Am I thinking in extremes?
>
> What is the likelihood of the worst thing happening?
>
> Even if the worst were to happen, can I imagine coping well with it?
>
> *What are the steps to problem solving?*

Allow students to generate the seven steps. For guidance, use Handout 18.1. Emotion Regulation: Problem Solving.

Homework Assignment (2 minutes)

Homework 18.3. Emotion Regulation: Practice with Problem Solving to Change Emotions

Explain:

> *During the week, you are to use your newly learned problem-solving skill for a situation that causes an unwanted emotion. Some of you have already started this as part of the class exercise. If you have, then you must follow through on the steps of putting your solutions into action and evaluating your outcomes. Remember that you can use Handout 18.2. Emotion Regulation: Putting Opposite Action and Problem Solving Together as a quick guide to determining whether your emotion fits the facts and whether you should use opposite action or problem solving.*

Diary Cards

Hand out the new diary cards to the students. Highlight that they have now learned problem solving, and that when they practice this skill for their homework, they are to circle the days and rate the skill use for the week on the diary card (along with the other skills that they have been taught).

Finally, do some troubleshooting: Ask students whether they have any questions about the homework or any obstacles to completing it. If so, answer the questions and address the obstacles. Obstacles may include, but are not limited to, the following: Students have no intention of doing the assignment, have too much other homework this week, are likely to forget, or don't understand the assignment. Help students to identify their obstacles, and work with them to make a plan to overcome them. Examples include encouraging a student to write down the assignment and set a reminder in a cell phone or calendar to complete it; discussing why a student has no intention of doing the homework, and working on increasing his or her motivation and the relevance of the assignment (e.g., grades); or clarifying any other points. Troubleshooting should be done each week after the homework is assigned.

Emotion Regulation

The A of ABC PLEASE

SUMMARY

Increasing positive emotions, reducing vulnerability to negative emotions, and staying out of emotion mind can be accomplished through practice of the skills summarized by the mnemonic ABC PLEASE. Today's lesson focuses on the A of ABC PLEASE. The goal of this lesson is to increase students' positive emotions in both the short term and long term. The lesson focuses on helping students increase their daily pleasurable activities in the short term and on teaching students to identify their personal values and their goals for living consistently with their identified values over the long term.

MAIN POINTS

1. The A in ABC PLEASE stands for Accumulating positive emotions.
2. Accumulating positive emotions includes both engaging in daily pleasurable activities in the short term and identifying values and goals in the long term.

MATERIALS

1. Handouts for this lesson:
   - Handout 19.1. Emotion Regulation: Overview of ABC PLEASE
   - Handout 19.2. Emotion Regulation: Accumulating Positive Experiences in the Short Term
   - Handout 19.3. Emotion Regulation: Pleasant Activities List
   - Handout 19.4. Emotion Regulation: Accumulating Positive Experiences in the Long Term

- Handout 19.5. Emotion Regulation: Wise Mind Values and Priorities List
- Homework 19.6. Emotion Regulation: Practice with Accumulating Positive Experiences (Short- and Long-Term)

2. Extra student skills binders, with pens or pencils, for students who attend class without materials.
3. Dry-erase markers or chalk for writing on the board.
4. Diary cards: Have new diary cards ready to distribute at the end of class. If possible, highlight the "Accumulating positives" skill.

PREPARATION

1. Review the lesson plan as well as handouts in student skills binder.
2. Arrange the desks in the classroom, if possible, in order for students to be able to see each other.

LESSON OVERVIEW AND TIMELINE

- Mindfulness exercise (5 minutes)
  - Participating: Storytelling (4 minutes)
  - Describing observations of the exercise (1 minute)
- Homework review (10 minutes)
  - Homework 18.1. Emotion Regulation: Practice with Problem Solving to Change Emotions
    - Sharing with partners
    - Sharing with class
  - Diary cards
- Introduction of main ideas (3 minutes)
  - Review of Handout 19.1. Emotion Regulation: Overview of ABC PLEASE
    - What is emotion mind?
    - ABC PLEASE skills decrease vulnerability to emotion mind.
- Discussion: Accumulating positive experiences in the short term (18 minutes)
  - Review of Handout 19.2. Emotion Regulation: Accumulating Positive Experiences in the Short Term (8 minutes)
    - Pleasant activities
    - Mindful of positive experiences
    - Be unmindful of worries
  - Review of Handout 19.3. Emotion Regulation: Pleasant Activities List (10 minutes)
    - Class exercise: Small-group activity with Handout 19.3
    - Identify and discuss possible pleasant activities to engage in.
- Discussion: Accumulating positive experiences in the long term (10 minutes)
  - Review of Handout 19.4. Emotion Regulation: Accumulating Positive Experiences in the Long Term (5 minutes)
  - Review of Handout 19.5. Wise Mind Values and Priorities List (5 minutes)
    - Students identify and prioritize their own wise mind values.

- Lesson summary (2 minutes)
  - Why is accumulating positives important to our emotions?
  - Why do we need to accumulate positives in the short term and long term? How?
- Homework assignment (2 minutes)
  - Homework 19.6. Emotion Regulation: Practice with Accumulating Positive Experiences (Short- and Long-Term)
    - Plan a pleasurable activity to complete each day.
    - Identify and take steps toward wise mind values and goals.
  - Diary cards

DETAILED LESSON PLAN

Mindfulness Exercise (5 minutes)

Participating: Storytelling (4 minutes)

Welcome the class and introduce today's mindfulness activity. Explain:

> *Today we are going to practice another mindfulness exercise that involves participating. In other words, everyone in the class will participate fully by doing just one thing in the moment. We are going to do what is called "storytelling."*
>
> *Here is how this works: We will start telling a story by having each of us say one word at a time. We will go around the room in order, each of us adding another word to the story. The key here is to practice participating one-mindfully by waiting for your turn to decide on your word. If you get ahead of the story, the word you choose may not be the word you want by the time it is your turn. This may result in judgments or disappointment. If that does occur, simply practice noticing it and then throwing yourself back into the moment and following the story. We will go around for 2 to 3 minutes, so we can see where our story takes us. We will do this exercise standing up and in a circle.*

For classes with more than 15 students, you may break the class up into two groups. Continue:

> *When I say 1, that's the signal to stand up and mindfully create a circle [or two circles, depending on class size]. I will let you take your positions before I say 2. When I say 2, that's the signal to take a deep breath. When I say 3, that's the signal for the group to begin. I will say the first word.*

Now start the practice by counting to 3.

> *1: Stand and mindfully create a circle. 2: Take a deep breath. 3: I will now say the first word.*

Say the first word, and then point to the student next to you to continue. (If there is more than one circle, appoint a student to begin the second circle.) After 3 minutes, say, "Stop," to end the exercise.

Describing Observations of the Exercise (1 minutes)

Highlight:

> *Our first goal in this exercise was to be one-mindfully participating in the story by waiting for our turn. The second goal was to be nonjudgmental—and if we were judgmental, to notice it, quickly let it go, and throw ourselves back into the exercise. What observations did you notice during the exercise?*

Have students share their observations of the mindfulness exercise. Provide feedback about observations as needed, ensuring that each statement consists of something a student can observe and describe nonjudgmentally (e.g., I noticed thoughts about where I wanted the story to go, I noticed a judgmental thought about myself for a word that didn't make any sense, I noticed stopping with each pause, I noticed a thought about how this was different from last week, I noticed a thought . . . , I noticed the sensation . . . , I noticed my mind wandering to other thoughts. I had lots of thoughts about how this could be helpful to me, I noticed I liked last week's practice better, I noticed I was uncomfortable so had to move . . .).

Homework Review (10 minutes)

Homework 18.3. Emotion Regulation: Practice with Problem Solving to Change Emotions

SHARING WITH PARTNERS

Have the students take out their completed copies of Handout 18.3. Instruct students to break into the same small groups they were in when they practiced the problem-solving skills during Lesson 18. Walk among the dyads to oversee and answer any questions and provide feedback. Explain:

> *You should each share with your group the problem and emotion that you used for problem solving during the week. Discuss the evaluation process, especially with the person whose example was worked on in class. It is important that you discuss each of the steps and troubleshoot any problems you encountered, along with what effects solving the problem had on your emotion.*

SHARING WITH THE CLASS

Ask for a couple of volunteers to share their experiences of problem solving. With each volunteer, specifically go through each of the steps, using the student's responses as teaching points and being sure to highlight how solving the problem affected their emotion. If there was no change in emotion, troubleshoot and discuss whether any of the steps in the process have to be reevaluated, especially identifying the problem that was causing the emotion.

Follow up with any students who did not complete the homework, and briefly discuss what interfered with the homework completion.

Diary Cards

Ask all students to turn in their diary cards and homework sheets to be reviewed. If you are not able to review homework with each student each lesson, then be sure to get to each student over the course of several lessons. Comment on the amount of skills use you see marked on the diary cards for students.

Introduction of Main Ideas (3 minutes)

Review of Handout 19.1. Emotion Regulation: Overview of ABC PLEASE

Begin by reviewing what it means to be in emotion mind. Ask:

What is emotion mind, and how does it affect us?

Elicit responses, which should be something like this (or say this):

Emotion mind is the state we are in when our emotions are high, and we are making decisions and engaging in behaviors based on our emotions rather than on our logic or wise mind.

Now explain:

All people are prone to emotional reactivity when they are under physical or environmental stress. Today and in the next lesson, we are going to learn how to increase our positive emotions, such as joy, pride, and self-confidence, and how to become less vulnerable to negative emotions, such as sadness, fear, and shame.

Have students turn to Handout 19.1. Because this handout is simply an overview of the skills that will be taught today and in the next lesson, spend only 1–2 minutes on reviewing it. Explain:

ABC PLEASE is a mnemonic, or memory helper, for the skills we will learn in order to decrease how vulnerable we are or how likely we are to end up in emotion mind. Today we will learn the A of the ABC PLEASE skills, which is Accumulating positive experiences. In the next lesson, we will learn the rest of these skills—which include Building mastery, Coping ahead with difficult situations, and the PLEASE skills for taking care of the mind by taking care of the body.

Ask a student to read the ABC points on Handout 19.1. Then go on:

In life we need to have balance, and one way of increasing our experience of positive emotions is to focus on having positive experiences in both the short and long term. An absence of pleasurable events will lead to an absence of positive emotions. It is also important to build up the positives because in the scale of life, if we have a buildup of positives, a negative that comes along will not tip the scale.

Discussion: Accumulating Positive Experiences in the Short Term (18 minutes)

Review of Handout 19.2. Emotion Regulation: Accumulating Positive Experiences in the Short Term (8 minutes)

Have students turn to Handout 19.2. Explain:

> *The A in ABC PLEASE is for Accumulating positive experiences. We do this in both the short term and the long term. Short-term positive events make us happy now, and long-term positive events give us a lasting sense of happiness. First we are going to focus on how to increase our positive emotions in the short term.*

Ask a student to read through "In the Short Term:" section of the handout. Then ask:

> *How many of you can say that you engage in some type of activity every day that brings you joy or pleasure?*

Reinforce those who say yes, and emphasize for everyone:

> *This is the goal of this skill. To make ourselves less vulnerable to emotions such as sadness, anger, fear, shame, and guilt, we need to make sure we are engaging in pleasurable activities every day in order to increase our positive emotions. Pleasant events are like vitamins; you need to take them daily. An absence of pleasant events can increase our sadness or other negative emotions.*

Add:

> *It is not effective to think about whether or not you deserve to have pleasant events in your life; thinking about deserving is judgmental thinking. We all need to engage in positive activities, even if we feel that we do not deserve them. In a few minutes, we will start identifying some pleasant events we can all engage in. First, though, let's finish reading through this handout.*

> Have a student read the "Be Mindful of Positive Experiences:" section of Handout 19.2. Then ask:

> *What do you think all this means? Give me an example of how you would do this.*

Since students have reviewed the mindfulness skills twice, this is an opportunity to have them generalize their use of the skills. Point out:

> *Just as it is important to plan pleasant events, it is equally important to be mindful when you are engaging in those events. If you are not fully engaged in a pleasant event, the event itself will have little effect on your overall emotions.*

Now have a student read through the "Be Unmindful of Worries:" section of Handout 19.2. Ask:

> *What do you think this means? What does it mean to be unmindful of worries? Give me an example of how you would do this.*

Elicit students' examples. If they have trouble coming up with examples, say:

> *Being unmindful of worries is like sitting on the beach during a vacation and not thinking about when your vacation will end and how sad or anxious you will be, or if you really deserve to be there, or if there is something else you should be doing at the moment. If you only focus on when an event or experience will end, or when "the other shoe is going to drop," you may end up missing the moment—and therefore not increasing your positive emotions.*
>
> *Another example is seeing an old friend who is visiting for the day. You have just that one day with the friend; you don't want to waste the day thinking about how he or she is leaving tomorrow.*

Ask:

> *Can you remember a time when you were having fun, but then stopped paying attention to the moment because you were thinking about when it would end, or whether you deserved it, or whether something else was expected of you?*

Elicit responses, and then ask:

> *So what do we need to do in these situations? How can we use our mindfulness skills to keep us unmindful of worries and mindful of positive experiences?*

Encourage students to share how they will practice focusing on just the activity of the moment, and how if they notice themselves thinking about the end or another activity, they will let go of those thoughts and bring their attention back to the moment. This is an opportunity for students to link the skills practiced in the mindfulness exercises at the beginning of each class to use in their daily lives.

Review of Handout 19.3. Emotion Regulation: Pleasant Activities List (10 minutes)

Have students turn to Handout 19.3. Explain:

> *The pages of this handout list lots of ideas for things you can do each day to help tip your life scale to the positive.*

Give students a moment to look over the handout.

CLASS EXERCISE: SMALL-GROUP ACTIVITY
WITH HANDOUT 19.3

Have the students break into groups of three or four. Instruct them:

> *Read through the list in Handout 19.3, and discuss the activities that you think you would enjoy. Circle the numbers of the activities that you think you would enjoy or have enjoyed in the past. Even if an activity you used to enjoy is something you don't think you would enjoy any more, circle the number of that activity as well.*
>
> *Not all activities will be pleasurable for every student, or even effective for every student. So this is an opportunity for you to all practice being nonjudgmental and learning about activities that you might not think you would enjoy. Of course, you may have valid reasons for not thinking you would enjoy some activities. For example, if one of your pets just recently died, taking care of your other pets might not be a pleasurable activity for you, or if you live in a tropical place, sledding might not be an option. Finally, if there are activities that you know you enjoy and they are not listed on the handout, add them in the blank spaces at the end.*

When students have finished going through the handout, ask for volunteers to share what they circled and what they added. Encourage students that if they hear something they think they might like, they should add it to their own list. Have students share whether they learned about any new pleasant activities from others in their group that they had not thought about.

Finally, explain that it is equally important to engage spontaneously in pleasurable activities and to plan ahead of time to do pleasant events. This list will help with both types of engagement.

Discussion: Accumulating Positive Experiences in the Long Term (10 minutes)

Review of Handout 19.4. Emotion Regulation:
Accumulating Positive Experiences in the Long Term (5 minutes)

Have students turn to Handout 19.4. Then ask these questions:

- *How many of you can tell me what your values are?*
- *What are some of your values?*
- *How many of you make decisions on a regular basis that are in line with your values?*

Pause after each question and elicit students' responses. Then say:

> *On the one hand, it is necessary for us to have positive things that we are going to put into our lives right now. On the other hand, it is also important to have goals that we are working toward—things that we really want in our lives. We want these goals to be in line with our wise mind values.*

Ask a student to read the "In the Long Term:" and "Work toward Goals Based on Your Values:" sections of Handout 19.4. Then say:

In a moment, we are going to identify some of our values. Once we know what our values are, we can set some goals for ourselves based on our values. In order to reach our goals, it is often most helpful to list the steps we need to take in order to accomplish those goals.

Now have a student read the "Pay Attention to Relationships:" section of the handout. Ask:

What does this mean?

Allow students to provide explanations, examples of relationships they could repair, or examples of relationships they should end. Add:

It is important to work toward building and maintaining relationships because relationships need attention. Like flowers in a garden, they need to be tended, watered, weeded, and fed.

Finally, it is important to avoid avoiding and to avoid giving up. How many of you have noticed a time in the past when you are avoiding something, like working on a project or talking to a friend who you think is mad at you or avoiding you? The key here is to avoid the avoiding of these activities. Mindfully notice when you are doing it, and then take opposite action.

Review of Handout 19.5. Emotion Regulation: Wise Mind Values and Priorities List (5 minutes)

Have students turn to Handout 19.5. Explain:

When we are determining our goals, often we first need to understand and know what our values and priorities are. Handout 19.5 is a list of common values that people have. As we read through this list, I want you to check off those that <u>you</u> value. Not everyone will share the same values, and that is OK. Learning what your values are is extremely important when it comes to making decisions and determining courses of action for yourself in difficult situations.

For example, if your values are to be responsible and to have fun, then you may struggle at times to decide between taking the next babysitting job offered to you or going to work on the weekend versus going to a sleepover or house party with your friends. Then you may have to <u>mindfully</u> identify which value is a higher priority for you or which one you haven't focused on in a while, in order to determine whether you should hang out with your friends or focus on working and earning money to help you become more independent.

A second example may be that your values are to be a part of a group and to build character. So what do you do when your friends start acting in ways that go against your wise mind value of building character, such as stealing, using drugs, or bullying? It's important that you can make sure you are living within your values and recognizing the consequences of engaging in behaviors that violate some of your values. Although you may prioritize belonging to a group over building character, are you ready to manage the consequences of how you feel about yourself if you violate your value of building character? The goal here is to help you to determine whether your actions are within your own wise mind values.

Now instruct the students:

Take the next few minutes to read through the values listed on the handout. Determine which items are your values. If you have more than one value (which you probably will), the next step is to put them in order, with 1 being your highest-priority value. Write the numbers next to each item once you have identified your values.

Allow 3–4 minutes for students to identify and prioritize values. Then ask:

What do you think the next step is, now that you have determined your wise mind values?

Allow students to answer. Then say:

Once you are able to identify and prioritize your values, the next step is determining whether or not you are living your life in a way that is within your own values. If you are not, you need to think about what you need to be doing so that you are. This is how you identify and set goals. The process of determining goals is important and needs to be consistent with your values.

I asked this question earlier, and now that we have started to learn about our values some more, I'll ask it again: How many of you would say that you are living a life that is in line with your values and that your goals are in line with your values?

Comment on whether or not the number of raised hands in the room has changed. Allow students to discuss, if desired, what has changed for them over the course of this lesson. Then say:

As part of your homework today, you will choose one of your values, and identify goals that you have that will help you come closer to living within your own values. Then you will determine some small beginning steps you can take to start working toward those goals. We will go over the homework in more detail in a few minutes.

Lesson Summary (2 minutes)

Have the students answer these questions:

- *Why is accumulating positives important to our emotions?*
- *Why do we need to accumulate positives in the short term? How can we do that?*
- *Why do we need to accumulate positives in the long term? How can we do that?*

Homework Assignment (2 minutes)

Homework 19.6. Emotion Regulation: Practice with Accumulating Positive Experiences (Short- and Long-Term)

Explain:

> *For homework, you are going to focus on accumulating positives in both the short and the long term. For the short term, engage in at least one pleasurable activity for each day of the next week, and rate your mood before and after each activity, using the scale of –5 through +5 that is described on the homework sheet.*

Ask students for questions about the first part of the homework. Then continue:

> *For the second part of your homework, from the list of prioritized values you made earlier, you are to determine one long-term goal associated with that value. Then identify the first step in reaching that goal that you can take in the next week. Once you have taken that first step, describe your experience. It may be helpful for you to list not only the first step you need to take, but multiple steps, so that you can identify your path. This will also help you to determine whether you need to break down any of the steps into smaller steps.*

Ask students for questions about this part of the homework.

Diary Cards

Hand out new diary cards to the students. Highlight that they have now learned the A in ABC PLEASE, and that when they practice this skill for their homework, they are to circle the days and rate the skill use for the week on the diary card (along with the other skills that they have been taught).

Finally, do some troubleshooting: Ask students whether they have any questions about the homework or any obstacles to completing it. If so, answer the questions and address the obstacles. Obstacles may include, but are not limited to, the following: Students have no intention of doing the assignment, have too much other homework this week, are likely to forget, or don't understand the assignment. Help students to identify their obstacles, and work with them to make a plan to overcome them. Examples include encouraging a student to write down the assignment and set a reminder in a cell phone or calendar to complete it; discussing why a student has no intention of doing the homework, and working on increasing his or her motivation and the relevance of the assignment (e.g., grades); or clarifying any other points. Troubleshooting should be done each week after the homework is assigned.

Emotion Regulation
The BC PLEASE of ABC PLEASE

SUMMARY

Lesson 19 has focused on increasing positive emotions, reducing vulnerability to negative emotions, and staying out of emotion mind through <u>A</u>ccumulating positive experiences in both the short term and long term; this is the A in ABC PLEASE. Today's lesson focuses on the remaining BC PLEASE skills. <u>B</u>uilding mastery is the skill of engaging in activities that are difficult but not impossible. By engaging in and completing difficult tasks on a regular basis, individuals can increase their overall sense of self-confidence and joy. <u>C</u>oping ahead is the skill of using imaginal practice to increase the ability to manage difficult emotions if they arise. Finally, the PLEASE skills focus on taking care of the body, such as maintaining a balanced diet and eating throughout the day, getting enough sleep, exercising daily, avoiding mood-altering substances, and taking care of any physical illnesses. By using the PLEASE skills, individuals can decrease their potential vulnerability to painful emotions. The students will work together to determine how many of the PLEASE skills they each engage in regularly to determine how well they are taking care of themselves in order to decrease their vulnerability to emotion mind.

MAIN POINTS

1. B is for <u>B</u>uilding Mastery.
2. C is for <u>C</u>oping ahead of time with emotional situations.
3. The PLEASE skills are as follows: treat <u>P</u>hysica<u>L</u> illness, balance <u>E</u>ating, <u>A</u>void mood-altering drugs, balance <u>S</u>leep, and get <u>E</u>xercise. Taking care of your body decreases vulnerability to negative emotions.

MATERIALS

1. Handouts for this lesson:
    -   Handout 20.1. Emotion Regulation: Building Mastery and Coping Ahead
    -   Handout 20.2. Emotion Regulation: PLEASE Skills
    -   Handout 20.3. Emotion Regulation: Food and Your Mood
    -   Handout 20.4. Emotion Regulation: 12 Tips for Better Sleep Hygiene
    -   Homework 20.5. Emotion Regulation: Practicing with Build Mastery, Cope Ahead, and PLEASE Skills
2. Extra student skills binders, with pens or pencils, for students who attend class without materials.
3. Dry-erase markers or chalk for writing on the board.
4. Diary cards: Have new diary cards ready to distribute at the end of class. If possible, highlight the "BC PLEASE" skills.

PREPARATION

1. Prepare a method to display the words to the song "Take Me Out to the Ball Game."
2. Review the lesson plan as well as handouts in student skills binder.
3. Arrange the desks in the classroom, if possible, in order for students to be able to see each other.

LESSON OVERVIEW AND TIMELINE

-   Mindfulness exercise (5 minutes)
    -   Participating: Singing "Take Me Out to the Ball Game" (3 minutes)
    -   Describing observations of the exercise (2 minutes)
-   Homework review (10 minutes)
    -   Homework 19.6. Emotion Regulation: Practice with Accumulating Positive Experiences (Short- and Long-Term)
        -   Sharing with partners
        -   Sharing with class
    -   Diary cards
-   Introduction of main ideas (2 minutes)
    -   B—Build mastery by doing difficult things.
    -   C—Cope ahead for difficult situations.
    -   Decrease vulnerability to emotions by taking care of your body: PLEASE
-   Discussion: Building mastery and coping ahead (15 minutes)
    -   Review of Handout 20.1. Emotion Regulation: Building Mastery and Coping Ahead
        -   Build mastery— do something difficult each day (5 minutes).
        -   Cope ahead— identify the threat and rehearse a plan (10 minutes).
            -   Class exercise: Small-group activity for coping ahead

- Discussion: Taking care of your body to take care of your mind (13 minutes)
  - Review of Handout 20.2. Emotion Regulation: PLEASE Skills (5 minutes)
    - Treat <u>P</u>hysica<u>L</u> illness.
    - Balance <u>E</u>ating.
    - <u>A</u>void mood-altering drugs.
    - Balance <u>S</u>leep.
    - Get <u>E</u>xercise.
  - Review of Handout 20.3. Emotion Regulation: Food and Your Mood (3 minutes)
    - Keep a food log for 1 week.
  - Review of Handout 20.4. Emotion Regulation: 12 Tips for Better Sleep (5 minutes)
    - Class exercise: Small-group discussion of Handout 20.4
- Lesson summary (3 minutes)
  - Review ABC PLEASE mnemonic by randomly calling on students.
  - Students share plans to incorporate BC PLEASE skills into their lives.
- Homework assignment (2 minutes)
  - Homework 20.5. Emotion Regulation: Practicing with Build Mastery, Cope Ahead, and PLEASE Skills
    - Identify two ways you practiced building mastery.
    - Practice two PLEASE skills.
  - Diary cards

DETAILED LESSON PLAN

Mindfulness Exercise (5 minutes)

Participating: Singing "Take Me Out to the Ball Game" (3 minutes)

Welcome the class and state that today's mindfulness activity will involve participating. Explain:.

> *We are going to sing mindfully today. All of us have different singing abilities and levels of comfort with singing. Today we are going to practice being nonjudgmental of ourselves and others, and participate fully in singing a song. The song we will sing is "Take Me Out to the Ball Game."*

Either write the words to the song up on the board before the lesson begins, or display them on a projector screen. They are as follows:

> Take me out to the ball game,
> Take me out with the crowd;
> Just buy me some peanuts and Cracker Jack,
> I don't care if I never get back.
> Let me root, root, root for the home team,
> If they don't win, it's a shame.
> For it's one, two, three strikes, you're out,
> At the old ball game.

Tell students:

> *Take a brief moment and imagine yourself singing the song with 100% participation, one-mindfully, and without judgment.*

Allow students about 15 seconds to imagine this, and then continue:

> *If you find yourself having judgmental thoughts about the exercise, such as "This is stupid," or judgmental thoughts about yourself, such as "I am terrible at this," just notice the thoughts, let them go, and return to the exercise.*

Remember that as the teacher, you are the role model for 100% participation, so you may want to practice singing this song prior to the class so that you can ensure you are throwing yourself in completely—regardless of what the class does! Now go on:

> *When I say 1, that's the signal to stand up and take a mindful position. When I say 2, that's the signal to take a deep breath. When I say 3, that's the signal to begin singing. We will stop and sit back down when the song is over.*

Now start the practice by counting to 3.

> *1: Stand up. 2: Take a deep breath. 3: Begin singing.*

Describing Observations of the Exercise (2 minutes)

State:

> *This is the kind of activity that moves fast, and if you stopped to have a judgmental thought about yourself, or someone else, or the activity, then you were no longer present in the moment, and the song was just about over. You may have missed the moment. This is what is meant by participating: being fully engaged, throwing yourself completely into what you are doing in the moment.*

Have a couple of students share an observation in the moment. Provide feedback about observations as needed, ensuring that each statement consists of something a student can observe and describe nonjudgmentally (.e.g., I noticed judgments about singing, I noticed a thought about how this was different from last week, I noticed a thought . . . , I noticed the sensation . . . , I noticed my mind wandering to other thoughts. I had lots of thoughts about how this could be helpful to me, I noticed I liked last week's practice better, I noticed I was uncomfortable so had to move . . .).

Homework Review (10 minutes)

Homework 19.6. Emotion Regulation: Practice with Accumulating Positive Experiences (Short- and Long-Term)

SHARING WITH PARTNERS

Have students take out their completed copies of Homework 19.6. Divide the students into dyads, and instruct them:

> Share with your partners the pleasant activities that you engaged in during the week, plus your goals and action steps taken. The partner who is not sharing at the moment is to ask whether the partner experienced any changes in his or her emotions during the week by accumulating more positive experiences or working on long-term goals.

Remind the class that adding pleasant activities and long-term goals helps to change emotions a little bit at a time. Students should not be discouraged if they did not notice any dramatic changes in their emotions over the course of the week.

SHARING WITH THE CLASS

Bring the class back together as a whole to review the long-term goals. Ask:

> Who would like to share a long-term goal with the class?

Follow up by asking what the student's first step in achieving the goal was and whether he or she has taken this first step.

Check in with students to see whether any of them had difficulty engaging in a pleasurable activity each day or completing their first action step. Reinforce students for completing their assignments, and add:

> After the homework review, we are going to move on to the next set of skills. It is important that you don't stop working on your goals just because we are moving on to another skill. I want you to keep working on engaging in daily pleasurable activities, as well as working toward your long-term goals and ensuring that they are in line with your values.

Troubleshoot with any students who did not complete the homework what may have been in their way and how they will complete the homework this week.

Diary Cards

Ask all students to turn in their diary cards and homework sheets to be reviewed. If you are not able to review homework with each student each lesson, then be sure to get to each student over the course of several lessons. Comment on students' use of skills during the week, to reinforce them for completing their diary cards and using skills. Encourage students who have low skill use ratings to practice weekly, and remind them that only with practice will the skills become more helpful and automatic.

Introduction of Main Ideas (2 minutes)

Say:

> *Stressors can lead to vulnerability to negative emotions and emotion mind. Last week we learned the A of ABC PLEASE, and this week we are going to learn the BC PLEASE skills, which give us more ways to decrease our vulnerability.*
>
> *You already know that A stands for Accumulating positive experiences. B is for Building mastery—that is, doing things that make you feel competent and effective. C is for Coping ahead of time with emotional situations by rehearsing a plan.*
>
> *This week we will also learn how to take care of our minds by taking care of our bodies with the PLEASE skills. PLEASE is a mnemonic (memory helper) for the following: treat PhysicaL illness, balance Eating, Avoid mood-altering drugs, balance Sleep, and get Exercise.*

Discussion: Building Mastery and Coping Ahead (15 minutes)

Review of Handout 20.1. Emotion Regulation: Building Mastery and Coping Ahead (5 minutes)

Have students turn to Handout 20.1. Explain:

> *Having confidence or a sense of competence, and being prepared for difficult emotional situations, will decrease your likelihood of experiencing negative emotions and will increase your use of skills in difficult situations. The next two skills will focus on each of these things: building confidence and competence (B), and preparing for difficult emotional situations (C).*

BUILDING MASTERY

Begin by stating:

> *It is important to do things that build a sense of confidence, control, and competence. This is what we call "building mastery."*

Have a student read through the first section in Handout 20.1, "Build Mastery." Then say:

> *There are two types of mastery activities you can engage in. The first type consists of activities that you may not enjoy while you are doing them (compared to pleasurable activities); however, once you have accomplished these tasks, you feel better. For example, you may not enjoy cleaning your room, but when you are done and you walk into a clean room, your emotions are more positive, and you feel better about your room and yourself. What other examples of this type of mastery can you think of?*

Elicit other examples from students: writing papers, athletic team practices, cleaning, organizing a school activity or function, cooking a meal, and so on. Then continue:

The second type of mastery activities consists of activities that leave you feeling effective and in control; they build confidence. Sometimes these activities are the same ones as we just gave examples for. The goal of this skill is to plan at least one activity a day to help build that feeling, to give you a sense of accomplishment. The trick is to plan something that is difficult and still possible. It is not very helpful to do extremely difficult or impossible things or things that are really easy to do. It needs to have an element of achievement. You want to plan for success, not failure. You can gradually increase the difficulty of what you are doing over time.

Ask students what things in their daily lives provide a sense of this sort of mastery. Be sure to highlight:

Mastery does not have to be a large event or reaching a huge goal. Mastery also does not necessarily have to be anything school-related. You can feel a sense of mastery from putting together a great outfit, doing an awesome makeup job, fixing your hair in a way that looks really good, making a tasty meal, solving a puzzle, or getting to the next level on a video game. These things may be difficult and also give you a sense of accomplishment. The key is to increase the level of difficulty gradually over time.

Have students fill in the blank for point 1 of "Build Mastery" on Handout 20.1.

COPING AHEAD (10 MINUTES)

Explain:

Coping ahead of time with a situation that is likely to prompt an intense unpleasant emotion is like rehearsing for a big event. You want to plan ahead so that you can cope effectively with the situation. You also want to plan ahead because some situations may raise your emotions so high that you forget your skills. It is extremely important to ask yourself, "What's the threat? What am I most worried will happen?" This is often what we want to cope ahead for: the threat.

    Athletes practice for a game or an event just the same way you want to practice for a stressful situation. If athletes are unable to get out to practice physically, they practice in their heads, with mental or imaginal rehearsing. It has even been found that in some cases, athletes who practiced in their heads by using imagery performed just as well as those athletes who got out and physically practiced. Imagining an activity affects many of the same brain regions as actually engaging in the activity does. The key is not only to practice the situation going really well, but, more important, to imagine the situation <u>not</u> going well and then rehearse how you will skillfully respond to it. It is like preparing for the best-case and worst-case scenarios, so that you are ready for anything that occurs. For instance, if Olympic divers focus on how to recover after a poor jump on the board, that may be helpful in regulating emotions for the next dive—but if what they are most fearful of is that the audience or their coaches will negatively judge them or they will judge themselves, then that may be the biggest threat, and the divers will want to prepare for that.

Knowing about imaginal practicing is good news for you since you most likely are not going to practice for a stressful event by engaging in an actual "practice" of the stressful event. Doing it in your head works just as well!

CLASS EXERCISE: SMALL-GROUP ACTIVITY FOR COPING AHEAD

Have students get into groups of two or three. Instruct them:

I want everyone to think of something coming up in your future that you may have difficulty dealing with effectively, and that you may need coping ahead for.

Elicit an example from one of the students. Using this example, read through the "Cope Ahead of Time . . ." section of Handout 20.1, and explain each of the four steps for coping ahead. After each step, have students work for 2–3 minutes in their small groups to talk about their own examples and walk through the steps.

For Step 1 ("Describe a situation that is likely to create negative emotions"), highlight:

This is where multiple skills are coming together. We need to describe the situation nonjudgmentally, and then use the skill of check the facts. Check the facts and describe the situation and emotions involved. Be sure to describe not only what the situation is, but also the different ways that you think you may react when it occurs. Ask yourselves, "What's the threat?"

For Step 2 ("Decide what coping or problem-solving skill you want to use in the situation"), say:

We haven't learned all of the skills yet, but of the ones we have learned, which ones would you use? Write it out.

For Step 3 ("Imagine the situation in your mind as vividly as possible"), say:

It is important to note that you need to imagine yourself in the situation, like divers who imagine the perfect dive that they are going to do. The divers do not imagine watching themselves; the divers see themselves in that situation. Imagine how you would cope effectively with the best and worst possible outcomes and the intense emotions. Talk it through with your group.

For Step 4 ("Rehearse in your mind coping effectively"), ask:

Do you think we need to do any troubleshooting? What might get in the way of your coping effectively in the moment?

Troubleshoot the class example, and have students troubleshoot in small groups. Add:

Let's go back to our example of the divers. They see the water, feel their bodies on the board, and feel how they are going to hold their bodies throughout the dive, while the whole audience watches from the side of the pool. The divers will imagine being really anxious on top of the board and imagine using coping skills to manage that anxiety. The divers will also imagine getting to the top of the board and feeling excited, and using coping skills to manage those emotions as well.

Explain:

It is important to understand that this skill is different from problem solving, which helps to avoid the worst possible outcome. Cope ahead is planning how to be skillful in case the worst possible outcome does occur.

Discussion: Taking Care of Your Body to Take Care of Your Mind (13 minutes)

Review of Handout 20.2. Emotion Regulation: PLEASE Skills (5 minutes)

Have students turn to Handout 20.2. Explain:

These are important skills for <u>everyone</u> to practice—adults, teenagers, parents, and teachers. All people need to be aware of how they are taking care of their bodies and how their bodies affect their minds and their vulnerabilities to negative emotions.

When people think they have been exposed to a virus, they might take supplements such as zinc or vitamin C in order to boost their immune systems and lower their vulnerability to catching the virus. This is how the PLEASE skills are used: They are like emotional vitamins and minerals. Taking care of your body makes you less vulnerable to negative emotions.

Name the PLEASE skills: treat <u>P</u>hysica<u>L</u> illness, balance <u>E</u>ating, <u>A</u>void mood-altering drugs, balance <u>S</u>leep, and get <u>E</u>xercise. As you discuss the skills, encourage students to bring up personal experiences with each one, and to highlight how much better they felt when they attended to each of the skills.

TREAT <u>P</u>HYSICA<u>L</u> ILLNESS

Point out:

Being sick lowers your resistance to negative emotions. It is important when you are sick to take care of your body.

Ask:

How many of you have ever been sick during the week, and there was a big party or game on Saturday that you really wanted to attend? You may have not felt completely better by Saturday, but you went to the event anyway. Did you notice that you may have been a bit more irritated or withdrawn than you usually would have been? This could be because you were more vulnerable to experiencing negative emotions, due to being sick.

BALANCE EATING

Say:

> It is important to try to eat the amounts and kinds of foods that help you feel good—not too much, and not too little. Eating too little can cause negative effects to your body and mind, like feeling weak or getting a headache. Eating too much can also cause negative effects to your body, like feeling sluggish or getting a stomachache.
>
> Have any of you ever noticed that you are more irritable when you are hungry or haven't had anything to eat in a while? This can be due to low blood sugar, and, again, it leaves you vulnerable to experiencing negative emotions. After we finish going over the PLEASE skills, we will go into more detail about steps toward healthier eating.

AVOID MOOD-ALTERING DRUGS

Explain:

> Alcohol and other drugs, like certain foods, can lower resistance to negative emotions. Alcohol is a depressant, which also lowers inhibitions, and lowering inhibitions can lead to quicker emotional reactions. Just think about a fight that occurs at a house party where people have been drinking. In addition, most people don't think of caffeine as a mood-altering drug, but it is. Caffeine will affect your mood by increasing adrenaline, cortisol (a stress hormone), and dopamine (a brain chemical), all of which can give you an energy boost or create an agitated state, but then lead to an energy fall and emotional low. Caffeine also affects your sleep.
>
> If you do drink coffee or caffeinated beverages daily, you may notice that when you don't have any caffeine, you feel more agitated, shaky, or lethargic. Once you have caffeine, those feelings go away. This can be also due to the fact that many people have caffeine addictions, and those symptoms you experience are withdrawal symptoms. Therefore, when you then have the caffeine, you are taking away your withdrawal symptoms.

BALANCE SLEEP

Continue:

> For teenagers, sleep can be a large problem because some teens have a tendency to stay up too late—working on homework, texting, following social media, or talking on the phone. School starts very early in the morning, and not going to bed and getting enough sleep can leave you particularly vulnerable to negative emotions. On the other hand, getting too much sleep can leave you feeling lethargic and depressed. Adolescents need 8–10 hours of sleep a night.
>
> Therefore, it is important to identify the amount of sleep you need to be fully functioning the next day. Then, based on when you have to wake up in the morning, you can determine the time you need to be in bed to sleep at night. This can be really hard, but it is really important to helping manage your emotions. In a few moments, we will also talk in more detail about how to get more sleep.

GET EXERCISE

Explain:

> *Exercise, done consistently, functions as an antidepressant. It also helps to reduce stress and can boost the immune system. Regular exercise can also build mastery. Too much exercise, though, can overexert the body and stress the immune system. Balanced exercise is the key—at least 20 minutes a day of exercise.*

Review of Handout 20.3. Emotion Regulation: Food and Your Mood (3 minutes)

Have students turn to Handout 20.3. Ask a few students to read aloud Steps 1–5. Ask students to consider the following questions:

> *How many of you think you already eat a balanced, healthy diet? How many of you think you need some help in improving your diet?*

Add:

> *Whether you already think you eat a healthy diet or need help, one way either to confirm that your diet is healthy or to improve it is to start a food diary. This means keeping track of everything you eat every day for at least 1 week. Once you have observed what you are eating, you can describe how it fits into a balanced diet and start to consider changes. Then make one or two small changes at a time.*

Ask for volunteers to share any ideas of things that they plan to change in their eating habits.

Review of Handout 20.4. Emotion Regulation: 12 Tips for Better Sleep Hygiene (5 minutes)

CLASS EXERCISE: SMALL-GROUP DISCUSSION OF HANDOUT 20.4

Have students get into groups of three. Then have them turn to Handout 20.4. Reemphasize the importance of the need for teenagers of getting a good night's sleep, and continue:.

> *Read through the 12 tips in your small groups and discuss the tips with which you have difficulty. How could you improve your sleep habits?*

Ask whether there are any questions or ideas that students are now going to try at night. Explain:

> *Because teenagers have such a difficult time with balancing sleep, we are going to spend a few minutes creating a plan for getting to sleep. Think about the things that you just read, and then write down what you plan to change. Some ideas might be not having a caffeinated soda before bed, or turning off your phone so you will not be distracted by text messages, or creating a new schedule for nighttime that will get you to bed earlier.*

Once you have completed your sleep plan, look over the other PLEASE skills (treating physical illness, balancing exercise, and avoiding mood-altering drugs). Discuss with your group how you can or will incorporate these skills into your schedule.

Lesson Summary (3 minutes)

Call on students to review what the letters ABC PLEASE stand for and why they are important. Have students volunteer to share their plans to incorporate the BC PLEASE skills into their lives as the lesson summary today.

Homework Assignment (2 minutes)

Homework 20.5. Emotion Regulation: Practicing with Build Mastery, Cope Ahead, and PLEASE Skills

Review the different parts of Homework 20.5 with the students. Explain:

Planning ahead to use your skills increases the likelihood that you will practice them and complete your homework. Take a minute to decide which two ways you will build mastery, and which two PLEASE skills you will focus on practicing this week. In addition, you may use the example for coping ahead you discussed today, or you can decide on another situation for practicing the skill this week.

Suggest also:

For the PLEASE portion of the homework, in addition to just checking off which PLEASE skills you practiced, you may make a note of what you did specifically for that skill.

Diary Cards

Hand out new diary cards to the students. Highlight that they have now learned the BC PLEASE skills, and that when they practice these skills for their homework, they are to circle the days and rate their skill use for the week on the diary card (along with the other skills that they have been taught).

Finally, do some troubleshooting: Ask students whether they have any questions about the homework or any obstacles to completing it. If so, answer the questions and address the obstacles. Obstacles may include, but are not limited to, the following: Students have no intention of doing the assignment, have too much other homework this week, are likely to forget, or don't understand the assignment. Help students to identify their obstacles, and work with them to make a plan to overcome them. Examples include encouraging a student to write down the assignment and set a reminder in a cell phone or calendar to complete it; discussing why a student has no intention of doing the homework, and working on increasing his or her motivation and the relevance of the assignment (e.g., grades); or clarifying any other points. Troubleshooting should be done each week after the homework is assigned.

Emotion Regulation
The Wave Skill—Mindfulness of Current Emotions

SUMMARY

Mindfulness of current emotions is also known as the "wave" skill. It is similar to the skill of mindfulness of current thoughts (allowing your mind), except that this one focuses on allowing your emotions. Mindfully experiencing an emotion, without pushing it away or holding on to it, is called "riding the emotion wave" by focusing on body sensations. This is the opposite of the distraction skills of ACCEPTS. As important as it is to be able to distract ourselves from our emotions at times, it is also important to be able to sit with and experience our emotions without pushing them away. Finally, this lesson also wraps up the entire Emotion Regulation module by revisiting the model of emotions and mapping each of the emotion regulation skills onto the model.

MAIN POINTS

1. At times it is effective to distract ourselves from our emotions, and at other times it is just as important to be able to sit with our emotions and allow them to come and go.
2. The specific emotion regulation skills are applicable to each component of the model of emotions.

MATERIALS

1. Handouts for this lesson:
    - Handout 21.1. Emotion Regulation: The Wave Skill—Mindfulness of Current Emotions
    - Handout 21.2. Emotion Regulation: Review of Skills for Components of the Emotion Model
    - Homework 21.3. Emotion Regulation: Practicing the Wave Skill
2. Extra student skills binders, with pens or pencils, for students who attend class without materials.

3. Dry-erase markers or chalk for writing on the board.
4. Diary cards: Have new diary cards ready to distribute at the end of class. If possible, highlight "Wave skill."

PREPARATION

1. Draw the original emotion regulation diagram (the model of emotions; see Handout 16.1) on the board.
2. Review the lesson plan as well as handouts in student skills binder.
3. Arrange the desks in the classroom, if possible, in order for students to be able to see each other.

LESSON OVERVIEW AND TIMELINE

- Mindfulness exercise (5 minutes)
  - Observe: Noticing urges (3 minutes)
  - Describing observations of the exercise (2 minutes)
- Homework review (10 minutes)
  - Homework 20.5. Emotion Regulation: Practicing with Build Mastery, Cope Ahead, and PLEASE Skills
    - Sharing with partners
    - Sharing with class
  - Diary cards
- Introduction of main ideas (4 minutes)
  - Experience an emotion without distracting or pushing away.
  - Opposite of distracting with the ACCEPTS skills
- Discussion: Mindfulness of current emotions (16 minutes)
  - Review of Handout 21.1. Emotion Regulation: The Wave Skill—Mindfulness of Current Emotions (11 minutes)
    - Experience your emotions.
    - Practice mindfulness of emotional body sensations.
    - Remember: You are not your emotions.
    - Don't judge your emotions.
  - Class exercise: Eye contact with a partner (5 minutes)
- Module overview (10 minutes)
  - Review of Handout 21.2. Emotion Regulation: Review of Skills for Components of the Emotion Model
    - Identify skills to use for each component of the model of emotions.
- Lesson summary (3 minutes)
  - When to use ACCEPTS versus the wave skill
- Homework assignment (2 minutes)
  - Homework 21.3. Emotion Regulation: Practicing the Wave Skill
    - Practice the wave skill and identify strategies used on homework sheet.
  - Diary cards

DETAILED LESSON PLAN

Mindfulness Exercise (5 minutes)

Observe: Noticing Urges (3 minutes)

Welcome the class and state that today's mindfulness activity will involve observing. Explain:

> *Today for our mindfulness exercise, we are going to notice our urges. Before any action, there is an action urge. We often believe that our behavior happens so quickly that we do not even notice the precipitating urge. For example, you may have the thought that if you have an itch, then you must scratch. Mindfulness, however, teaches us that we can notice thoughts, feelings, and urges to engage in a behavior without having to act upon the urges. So today we are going to practice simply noticing our urges without acting on them. During the practice, you are going to focus on noticing any urges that you may have: urges to open or close your eyes, to shift your position, to scratch an itch, or to do something else. For this practice, we are going to begin with following our breath. Then we will notice any urges that arise, and continue to observe the urges without acting on them. Tolerate the urges, and do not engage in the behaviors. If the urge goes away, you can bring your attention back to your breath and then notice if another urge arises. As with all of our mindfulness exercises, if you notice the urge to blink or swallow, you can allow it, as those urges are natural.*

Continue:

> *When I say 1, that's the signal to sit in the mindful/wide-awake position we are pretty familiar with by now. As usual, this means keeping our feet flat on the floor, sitting up straight, and putting our hands in our laps. For this exercise, we will keep our eyes open with a soft gaze, looking forward and down, but at nothing in particular. If you notice any urges to move, other than blinking or swallowing, notice it without acting on it, and return to your breath. When I say 2, that's the signal to take a deep breath. When I say 3, that's the signal to begin the practice and start observing any urges that arise. I'll say, "Stop," to end.*

Now start the practice by counting to 3.

> *1: Get yourself into the mindful/wide-awake position. 2: Take a deep breath. 3: Begin the practice.*

Have students observe for 2 minutes, and then say, "Stop."

Describing Observations of the Exercise (2 minutes)

Have several students share an observation about any urges, emotions, or sensations that occurred. Provide feedback about observations as needed, ensuring that each statement consists of something a student can observe and describe nonjudgmentally (e.g., I noticed the urge to cross my legs, I noticed the urge to look around, I noticed I had memories about a past event, I noticed a thought about how this was different from last week, I noticed a thought . . . , I noticed the sensation . . . , I noticed my mind wandering to other thoughts. I had lots of thoughts about how this could be helpful to me, I noticed I liked last week's practice better, I noticed I was uncomfortable so had to move . . .).

Homework Review (10 minutes)

Homework 20.5. Emotion Regulation: Practicing with Build Mastery, Cope Ahead, and PLEASE Skills

SHARING WITH PARTNERS

Divide the students into dyads. Explain:

> *Each of you will share with your partner the two ways that you built mastery during the week and an emotional situation with which you coped effectively. Discuss any difficulties you had and any successes you had.*

SHARING WITH THE CLASS

Ask:

> *Let's go through some examples that you all completed. Who can share how they built mastery this week?*

Provide corrective feedback as needed, and reinforce students for doing homework and participating. Then ask:

> *Who practiced coping ahead this week?*

Again, provide corrective feedback as needed, and reinforce students for participating. Finally, review the PLEASE skills with the class by talking through one skill at a time and asking for examples from the class.

Diary Cards

Ask all students to turn in their diary cards and homework sheets to be reviewed. If you are not able to review homework with each student each lesson, then be sure to get to each student over the course of several lessons. Comment on the amount of skills use you see marked on the diary cards for students.

Introduction of Main Ideas (4 minutes)

Explain:

> *Today we will learn how to allow ourselves to experience emotions like a wave by being mindful of how they begin, build to a peak, and then go down—without trying to control them.*

Ask:

How many of you allow yourself to feel all of your emotions all of the time?

Elicit responses, and then go on:

In the Distress Tolerance module, we learned the importance of using our ACCEPTS skills to distract ourselves from painful emotions. If we are supposed to distract ourselves skillfully, why should we also pay attention to our emotions and let them hang around?

Allow students to generate answers before continuing:

On the other side of the dialectic, it is equally important to be able to sit with and experience emotions without pushing them away. Many times in our lives, we may have been told not to be anxious about something, or someone may have said that even though we are sad, we still have to do something. From this, we may have learned the need to push emotions away through either distraction or avoidance. What we may not have learned is that it is just as important to allow ourselves to be sad or anxious and that we can tolerate those emotions as well. A moderate amount of anxiety can be quite effective in motivating us to complete different tasks; however, we have to be able to tolerate that moderate amount of anxiety. Today's lesson will focus on how to tolerate and experience emotions by focusing on them rather than distracting ourselves.

Add:

Toward the end of the lesson today, we will also return to the diagram of the components of emotions that we used at the beginning of the module. This time, we will take a more thorough approach to viewing it.

Discussion: Mindfulness of Current Emotions (16 minutes)

Review of Handout 21.1. Emotion Regulation:
The Wave Skill—Mindfulness of Current Emotions (11 minutes)

Have students turn to Handout 21.1. State:

Mindfulness of our emotions is important, so that we can both notice and experience an emotion without trying to control it, either by holding on to it and making it last longer or by trying to push it away. Ignoring or suppressing emotions does not make them go away; they just come back later, sometimes more strongly. In other words, we need to practice radically accepting our emotions, just as we practiced radical acceptance of other things when we went through the Distress Tolerance module. "Mindfulness of current emotions" is allowing emotions to occur without trying to push them away or making them stronger.

Ask the class:

Which two mindfulness skills do you think we will want to use if we are going to be mindful of our emotions?

Elicit these answers: observe and describe. Then go on:

Remember what we discussed about suffering and pain when we learned about radical acceptance? Pain is inevitable, but suffering is optional. So mindfulness to current emotions is about learning to allow the pain. We all know that at points in our lives we are going to feel sad, angry, or anxious, and we need to be able to tolerate having those emotions.

Now ask:

If you are going to practice observing and describing your emotions, what will you be observing?

Elicit these answers: thoughts, physical sensations, and urges. Then continue:

We have already learned the distress tolerance skill of mindfulness to current thoughts, which focuses on observing and describing our thoughts, so today we are going to focus on observing our physical sensations and urges. By being able to observe and describe these different components, we can gain distance from our emotions—and, ultimately, this can help us to have an easier time with problem solving. The more we allow ourselves to experience emotions, the more we will also be teaching our brains that emotions are not something to fear. How many of you have ever had thoughts like these cross your mind: "Emotions are for the weak," "I can't stand feeling sad," "I don't do emotions," and so on?

Allow students to answer and provide examples. Then say:

By becoming mindful of your emotions, you can begin challenging some of these myths and allowing yourself to feel.

EXPERIENCE YOUR EMOTIONS

Have a student read the bullet points in the first box in Handout 21.1. Ask:

Have any of you ever experienced an intense emotion, and your first reaction was to push it away and forget about it or distract from it?

Gather answers and examples from students, and then ask:

What happened when you tried to push it away? Was it helpful in the short term? Was it helpful in the long term?

Again, elicit examples. Then explain:

As we learned with the ACCEPTS skills in the Distress Tolerance module, it is useful to distract yourself from your emotions at times. The problem comes in when you distract yourself from your emotions <u>all</u> the time. When you are just about to take a test, and you have just found out that your boyfriend or girlfriend is breaking up with you, then this would be a good time to distract. However, at the end of the day when you get home and nothing is pressing on you for a period of time, it will be important to allow yourself to be sad, embarrassed, angry, or whatever emotion you are experiencing. Again, think of emotions as waves: They come and they go. Just let your emotion flow. By exposing yourself to emotions, you will find that they are not catastrophic and that you can manage and tolerate them. The key here is allowing yourself to experience the emotions and physical sensations without acting on them.

Continue:

What is the hardest part of an emotion to tolerate? For many people, the most uncomfortable parts of the emotion are the physical sensations associated with the emotion—the pit in the bottom of the stomach, the tension in the shoulders, or the heaviness in the chest. Have you ever noticed that when you are trying to get away from an emotion, you are often trying to get away from your thoughts and your body sensations?

PRACTICE MINDFULNESS OF EMOTIONAL BODY SENSATIONS

Ask a student to read the bullet points in the second box in Handout 21.1. Explain:

Practicing mindfulness of your emotional body sensations will allow you to experience an emotion. It is a way of not blocking out or suppressing an emotion by focusing fully on the physical sensation of it. The physical sensation of an emotion is one of the most prominent ways in which we experience emotions.

I am now going to ask you a series of questions. On your handout somewhere, I want you to answer these questions.

Allow students a few moments to write down their answers between questions.

- *When you are anxious, where do you feel it in your body?*
- *When you are sad, where do you feel it in your body?*
- *When you are excited, where do you feel it in your body?*
- *When you are angry, where do you feel it in your body?*

Ask students to share their answers. Then ask:

Do you always like those sensations in your body? Often it can be those physical sensations that make us feel uncomfortable, and we want to avoid those sensations by avoiding our emotions. So if you can learn to experience and tolerate the sensations, you can also learn that you can experience and tolerate your emotions. As a result, you will be more likely to <u>allow</u> an emotion to come in, go up, and then go down like a wave, while not pushing *it away and inadvertently making it last longer or get stronger. Remember, research tells us that emotions only last for a total of about 60–90 seconds. And the reason they seem to last so much longer is because of continual refiring of neurons in our brains. It can be thoughts, images, or behaviors that are causing the refiring of an emotion. So by mindfully focusing all of our attention on the physical sensations and effectively distracting from our thoughts and images, we are also stopping the continual refiring and allowing ourselves to experience the sensations and ride the wave.*

REMEMBER: YOU ARE NOT YOUR EMOTIONS

Ask a student to read the bullet points in the third box in Handout 21.1. Explain:

You do not have to act on every emotion that you experience. Remember that when we learned the components of the model of emotions, we discussed that there is a difference between an emotion action and an emotion action urge. You can have the emotion and tolerate the urge to act on it. You are not your emotions.

DON'T JUDGE YOUR EMOTIONS

Ask a student to read the bullet points in the fourth box in Handout 21.1. Explain:

Accepting your emotions allows you to do something about them. By allowing yourself to accept and experience your emotions, you decrease the likelihood that you will experience emotional suffering. Remember, radical acceptance is a way of decreasing suffering. We don't have to be afraid of experiencing emotions. We can embrace them and recognize that emotions are inevitable, so we must learn to experience them rather than push them away.

CLASS EXERCISE: EYE CONTACT WITH A PARTNER (5 MINUTES)

Have students get into pairs, preferably with someone who is not a close friend. State:

In a moment we are going to practice mindfulness of current emotions. I want each of you to notice the physical sensations that arise within your body, notice any urges to move or look away from the other person, and don't act on the urges. Notice any judgments, and then let them go and bring your attention back to the practice and noticing your emotions (sensations).

Continue:

When I tell you to, I want you to stand up and put about 6–12 inches of space between you and your partner. Then you are to look directly at your partner and hold eye contact with the partner throughout the practice. Often, when we hold eye contact with another person in close proximity to us, a variety of emotions may arise. Remember to observe each emotion as it arises, notice any urges to look away, laugh, smile, etc., and tolerate the urges, without acting on them. Experience the emotion like a wave, going up and then down. Let go of any judgments and accept the emotion. Focus on your body sensations.

Now begin the exercise. Have students maintain the eye contact for 1–2 minutes, and then ask them to sit down when the time is over. Instruct students to take a moment to observe and describe the experience to themselves, and to write this down.

Have a few students share what they noticed. If any students had difficulty with the exercise, go over what they struggled with and what they could practice in order to use this skill in the future. Highlight whether any students comment on noticing an urge to look away in order to avoid some aspects of the emotion (e.g., physical sensations, thoughts, urges). Emphasize that being able to continue making eye contact rather than avoiding it is practicing mindfulness to current emotions.

Module Overview (10 minutes)

Review of Handout 21.2. Emotion Regulation: Review of Skills for Components of the Emotion Model

Have students turn to Handout 21.2. State:

> *This diagram looks similar to Handout 16.1, which we examined at the beginning of this module. Now you can see the specific skills that apply to the components that are part of the emotional experience. Let's go over the model of emotions and review the skills that are most useful for each component. Notice that although many of these are skills you have learned in the Emotion Regulation module, some are skills you learned in the Distress Tolerance module.*

Have students look at Handouts 16.1 and 21.2 side by side. Or draw or post the original diagram on the board, and refer back to it as you read through Handout 21.2. Encourage the class to ask questions about any points that they may be confused about. Emphasize how useful it will be for them in their day-to-day lives to have a firm grasp and understanding of where to apply which skills.

As you go through Handout 21.2, ask students to generate examples of how they would use each skill with each component of the model. Or use the examples listed below. Proceed as follows by drawing each component on the board in the order detailed below:

> *Reduce emotional vulnerability factors by using the PLEASE skills.*

Examples:

> *Focus on making sure you eat three to five nutritional meals per day in order to feel less agitated and emotionally sensitive. Get enough sleep and nutrition the night before a big game or prom, so that you are less emotionally sensitive.*
>
> *Change thoughts about the event by using check the facts and using mindfulness of current thoughts.*

Example:

> *You saw your boyfriend talking to another girl after school, and you thought he was flirting with her. Check the facts to find out what was really going on: She was telling him the homework assignment for a class he missed earlier in the day.*

> *Deal with emotion-generating events ("Prompting Events 1 and 2" in the model) by using ABC skills and problem solving.*

Example:

> *You are really scared and angry, because you failed the last three chemistry tests and you are not sure if you are going to pass. The emotions do fit the facts. Problem solving would be to tell your parents and hire a tutor or get extra help from the teacher or another student.*

> *Reduce body changes and physical sensations and tolerate action urges by using TIP, the wave skill, and other crisis survival strategies.*

Example:

> *Your father just told you he doesn't feel like driving you over to your friend's house after you spent an hour getting ready. You want to scream and throw things across your room. The wave skill would include mindfully focusing on those urges and riding them out like a wave, without distracting from them—just simply and painfully watching them. If you were not able to tolerate those sensations or urges and were in jeopardy of making the situation worse, you can use the TIP skills.*

> *Change your emotional reactions ("Expressions, Actions, Behaviors" in the model) by taking opposite action.*

Example:

> *You just broke up with your girlfriend and you are really sad, so you don't want to go out and do anything. Opposite action would be making plans with friends or family members for the weekend to do something fun.*

> *Put names to emotions ("Emotion Name" in the model) by describing emotions.*

Example:

> *You just found out that your boyfriend was accepted into a summer school program in another state. He will be there for 3 weeks, and you won't be able to see each other. You are not sure how you feel about it. You think it is great that he was accepted, but you also think that he will meet a lot of people there and be too busy to think about you. Maybe you are both happy and scared. You can look at the list of different emotions in Handout 16.2 and figure out which one matches your current thoughts and body sensations.*

Tolerate Consequence of Actions by using distress tolerance skills. Depending on the situation, determine if crisis survival or accepting reality skills are needed.

Example:

You have plans to go to a concert with your friends this weekend and have been planning this for months. Your parents just told you that your aunt is very sick, and the family is going to visit her for the weekend because this may be the last chance to see her and you won't be able to go to the concert. You may need to practice crisis survival skills so that you don't start engaging in behaviors that get you in trouble or make things harder on your parents. And you may need to practice radical acceptance that you won't be able to go to the concert and allow yourself to be sad about that.

Finally, reemphasize:

We all have emotions; they are natural parts of being human. Emotions are hard-wired into our brains. Even if we try to deny or ignore an emotion, our bodies still know that it is there. We cannot prevent having an emotion. Emotions happen for a reason—an emotion has to be triggered—but the automatic thoughts and interpretations that accompany the emotion do not make it a fact. As you can see, when you are having a negative emotion, there are many points at which you can use skills to intervene by stopping or decreasing the emotion once it starts or by stopping the unwanted emotion from even starting in the first place.

Lesson Summary (3 minutes)

After congratulating the class for completing the Emotion Regulation module, ask for a volunteer to review what it means to use the wave skill. Then ask:

When should you distract with the ACCEPTS skills versus be mindful of your emotion with the wave skill?

Elicit responses, or say:

In the moment that you are struggling with the urges to act on your emotion and you are afraid you will make things worse, use the ACCEPTS skills. In small increments, at first, you may start practicing being mindful to lower-level emotions, so you can observe and describe the sensations that accompany an emotion. Sometimes it is safer to allow yourself to experience an emotion when you know you are with a trusted person like a parent or close friend, who will keep you from acting impulsively on your emotion.

Homework Assignment (2 minutes)

Homework 21.3. Emotion Regulation: Practicing the Wave Skill

Instruct students:

> At some time during the week when you have an emotion, follow and complete Homework 21.3 for practicing mindfulness of current emotions, also known as the wave skill. Check off on the homework sheet how you practiced mindfulness of current emotions. The sheet lists several strategies that you can use to practice the wave skill.

Ask a student to read the strategies to the class.

Diary Cards

Hand out the new diary cards to the students. Highlight that they have now learned mindfulness of current emotions or the wave skill, and that when they practice this skill for their homework, they are to circle the days and rate the skill use for the week on the diary card (along with the other skills that they have been taught). Remind students that the Emotion Regulation Test will be given in the next lesson, so they should also be studying all of their emotion regulation skills.

Finally, do some troubleshooting: Ask students whether they have any questions about the homework or any obstacles to completing it. If so, answer the questions and address the obstacles. Obstacles may include, but are not limited to, the following: Students have no intention of doing the assignment, have too much other homework this week, are likely to forget, or don't understand the assignment. Help students to identify their obstacles, and work with them to make a plan to overcome them. Examples include encouraging a student to write down the assignment and set a reminder in a cell phone or calendar to complete it; discussing why a student has no intention of doing the homework, and working on increasing his or her motivation and the relevance of the assignment (e.g., grades); or clarifying any other points. Troubleshooting should be done each week after the homework is assigned.

Emotion Regulation
Emotion Regulation Test

SUMMARY

This lesson includes a mindfulness exercise, homework review, and a brief time to answer questions from the students about the mindfulness and emotion regulation skills. The students will spend the majority of the class time on taking the Emotion Regulation Test. The purpose of the test is for students to demonstrate what they have learned in this module and to assess for any areas of weakness that may need further review.

MATERIALS

1. There are no handouts for this lesson.
2. Emotion Regulation Test (make enough copies for the whole class).
3. Dry-erase markers or chalk for writing on the board as needed.
4. Diary cards: Have new diary cards ready to distribute at the end of class.
5. Extra student skills binders, with pens or pencils, for students who attend class without materials.

PREPARATION

1. Arrange desks as usual for taking exams.
2. Review the Emotion Regulation Test in order to be able to answer any questions students may have.

LESSON OVERVIEW AND TIMELINE

- Mindfulness exercise (5 minutes)
  - Observe/wise mind: Breathing in "Wise," breathing out "Mind" (3 minutes)
  - Describing observations of the exercise (2 minutes)
- Homework review (10 minutes)
  - Homework 21.3. Emotion Regulation: Practicing the Wave Skill
    - Sharing with class
  - Diary cards

- Homework assignment (2 minutes)
  - Diary cards
- Module and test review (5 minutes)
- Administration of test (28 minutes)

DETAILED LESSON PLAN

Mindfulness Exercise (5 minutes)

Observe/Wise Mind: Breathing in "Wise," Breathing out "Mind" (3 minutes)

Welcome the class and introduce the mindfulness exercise.

> *Today, since it is the day for our module exam, we are going to do a mindfulness exercise we have done before to observe our breath and access wise mind. We are going to try to find that still point within us, focusing on the present moment. We are going to breathe the word "Wise" in and the word "Mind" out. So breathing in, say to yourself, "Wise"; breathing out, say, "Mind." Speak slowly in your mind, using the entire breath. Fold your entire attention into each word as you say it. Again, if thoughts come up, notice them and then just let them go, returning to your breathing.*
>
> *When I say 1, that's the signal to sit in the mindful/wide-awake position we know pretty well by now. This means keeping our feet flat on the floor, sitting up straight, and putting our hands in our laps. This time, we will keep our eyes open with a soft gaze, looking forward and down, but at nothing in particular. If you notice any urge to move, other than blinking or swallowing, notice it without acting on it, and return to your breath. When I say 2, that's the signal to take a deep breath. When I say 3, that's the signal to begin the practice. I'll say, "Stop," to end it.*

Now start the practice by counting to 3.

> *1: Get yourself into the mindful/wide-awake position. 2: Take a deep breath. 3: Begin the practice.*

Have students breathe for 2 minutes, and then say, "Stop."

Describing Observations of the Exercise (2 minutes)

Have several students share an observation about accessing wise mind or observing their breath as they breathed the words. Provide feedback about observations as needed, ensuring that each statement consists of something a student can observe and describe nonjudgmentally (e.g., I noticed a sense of centeredness in my body, I noticed I forgot the words, I noticed the urge to cross my legs, I noticed the urge to look around, I noticed I had memories about a past event, I noticed a thought about how this was different from last week, I noticed a thought . . . , I noticed the sensation . . . , I noticed my mind wandering to other thoughts. I had lots of thoughts about how this could be helpful to me, I noticed I liked last week's practice better, I noticed I was uncomfortable so had to move . . .).

Homework Review (10 minutes)

Homework 21.3. Emotion Regulation: Practicing the Wave Skill

SHARING WITH THE CLASS

Have the students take out their completed copies of Homework 21.3. Review the homework with the class as a whole by first asking for volunteers who completed the homework. Ask these students:

> *Please share the emotion you were experiencing and what strategies you used to practice mindfulness of current emotions. What was your experience in riding the wave of your emotion?*

As students share the strategies used, involve other students by asking who used similar strategies and allowing them to share as well. Then check with other students who completed the homework and used different strategies. End the review by highlighting:

> *As we learned last week and you practiced last week, there are several different strategies you can use to practice the wave skill. The ultimate goal is to allow yourself to experience an emotion without either pushing it away or acting on it.*

Follow up with any students did not complete the homework and briefly discuss what interfered with homework completion.

Diary Cards

Ask all students to turn in their diary cards and homework sheets to be reviewed. If you are not able to review homework with each student each lesson, then be sure to get to each student over the course of several lessons. Comment on the amounts of skills use you see marked on the diary cards for students. Encourage students who have low skills use to practice weekly, and remind them that only with practice will the skills become more helpful and automatic.

Homework Assignment (2 minutes)

Distribute new diary cards to the students. State:

> *You have now learned all of the core mindfulness, distress tolerance, and emotion regulation skills. Circle the skills you practiced on the diary card this week.*

Module and Test Review (5 minutes)

Answer students' questions about the skills presented in the Emotion Regulation module (and remind them that the test will also include a few questions about the Mindfulness module). Remind them that the next two lessons return to reviewing the core mindfulness skills.

Administration of Test (28 minutes)

Administer the Emotion Regulation Test.

Mindfulness
Wise Mind Review

SUMMARY

Mindfulness skills are central to other skills, which is why "refresher" lessons on these skills are interspersed with the other modules in DBT STEPS-A. Today's lesson focuses on leading the class through a wise mind practice and then generating both small- and large-group discussions about the importance and use of wise mind. Furthermore, students will have one final opportunity to generate and discuss difficult situations that they may be experiencing in reasonable or emotion mind and solutions for accessing wise mind.

MAIN POINTS

1. Mindfulness is learning to be in control of our own minds.
2. There are three states of mind: reasonable mind, emotion mind, and wise mind.
3. Mindfulness skills require regular practice.

MATERIALS

1. Handouts for this lesson:
   - Handout 3.3. Mindfulness: Practicing Wise Mind
   - Homework 23.1. Mindfulness: Getting into Wise Mind
2. Extra student skills binders, with pens or pencils, for students who attend class without materials.
3. Dry-erase markers or chalk for writing on the board.
4. Three to four tennis balls (or balls of a similar type) for the mindfulness exercise. If the class has more than 14 students, you may want to form two groups; in this case, you will need six to eight balls.
5. Diary cards: Have new diary cards ready to distribute at the end of class.

PREPARATION

1. Review the lesson plan as well as handouts in student skills binder. In addition, review teaching points in Lessons 3 and 13 on mindfulness and wise mind.
2. Make enough copies of Figure L23.1 to hand out to small groups of students.
3. Arrange the desks in the classroom, if possible, in order for students to be able to see each other.

LESSON OVERVIEW AND TIMELINE

- Mindfulness exercise (7 minutes)
  - Participating: Group juggling (5 minutes)
  - Describing observations of the exercise (2 minutes)
- Test review (10 minutes)
- Introduction of main ideas (3 minutes)
- Discussion: Wise mind (25 minutes)
  - Review of the three states of mind (3 minutes)
    - Class exercise: Is this wise mind? (5 minutes)
    - Class exercise: Small-group discussions and presentations (17 minutes)
- Lesson summary (2 minutes)
- Homework assignment (3 minutes)
  - Handout 3.4. Mindfulness: Practicing Wise Mind
  - Homework 23.1. Mindfulness: Getting into Wise Mind
  - Diary cards

DETAILED LESSON PLAN

Mindfulness Exercise (7 minutes)

Participating: Group Juggling (5 minutes)

Welcome the class and state that today's mindfulness exercise will involve participating. Explain:

> Today we are going to do group juggling as a form of participating. This is how this exercise will work: I will say a person's name, and throw the ball to him or her. That person will pick another student (who does not have to be the student next to him or her), say that student's name, and throw the ball to him or her. That person will pick another student, say his or her name, and then throw the ball. We will not throw the ball to someone who has already had it thrown to him or her. Once everyone has been thrown the ball, we will go through the process again: Each person will throw to the same person as before, saying that person's name before throwing the ball. But this time I will add a second ball, and on the next round I will add a third. If someone drops the ball, anyone else can pick up the ball and start again by throwing the ball to the next person.

If you find yourself having judgmental thoughts about this exercise, such as "This is stupid," or judgmental thoughts about yourself, such as "I am terrible at this," notice the thoughts, let them go, and return to the activity.

If there are more than 14 students in your class, divide the class into two groups and run the practice simultaneously in both groups. For this exercise, as the teacher you will not participate if there is more than one group. Instead, you will mindfully observe so that you can add a second ball to both groups after one rotation and a third ball after another rotation. Continue:

First, let's go around the circle and all say our names, just to be sure that we all know each other by now.

Once all group members have introduced themselves, explain:

When I say 1, that's the signal to stand up and quietly move into a circle [or two circles, depending on the number of students]. I will let you take your places before saying 2. When I say 2, that's the signal to take a deep breath. When I say 3, that's the signal to begin the group juggling. I'll say, "Stop," to end it.

Now start the practice by counting to 3.

1: Get yourself quietly into a circle. 2: Take a deep breath. 3: Begin juggling.

After the ball has gone to each person in the group one time, then add a second ball after the first ball has been thrown to a few people in the second round. Then add a third ball and a fourth ball at appropriate intervals as well. Stop the exercise after 2 minutes.

Describing Observations of the Exercise (2 minutes)

Have a couple of students share an observation in the moment. Provide feedback about observations as needed, ensuring that each statement consists of something a student can observe and describe nonjudgmentally (e.g., I noticed judgments about my throwing or catching, I noticed a thought about how this was different from last week, I noticed a thought . . . , I noticed the sensation . . . , I noticed my mind wandering to other thoughts. I had lots of thoughts about how this could be helpful to me, I noticed I liked last week's practice better, I noticed I was uncomfortable so had to move . . .).

Test Review (10 minutes)

Return the graded Emotion Regulation Tests to students. Review any commonly missed questions and clarify the answers through group discussion. Repeat this process for any additional questions students have.

Introduction of Main Ideas (3 minutes)

State:

> *Mindfulness is learning to be in control of our own minds, instead of letting our minds be in control of us. It is about putting our minds where we want them to be.*

Ask students to provide their own explanations of mindfulness. The goal is to generate answers such as these: being present in the moment; paying attention on purpose, controlling where we focus our minds, and being aware of what we are experiencing right now. Then ask:

> *Please share examples of when and how you have practiced mindfulness since the DBT STEPS-A curriculum began. How have these examples been different from how you were doing things in the past?*

Discussion: Wise Mind (25 minutes)

Review of the Three States of Mind (3 minutes)

Ask students to name the three states of mind (reasonable mind, emotion mind, and wise mind). Draw the circle diagram of these three states on the board. Then ask:

> *Who can define each state of mind and the differences between the three states?*

Elicit students' responses, and elaborate on these as necessary:

> *Reasonable mind is cool, rational, logical, calculated, and task-focused. Emotion mind is when your emotions are in control—when they influence and control your thinking, behavior, and urges to do or say things. Facts and logic are not important, and there is no balance of reason to your emotions. Wise mind is intuitive; it's a balance of emotion and reason. Wise mind is the part of each person that knows and experiences truth. It is almost always quiet. It is where a person knows something in a centered way.*

CLASS EXERCISE: IS THIS WISE MIND? (5 MINUTES)

Students should clear their desks. State:

> *It is important to practice mindfulness every day. It will work best if you find a mindfulness exercise that fits for you. Today we are going to briefly practice another wise mind exercise for about 3 minutes.*

If you think 3 minutes will be too long for many of your students, then begin with 2 minutes. If you think your students can practice for longer periods of time, then increase the time to 4 or 5 minutes. Or say:

When you practice at home, you may choose to begin with practicing for 3 minutes, but ideally you will want to build up to longer stretches of time. It is important to know that it is more effective to sit every day for 3–5 minutes than to sit once per week for 30 minutes.

Now continue:

In previous lessons, we have practiced breathing in the word "Wise" and breathing out the word "Mind." Today we are going to practice asking wise mind a question and waiting for the answer. This exercise is item 4 on Handout 3.4. Practicing Wise Mind. When you breathe in, you will ask yourself, "Is this [action, thought, behavior, plan, etc.] wise mind?" When you exhale, you will listen for the answer that comes from within yourself. Don't force the answer; listen for it. With each inhale, ask the same question and listen for the answer. If no answer comes today, then try again another time, until your answer does come from your wise mind. For example, when I go out to dinner tonight, just before I order my meal, I might ask myself, "Is my dinner choice a wise mind decision?" and then I would wait for the answer before I order. Any questions?

Go on:

When I say 1, that's the signal to sit in the mindful/wide-awake position we are familiar with by now. This means keeping our feet flat on the floor, sitting up straight, and putting our hands in our laps. For this exercise, we will keep our eyes open with a soft gaze, looking forward and down, but at nothing in particular. If you notice any urges to move, other than blinking or swallowing, notice each urge without acting on it, and return to your breath. When I say 2, that's the signal to take a deep breath. When I say 3, that's the signal to begin the practice. After 3 minutes, I'll say, "Stop," to end the practice.

Now start the practice by counting to 3.

1: Get yourself into the mindful/wide-awake position. 2: Take a deep breath. 3: Begin the practice.

Have students breathe for 3 minutes, and then say, "Stop." Then ask students to share their observations of this practice:

Which students heard a wise mind answer to their question? Please share.

Let these students respond, and then ask:

Who did not hear any answer? Will you continue to practice this until you do?

CLASS EXERCISE: SMALL-GROUP DISCUSSIONS AND PRESENTATIONS (17 MINUTES)

Divide the students into four or five groups, depending on class size (approximately five people per group for large classes). Each group will work through a set of discussion questions listed in Figure L23.1.

Then the members of each group should work together to create a scenario for the last item in Figure L23.1 and generate solutions to accessing wise mind. After 10 minutes, each group will present its scenario and solutions to the class. Allow other groups to provide feedback and additional suggestions.

As time allows, continue the large-group discussion with the first six questions on the list. Answers are provided for questions 1 and 3 only because those two questions have specific answers.

Lesson Summary (2 minutes)

Repeat that mindfulness is being aware of the present moment and putting our minds where we want them to be. Then ask:

How do you know for yourself when you are in emotion mind? How will you get yourself to reasonable mind or wise mind?

- Does everyone have a wise mind?

  Answer: Yes, sometimes it takes practice finding and listening to your Wise Mind.

- What practice exercises are helpful to you in reaching wise mind?

- Do you always want to be in wise mind?

  Answer: No, you don't always have to be in Wise Mind; sometimes it is helpful to be in reasonable mind, especially when we are working on something that needs a lot of focus and logic. Sometimes, you want to experience your emotions and enjoy them. The key is to not live in the extremes of Emotion Mind or Reasonable Mind.

- What are your biggest struggles in finding wise mind?

- When do you think it is the most difficult to access wise mind?

- What do you think would help you to access wise mind?

- Create a scenario of when it might be really hard to notice that you are in emotion mind or reasonable mind and what you would do to get to wise mind. Describe what both reasonable mind and emotion mind would look like. What strategies did you use to access wise mind? What would wise mind look like?

FIGURE L.23.1. Questions for small groups.

Homework Assignment (3 minutes)

Handout 3.4. Mindfulness: Practicing Wise Mind
Homework 23.1. Mindfulness: Getting into Wise Mind

Instruct students:

> *For the next week, you are to do any of the other practice exercises from Handout 3.4 for homework at least three times during the week, for 3–5 minutes each time. You are to check off the box next to the exercise each time you complete a practice. Furthermore, please answer the questions in Homework 23.1 about one situation in which you experienced emotion mind, one in which you experienced reasonable mind, and one in which you experienced wise mind.*

Diary Cards

Distribute the new diary cards to the students. Remind them that they now know all of the mindfulness, distress tolerance, and emotion regulation skills. Instruct them to circle the days and rate their use of these skills for the week on the diary card.

Finally, do some troubleshooting: Ask students whether they have any questions about the homework or any obstacles to completing it. If so, answer the questions and address the obstacles. Obstacles may include, but are not limited to, the following: Students have no intention of doing the assignment, have too much other homework this week, are likely to forget, or don't understand the assignment. Help students to identify their obstacles, and work with them to make a plan to overcome them. Examples include encouraging a student to write down the assignment and set a reminder in a cell phone or calendar to complete it; discussing why a student has no intention of doing the homework, and working on increasing his or her motivation and the relevance of the assignment (e.g., grades); or clarifying any other points. Troubleshooting should be done each week after the homework is assigned.

Mindfulness

"What" and "How" Skills Review

SUMMARY

This lesson focuses on briefly reviewing the "what" and "how" skills. Specifically, it includes a review of the different types of judgments (discriminant and evaluative) and a focus on observing and describing. Students will role-play different scenarios, while the rest of the class practices observing and describing what they see nonjudgmentally. This lesson is the last time the class reviews the mindfulness materials.

MAIN POINTS

1. Mindfulness skills are divided into the "what" and "how" skills.
2. The "what" skills are observing, describing, and participating.
3. The "how" skills are nonjudgmentally, one-mindfully, and effectively.

MATERIALS

1. Handouts for this lesson:
   • Homework 24.1. Mindfulness: Observing, Describing, Participating Checklist
   • Homework 24.2. Mindfulness: Nonjudgmentalness, One-Mindfulness, Effectiveness Checklist
2. Extra student skills binders, with pens or pencils, for students who attend class without materials.
3. Dry-erase markers or chalk for writing on the board.
4. Diary cards: Have new diary cards ready to distribute at the end of class.
5. A scented candle, preferably with a strong scent (e.g., evergreen or cinnamon), for the

mindfulness exercise. If necessary because of open-flame restrictions, substitute a strong air freshener.

6. Class exercise scenarios, each written on an individual sheet of paper, to be distributed to dyads during lesson for role plays.

PREPARATION

1. Review the lesson plan as well as handouts in student skills binder. In addition, review teaching points in Lessons 4, 5, and 14 on the "what" and "how" skills.

2. Arrange desks in the classroom, if possible, in order for students to be able to see each other.

LESSON OVERVIEW AND TIMELINE

- Mindfulness exercise (5 minutes)
  - Observing: Scent (3 minutes)
  - Describing observations of the exercise (2 minutes)
- Homework review (10 minutes)
  - Handout 3.4. Mindfulness: Practicing Wise Mind
  - Homework 23.1. Mindfulness: Getting into Wise Mind
    - Sharing with class
  - Diary cards
- Introduction of main ideas (5 minutes)
  - Review "What" and "How" skills
- Discussion: Nonjudgmental stance (5 minutes)
  - Evaluative judgments
  - Discriminant/differentiating judgments
- Class exercise: Dyadic role-play scenarios (20 minutes)
  - Practicing observing and describing nonjudgmentally
- Lesson summary (3 minutes)
  - Purpose of the "What" and "How" skills
    - To be able to observe and describe which state of mind we are in, especially if we are in emotion mind.
    - To increase our ability to be mindful of the moment.
    - To keep us actively engaged in the present moment.
    - To help us stay focused on our long-term goals.
- Homework assignment (2 minutes)
  - Homework 24.1. Mindfulness: Observing, Describing, Participating Checklist
    - Practice three "What" skills.
  - Homework 24.2. Mindfulness: Nonjudgmentalness, One-Mindfulness, Effectiveness Checklist
    - Practice three "How" skills.
  - Diary cards

DETAILED LESSON PLAN

Mindfulness Exercise (5 minutes)

Observing: Scent (3 minutes)

Have the scented candle lit (or use the air freshener if it is not possible to light a candle in the classroom because of open-flame restrictions) before the students arrive. Welcome the class and state that today's mindfulness activity will involve observing. Explain:

> *Today we are going to do an observing exercise where we focus on our sense of smell. We are going to let go of any distractions and nonjudgmentally observe the smell of this scented candle [or air freshener]. We are going to just notice the emotions, thoughts, and sensations that arise. If you find yourself having judgments, either positive or negative, about the scent, just notice each thought as a judgment, let it go, and bring your attention back to the scent.*

Continue:

> *When I say 1, that's the signal to sit in the mindful/wide-awake position we know quite well by now. This means keeping our feet flat on the floor, sitting up straight, and putting our hands in our laps. For this exercise, we will keep our eyes open with a soft gaze, looking forward and down, but at nothing in particular. If you notice any urges to move, other than blinking or swallowing, notice it without acting on it, and return to your breath. When I say 2, that's the signal to take a deep breath. When I say 3, that's the signal to begin the practice and start observing the scent of the candle. I'll say, "Stop," to end the practice.*

Now start the practice by counting to 3.

> *1: Get yourself into the mindful/wide-awake position. 2: Take a deep breath. 3: Begin the practice.*

Have students smell the candle (or air freshener) for 2 minutes, and then say, "Stop."

Describing Observations of the Exercise (2 minutes)

Have several students share an observation about the scent of the candle (or air freshener), or about the thoughts, emotions, or sensations that they had. Provide feedback about observations as needed, ensuring that each statement consists of something a student can observe and describe nonjudgmentally (e.g., I noticed thoughts about a campfire come up, I noticed I had memories about a past event, I noticed a thought about how this was different from last week, I noticed a thought . . . , I noticed the sensation . . . , I noticed my mind wandering to other thoughts. I had lots of thoughts about how this could be helpful to me, I noticed I liked last week's practice better, I noticed I was uncomfortable so had to move . . .).

Homework Review (10 minutes)

Handout 3.4. Mindfulness: Practicing Wise Mind
Homework 23.1. Mindfulness: Getting into Wise Mind

SHARING WITH THE CLASS

Have students take out their copies of Handout 3.4 and Homework 23.1. State:

> *Wise mind is the synthesis of reason mind and emotion mind.*

Go around the class and ask several students to share with the class what they practiced for wise mind from Handout 3.4. As students share their practice exercises, ask whether other students practiced the same exercise. If so, were their experiences similar or different? Be sure to elicit a variety of different exercises from students who share their homework. In addition, ask some students to share their examples of reasonable mind, emotion mind, and wise mind from Homework 23.1.

After a student has shared his or her mindfulness practice, inquire about any observations that the student may have noticed while practicing or any changes in his or her life during the week related to having been in wise mind.

Troubleshoot with any students who did not complete the homework what may have been in their way and how they will complete the homework this week.

Diary Cards

Ask all students to turn in their diary cards and homework sheets to be reviewed. If you are not able to review homework with each student each lesson, then be sure to get to each student over the course of several lessons. Comment on the amounts of skills use you see marked on the diary cards for students. Encourage students who have low skill use to practice more, and remind them that only with practice will the skills become more helpful and automatic.

Introduction of Main Ideas (5 minutes)

State:

> *Today's lesson is going to be all about the "what" and "how" skills. For the final time in this curriculum, we will review these skills.*

Ask a student volunteer to name the three "what" skills (what to do to be in wise mind) and the three "how" skills (how to do the "what" skills). Write the words on the board as they are listed:

What	How
Observe	*Nonjudgmentally*
Describe	*One-mindfully*
Participate	*Effectively*

Call on different students to describe each of the six skills. Allow students to assist one another if the main points from Lessons 4 and 5 (Handouts 4.1 and 5.1) are not covered. Review in more detail any of the "what" and "how" skills that students may not understand.

Discussion: Nonjudgmental Stance (5 minutes)

Explain:

> Today we are going to focus on practicing the skills of observing, describing, and participating nonjudgmentally.

Ask the class: *What are the two types of judgments that can be made? This is an important distinction that we want to review.*

Elicit from students that the two types are evaluative or evaluating judgments and discriminant or discriminating/differentiating judgments.

Evaluative Judgments

Remind students of the points below if not generated:

> Judgments as evaluations are based on opinions, ideas, and values, and are not based on fact or reality. Often these judgments describe things as "good or bad," "valuable or not valuable," "right or wrong." Evaluative judgments can often be considered a shorthand way of describing something. For example, we can label a piece of fruit "bad" as a way of explaining that it is inedible, brown, and full of bugs.

Discriminant/Differentiating Judgments

Continue:

> Discriminant/differentiating judgments are based on the facts of reality. They determine whether or not two or more things are the same or different, or whether or not something meets a predetermined set of standards. For example, a judge discriminates by stating whether something is within the boundaries of the law or against the law. A teacher discriminates or judges whether an answer on a test is correct or incorrect. This is not a judgment of "good or bad"; it is simply a statement determining whether or not something fits within certain predetermined parameters. Discrimination is based on facts and essential to life. We do not want to get rid of discriminating judgments. Remember we also discussed in Lesson 5 that discriminant judgments are based on a set of established standards, such as laws. This should not be confused with judging people as good versus bad or discrimination against others based on race, gender, age, or sexual orientation.

Now state:

The goal of taking a nonjudgmental stance is to decrease the number of evaluative judgments we make. We want to get rid of the judgmental thoughts that are based on our perceptions or opinions, rather than on facts in reality. For example, I hate olives. I think they are bad. "Bad" is my evaluative judgment. To others, olives are great. Rather than describe them as "bad" or "great," we want to describe that they are "soft or firm," "black, green, or purple," "salty," and so on.

Class Exercise: Dyadic Role-Play Scenarios (20 minutes)

Explain to students:

You are going to split up into pairs. I am going to give each pair a scenario to role-play for the class. While the students in each pair are role-playing their scenario, the rest of you are going to practice observing and describing what you see nonjudgmentally by writing down what you see. Once all the scenarios have been acted and you have all written down your observations after each scenario, we will discuss them as a class.

Now ask students to pair off. Once they have done so, assign each dyad one of the scenarios listed below. Depending on the size of the class, some dyads may need to be assigned the same scenario, or you can develop additional scenarios. Each dyad will act out a scenario. The remaining students will then practice writing down and describing nonjudgmentally what they observe.

Once students write down their observations after each scenario, the class will begin discussing what they observed as a group. For example, a student may state, "I observed that Billy was really angry at Andy." Ask this student, "How do you know Billy was angry? What did you observe?" Guide students in making observations such as "His hands were clenched," "His voice was raised," "His face was tense," or "His eyes were staring directly at Andy."

Discuss how these actions together may be interpreted as anger, and that, as with all interpretations, we have the possibility of being wrong; this possibility intensifies the need to check the facts in any situation. Furthermore, be sure to highlight that we also cannot observe a person's intent (e.g., "He was trying to push my buttons," "She is trying to make me feel guilty," "He is just acting like he does not know what I am talking about").

Use the number of students in the class to determine how much time will be allowed for acting and discussing each scenario. The scenarios are as follows; again, you may develop additional scenarios as needed.

• There is a big math test tomorrow, and you haven't studied for it at all because you have been so busy lately. You beg your best friend to let you cheat off him or her on the test, because if you fail, your parents will punish you and you won't be able to go to your best friend's birthday party next week.

• You just arrived home from school, and you are so excited to tell your parents about the A you earned on your biology test. Your parents are really proud of you.

- You just arrived home from school, and you are so excited to tell your parents about the B you earned on the biology test. Your parents are disappointed that you didn't earn a better grade.

- You and your friend Marisa have both been talking about trying to be skinny and restricting what you eat. When you start telling your friend that you think you ate too much today, she says she thinks it is unhealthy for you to be supporting each other in unhealthy behaviors, and she wants your conversations to focus on recovery and healthy eating.

- You and your partner have been dating for 2 months, and you really want to move beyond kissing. You start telling your partner why becoming more sexually active with each other will make your relationship so much better. Your partner is resistant and scared you will break up.

- Your teacher asks you to stay after class to discuss your grades and tells you that you will never get into a good college if you don't get your act together and start studying. You get angry at the teacher and say that you don't care what he or she thinks about you.

- Your teacher asks you to stay after class to discuss your grades and tells you that he or she is afraid you might fail the class if you don't start turning in your assignments. The teacher is trying to be supportive and help you problem-solve. You get embarrassed and worried that you are going to fail.

- You are hanging out at your boyfriend's or girlfriend's house, and he or she is watching a sports game on TV. You don't care about the game, and you are trying to have a conversation about what happened at school with your friends on Friday. Your boyfriend or girlfriend is ignoring you, and you think it means that he or she doesn't really like you.

- You hear that another person has been flirting with your boyfriend or girlfriend, and you are really angry. You confront this person. The other person reacts in an angry and defensive manner and says that you are wrong because they were only studying together.

- You hear that another person has been flirting with your boyfriend or girlfriend, and you are really angry and hurt. You confront this person. The other person reacts in a surprised and apologetic manner and states that they were only studying for their exam together.

Lesson Summary (3 minutes)

Congratulate students for their excellent role plays and practicing their mindfulness skills. Ask:

What is the purpose of practicing these "what" and "how" skills?

Elicit answers such as these:

- *To be able to observe and describe which state of mind we are in, especially if we are in emotion mind.*
- *To increase our ability to be mindful of the moment.*
- *To keep us actively engaged in the present moment.*
- *To help us stay focused on our long-term goals.*

Homework Assignment (2 minutes)

Homework 24.1. Mindfulness: Observing, Describing, Participating Checklist
Homework 24.2. Mindfulness: Nonjudgmentalness, One-Mindfulness,
Effectiveness Checklist

Explain:

> *You are to practice at least three of the exercises listed on Homework 24.1 and three of the ones listed on Homework 24.2, and report back next week. Consider these questions: Are you able to be more mindful of both your internal experiences and the things around you with more practice? What impact, if any, on your day-to-day experiences has practicing and increasing your ability to be mindful had for you?*

Diary Cards

Distribute new skills diary cards to the students. Remind them that they now know all of the mindfulness, distress tolerance, and emotion regulation skills. Instruct them to circle the days and rate their use of the skills for the week on the diary card.

Finally, do some troubleshooting: Ask students whether they have any questions about the homework or any obstacles to completing it. If so, answer the questions and address the obstacles. Obstacles may include, but are not limited to, the following: Students have no intention of doing the assignment, have too much other homework this week, are likely to forget, or don't understand the assignment. Help students to identify their obstacles, and work with them to make a plan to overcome them. Examples include encouraging a student to write down the assignment and set a reminder in a cell phone or calendar to complete it; discussing why a student has no intention of doing the homework, and working on increasing his or her motivation and the relevance of the assignment (e.g., grades); or clarifying any other points. Troubleshooting should be done each week after the homework is assigned.

Interpersonal Effectiveness
Goals and Overview

SUMMARY

Interpersonal effectiveness emphasizes effective strategies for asking for what one needs, saying no, and coping with interpersonal conflict, as well as maintaining relationships and maintaining self-respect. Today's lesson includes an introduction to the module, an explanation about clarifying priorities and goals of interpersonal interactions, and an examination of worry thoughts or myths that cause problems during interactions with others.

MAIN POINTS

1. It is important to recognize the goals involved in any interpersonal situation.
2. Goals can be divided into three categories: objectives effectiveness, relationship effectiveness, and self-respect effectiveness. It is also important to recognize and challenge the myths and worry thoughts that can interfere with achieving personal goals.

MATERIALS

1. Handouts for this lesson:
   - Handout 25.1. Interpersonal Effectiveness: Overview of Building Interpersonal Effectiveness.
   - Handout 25.2. Interpersonal Effectiveness: What Is Your Goal?
   - Handout 25.3. Interpersonal Effectiveness: What Stops You from Achieving Your Goals?
   - Homework 25.4. Interpersonal Effectiveness: Clarifying Priorities in Interpersonal Situations
2. Extra student skills binders, with pens or pencils, for students who attend class without materials.
3. Dry-erase markers or chalk for writing on the board.
4. Diary cards: Have new diary cards available to distribute at the end of class. If possible, highlight the "Ranking priorities" skill.

PREPARATION

1. Review the lesson plan as well as handouts in student skills binder.
2. Arrange desks in the classroom, if possible, in order for students to be able to see each other.

LESSON OVERVIEW AND TIMELINE

- Mindfulness exercise (5 minutes)
  - Observing: Mindful walking (3 minutes)
  - Describing observations of the exercise (2 minutes)
- Homework review (10 minutes)
  - Homework 24.1. Mindfulness: Observing, Describing, Participating Checklist
  - Homework 24.2. Mindfulness: Nonjudgmentalness, One-Mindfulness, Effectiveness Checklist
    - Sharing with class
  - Diary cards
- Introduction of main ideas (10 minutes)
  - Review of Handout 25.1. Interpersonal Effectiveness: Overview of Building Interpersonal Effectiveness
  - Asserting your rights: DEAR MAN
  - Building and maintaining relationships: GIVE
  - Building and maintaining self-respect: FAST
  - Clarifying priorities
  - Factors to consider
- Discussion: Clarifying priorities and goals (10 minutes)
  - Review of Handout 25.2. Interpersonal Effectiveness: What Is Your Goal? (5 minutes)
    - Relationship effectiveness
    - Objectives effectiveness
    - Self-respect effectiveness
  - Class exercise: Practice exercise from Handout 25.2 (5 minutes)
- Discussion: What stops you from achieving your interpersonal goals? (10 minutes)
  - Review of Handout 25.3. Interpersonal Effectiveness: What Stops You from Achieving Your Goals?
    - Lack of skill
    - Worry thoughts
    - Emotions
    - Can't decide
    - Environment
- Lesson summary (3 minutes)
    - Relationship effectiveness
    - Objectives effectiveness
    - Self-Respect effectiveness
- Homework assignment (2 minutes)

- Homework 25.4. Interpersonal Effectiveness: Clarifying Priorities in Interpersonal Situations
    o Identify prompting event.
    o Rank priorities for interpersonal situations.
- Diary cards

DETAILED LESSON PLAN

Mindfulness Exercise (5 minutes)

Observing: Mindful Walking (3 minutes)

Welcome the class and state that today's mindfulness activity will involve observing. Explain:

> Today for mindfulness, we are going to do something that we all do, yet pay very little attention to the act of doing it. We are going to practice observing by mindfully walking. Most of us walk without being aware. It is only when the ground is icy or we have had a recent injury that we slow down and notice where we are putting our feet or the way that we are moving our legs.
>
> We are all going to stand up and walk mindfully around the desks. I want you to notice the act of walking. Be aware of your body. While breathing in, lift a foot and step forward. While breathing out, let the foot touch the floor. Breathe in and lift the other foot, and so on.
>
> You will want to keep your eyes open, so that you can see where you are going and not lose your balance, but keep a soft gaze and do not look at any one thing in particular. Let your arms hang naturally and loosely by your body. Place your full attention on the act of walking. Notice the sensations in your feet and legs as your muscles work to lift the leg and the impact of your foot upon the floor. If you notice your mind wandering from the exercise, or if you notice judgmental thoughts, just notice them and then gently bring yourself back to the walking.

Continue: *When I say 1, that's the signal to stand up next to your desk and push in any chairs around you.*

If the students are not already sitting in a circle, direct the students during the instructions for the pattern in which they are to join the line. Then go on:

> When I say 2, that's the signal to take a deep breath. When I say 3, that's the signal to begin the practice of observing while walking. I will lead the walk. I'll say, "Stop," to end it.

Now start the practice by counting to 3.

> 1: Stand up and move the chairs in around you. 2: Take a deep breath. 3: Begin mindfully walking.

Stop the exercise after 2 minutes or after the students have had ample time to walk mindfully around the room.

Describing Observations of the Exercise (2 minutes)

After students return to their seats, have a couple of students share an observation in the moment. Provide feedback about observations as needed, ensuring that each statement consists of something a student can observe and describe nonjudgmentally (e.g., I noticed judgments about this exercise, I noticed difficulty with my balance, I noticed a thought about how this was different from last week, I noticed a thought . . . , I noticed the sensation . . . , I noticed my mind wandering to other thoughts. I had lots of thoughts about how this could be helpful to me, I noticed I liked last week's practice better, I noticed I was uncomfortable so had to move . . .).

Homework Review (10 minutes)

Homework 24.1. Mindfulness: Observing, Describing, Participating Checklist
Homework 24.2. Mindfulness: Nonjudgmentalness, One-Mindfulness, Effectiveness Checklist

SHARING WITH THE CLASS

Have students take out their completed copies of Homework 24.1 and Homework 24.2. Remind students:

> *The "what" and "how" skills are the way in which we practice mindfulness and get to wise mind.*

Go around the class and ask several students to share with the class what they practiced for the "what" and "how" skills. As students share their practice exercises, ask whether other students practiced the same exercise. If so, were their experiences similar or different? Be sure to elicit a variety of different practice exercises from students who share their homework.

After a student has shared his or her mindfulness practice, inquire about any observations that he or she may have made while practicing or any changes in his or her life during the week related to having been mindful.

Troubleshoot with any students who did not complete the homework what may have been in their way and how they will complete the homework this week.

Diary Cards

Ask all students to turn in their diary cards and homework sheets to be reviewed. If you are not able to review homework with each student each lesson, then be sure to get to each student over the course of several lessons. Comment on the amount of skills use you see marked on the diary cards for students. Encourage students who have low skill use to practice more, and remind them that only with practice will the skills become more helpful and automatic.

Introduction of Main Ideas (10 minutes)

Review of Handout 25.1. Interpersonal Effectiveness: Overview of Building Interpersonal Effectiveness

Have students turn to Handout 25.1. State:

We all know what it can be like not to be skillful—to ask for something from parents or teachers in a way that almost guarantees they will say no, or telling friends that we don't want to do something with them in a way that hurts their feelings or makes them angry. There can be unpleasant consequences of not being interpersonally skillful.

Ask:

What types of skills do you think we will learn or need to learn in the Interpersonal Effectiveness module?

Allow students to generate a list of areas or types of skills they think they will learn. As they generate ideas, write these ideas on the board and organize them into four columns with the following headings. Examples of each category are also listed below:

- <u>Asserting Your Rights</u>: (e.g., saying no, asking for help with homework, asking for a ride home, asking someone to stop picking on you or someone else);
- <u>Building and Maintaining Relationships</u> (e.g., hanging out with friends at lunch or on the weekend; keeping good relationships with parents, siblings, or other family members);
- <u>Building and Maintaining Self-Respect</u> (e.g., feeling good about yourself, acting in a way you think is right);
- <u>Intensity of How to Ask for Things</u> (e.g., ranging from demanding someone do something for you to hinting at it all the way to not asking at all).

Note that although there is no separate column for "Clarifying Priorities," the students will also eventually learn how to prioritize which areas are most important in any given situation.

Now explain:

Interpersonal skills are a huge part of our lives because relationships are a key aspect of being human. Sometimes there are things that we may want, but we don't know how to ask for them. There may be things that we don't want to do, but we don't know how to say no. What are some situations in your own lives where you have interpersonal difficulties? Do you have a hard time asking for things? Do you have a hard time saying no? Do you sacrifice what you want in order to keep another person happy or not make waves in the relationship?

Over the corresponding column ("Asserting Your Rights") on the board, write DEAR MAN. Say:

We are going to learn a set of skills called DEAR MAN to assist us in asking for things we want and saying no to things we don't want. Who thinks this might be helpful for them?

Elicit responses, and continue:

There also may be times when keeping someone else happy is the most important thing to us, or when ensuring the person still wants to be in a relationship with us after the interaction has ended is our major goal.

Write GIVE over the corresponding column ("Building and Maintaining Relationships") on the board, and explain:

We are also going to learn a set of skills called GIVE to build and maintain relationships.

Go on:

And still at other times, the most important thing is maintaining our own self-respect or feeling good about ourselves after the interaction has ended.

Write FAST over the corresponding column ("Building and Maintaining Self-Respect") on the board, and explain:

FAST skills are the skills we will learn to improve how we feel about ourselves.

Continue:

We will also learn skills that help us clarify which is most important for us. Look at the "Clarifying Priorities" section at the top of Handout 25.1. These skills are important because you need to figure out what you actually want in a situation. Is it most important to get what you want? Is it most important to save the relationship? Is it most important to maintain your own self-respect? Finally, we may also need to learn how to determine the intensity we should be using when asking for things or saying no. Look at the "Factors to Consider" at the bottom of Handout 25.1. All of these things require interpersonal effectiveness skills. Therefore, we are going to begin learning these skills today.

Discussion: Clarifying Priorities and Goals (10 minutes)

Review of Handout 25.2. Interpersonal Effectiveness: What Is Your Goal?

Have students turn to Handout 25.2. State:

Goals can be divided into three categories: "relationship effectiveness," "objectives effectiveness," and "self-respect effectiveness."

As you go over each category, write each of these terms over the corresponding column that was already created on the board. Have a student read the first box in Handout 25.2 to the class, and then clarify:

Relationship effectiveness is for keeping and maintaining healthy relationships while trying to get what you want. This is your goal when you use GIVE skills. These skills are for use when it is important to you how the other person thinks and feels about you after the interaction is over. Do any of you think you could benefit from improving your relationships?

Elicit responses. Then have a student read the second box in Handout 25.2 to the class and clarify:

INSTRUCTOR INFORMATION, LESSON PLANS, AND TESTS

Objectives effectiveness is for getting somebody to do what you want or saying no to someone. This is your goal when you use the set of skills called DEAR MAN skills. They are for when you want a specific result. Do any of you have difficulty asking people for things or saying no to people when a request is made of you?

Again, elicit responses. Then have a student read the third box in Handout 25.2 to the class and clarify:

Self-respect effectiveness is for building and maintaining your self-respect during and after an interaction with someone else. For this, we will learn the set of skills called the FAST skills. They help you to stick to your beliefs and values. Giving up your beliefs for approval, or acting helpless when you are not, can hurt your self-respect. This skill will tie in with the work on identifying values we did during the Emotion Regulation module.

Now continue:

All three categories of effective behavior should be considered in any interpersonal inter- action. You need to decide the order of importance for these three areas in order to determine how much of each skill will be most effective for you. Which type is the most important for your specific situation, and how should you order your priorities? Ordering priorities does not mean that you completely give up one area for another, such as "My relationship with my best friend is most important, so I will do whatever he or she asks." Ordering priorities helps us to identify our goals in each interaction, so that we don't com- pletely give up one for another.

CLASS EXERCISE: PRACTICE EXERCISE FROM HANDOUT 25.2 (5 MINUTES)

Instruct students:

At the bottom of Handout 25.2 is a practice exercise. I want all of you to take a minute and think about an interaction that you will have with someone today. Not every interpersonal interaction involves trying to achieve a goal, so be sure to try to think of one that fits the following criteria.

Think about a situation in which your rights or wishes are not being respected, you want someone to do something or give you something, you want to say no to something, you want to get your point of view taken seriously, you have a conflict with someone, or you want to improve your relationship with someone. It could be meeting up with your friends for lunch and deciding where to go eat, or a conversation about increasing your allowance that you know you will be having with your parents tonight.

You can use the following as an example:

I really want to see the new movie that is opening this weekend. My friend Lexa wants to see a different movie. I need to consider how much I want to see this movie versus mak- ing my friend happy and maintaining that relationship. But maybe I always see the movies that she wants, and now my self-respect has been damaged and I need to balance that with letting her have her way. These are the types of things to consider when making your decisions. Think about what is the most important thing to you: keeping the relationship, getting what you want, or keeping your self-respect. Then rank those lines at the bottom of Handout 25.2 accordingly.

After students have had a minute to fill out the Handout 25.2 practice exercise, ask for volunteers to share their rankings and to explain why they gave those rankings. Highlight that although relationship effectiveness is important, it can't always be a person's highest priority, because always sacrificing personal goals and objectives to maintain relationships, approval, and liking is eventually ineffective. Many times this leads to a buildup of frustrations that may erupt into a fight or ending a relationship completely or to a decrease in the person's own self-respect over time.

Discussion: What Stops You from Achieving Your Interpersonal Goals? (10 minutes)

Review of Handout 25.3. Interpersonal Effectiveness: What Stops You from Achieving Your Goals?

Have students turn to Handout 25.3. Ask:

What do you think gets in the way of your being as interpersonally skilled as you would like to be?

Allow students to generate answers and discuss. Then state:

In general, there are five areas that get in people's way when they try to achieve their goals: lack of skill, worry thoughts, emotions, not being able to decide, and environment. Let's go through each of these on Handout 25.3, and determine whether the things you just discussed fit into these categories.

As you go through each area on the handout, call on students to read the information in the boxes one at a time, and elaborate with the explanations below. Highlight for "lack of skill":

For any of the interpersonal effectiveness skills, the skills need to be overlearned so that they become automatic. This requires practice and feedback. Many people don't learn these skills as they are growing up, so this is why we are learning them now. As with all the skills in this class, these are important for the rest of our lives. Have any of you ever seen an interaction among adults that didn't seem to be an effective style of communication? Do you think those adults could benefit from learning some skills on how to communicate better? We are lucky that we are learning them now.

Highlight for "worry thoughts":

All people have some worries about asking for what they want, standing up for themselves, or saying no. People can also be susceptible to interpersonal myths. One way to counteract these worries is to challenge these myths or worry thoughts logically. There is an additional lesson that focuses on the skill of myth busting, which we will get to later.

Highlight for "emotions":

Sometimes a person can have a skill, but emotions get in the way and inhibit skillful action. An example of this is trying to talk to the person that you have a crush on, or trying to ask your parents to take you to the mall after you just broke up with your girlfriend or boyfriend. Your emotions, such as anxiety and excitement or sadness and anger, are so high that even a simple conversation becomes difficult. Or maybe you feel shame and don't think you deserve to ask for what you want. This is how the skills that we just learned in the Emotion Regulation module can relate to interpersonal effectiveness.

Ask the students to generate additional examples of when emotions could impair their ability to interact effectively with someone.

Highlight for "not being able to decide":

It is common for indecision or ambivalence to get in our way. Sometimes we are just not sure of what we really want. This is also why the mindfulness skills are important, and it helps to understand how to determine our priorities.

Ask the class to generate examples of when being indecisive may interfere with interpersonal communication. What impact might this have on a relationship or self-respect?

Highlight for "environment":

Even the most skilled people cannot always get what they want when other people are too powerful. As teenagers, this is one that you know all too well, with your parents and teachers holding so much power. Or sometimes you just cannot help but being disliked by someone else, and there is nothing that you can do about it. And sometimes the only way to get what you want is to sacrifice your self-respect. Radical acceptance and acting effectively (mindfulness How skill) are important skills when you are faced with this kind of a situation.

Ask for an example of a situation in which a person might need to practice radical acceptance because no matter how interpersonally skilled that person is, the individual might not get what he or she wants. Or use this example:

Let's say you came to school late on a game day, and the rules say you have to be on time in order to play in the game. You want to ask the coach and principal to let you play because your mother scheduled this doctor's appointment for you without your knowing about it and said you couldn't miss it. This is a situation where the coach and principal may not be willing to bend the rules, regardless of how skillfully you ask.

Next, take a few minutes to let the students review this handout and think about how it applies to them. State:

Now you are going to spend the next few minutes working independently. Review the five points on Handout 25.3, and decide which area or areas you struggle with the most. Is it that you don't know what to do? Do you worry too much? Do your emotions get in the way? Do you have a hard time making decisions? Or does your environment block you from reaching your goals? There may not be any one answer that covers everything, so think about how different things may block your goals, depending on the different situations or relationships in your life.

Finally, once you have decided what stops you from reaching your interpersonal goals, I want you to take a minute to make a wise mind commitment to yourself to work on these areas. Notice if any emotions come up with you and acknowledge them. Allow yourself to sit with wise mind and your wise mind commitment.

Lesson Summary (2 minutes)

Review the three goals of interpersonal effectiveness—objectives effectiveness, relationship effectiveness, and self-respect effectiveness—as well as the importance of clarifying priorities in each interaction.

Homework Assignment (3 minutes)

Homework 25.4. Interpersonal Effectiveness: Clarifying Priorities in Interpersonal Situations

Have students turn to Homework 25.4. Explain:

Your homework will be similar to what we did in class today when determining our priorities: You should do this again on Homework 25.4 with another example. You will describe the prompting event, list your goals for each of the priority areas, and then describe how you prioritized your objectives, relationship, and self-respect.

Diary Cards

Hand out new diary cards to the students. Highlight that they have now learned ranking priorities, and that when they practice this skill for their homework, they are to circle the days and rate the skill use for the week on the diary card (along with the other skills that they have been taught).

Finally, do some troubleshooting: Ask students whether they have any questions about the homework or any obstacles to completing it. If so, answer the questions and address the obstacles. Obstacles may include, but are not limited to, the following: Students have no intention of doing the assignment, have too much other homework this week, are likely to forget, or don't understand the assignment. Help students to identify their obstacles, and work with them to make a plan to overcome them. Examples include encouraging a student to write down the assignment and set a reminder in a cell phone or calendar to complete it; discussing why a student has no intention of doing the homework, and working on increasing his or her motivation and the relevance of the assignment (e.g., grades); or clarifying any other points. Troubleshooting should be done each week after the homework is assigned.

Interpersonal Effectiveness
DEAR MAN Skills

SUMMARY

This lesson focuses on the skills for objectives effectiveness. These are called the DEAR MAN skills. Many students struggle with being able to obtain their goals in interpersonal situations due to lack of assertiveness skills in effective communication. The DEAR MAN skills are the basic assertiveness skills that individuals need in order to ask effectively for things they want and to say no to things they do not want. Using skills does not guarantee that people will be successful; it only increases the likelihood that they will be successful. This lesson uses the DEAR MAN cards teaching aid to assist students in remembering the mnemonic.

MAIN POINTS

1. If the goal of an interaction is objectives effectiveness, then the DEAR MAN skills should be used.
2. The DEAR skills involve "what to do" (Describe, Express, Assert, Reinforce), and the MAN skills involve "how to do it" ([be] Mindful, Appear confident, Negotiate).

MATERIALS

1. Handouts for this lesson:
   - Handout 26.1. Interpersonal Effectiveness: Getting Someone to Do What You Want
   - Handout 26.2. Practice Cards for Learning the DEAR MAN Skills
   - Homework 26.3. Interpersonal Effectiveness: Practicing DEAR MAN Skills
2. Extra student skills binders, with pens or pencils, for students who attend class without materials.
3. Dry-erase markers or chalk for writing on the board.
4. Diary cards: Have new diary cards available to distribute at the end of class. If possible, highlight the "DEAR MAN" skills.

PREPARATION

1. Review the lesson plan as well as handouts in student skills binder.
2. Practice singing "Row, Row, Row Your Boat" with 100% participation, including a loud voice and body movements, in order to model for the class.
3. Arrange desks in the classroom, if possible, in order for students to be able to see each other.

LESSON OVERVIEW AND TIMELINE

- Mindfulness exercise (5 minutes)
  - Participating: Singing "Row, Row, Row Your Boat" (3 minutes)
  - Describing observations of the exercise (2 minutes)
- Homework review (10 minutes)
  - Homework 25.4. Interpersonal Effectiveness: Clarifying Priorities in Interpersonal Situations
    - Sharing with class
  - Diary cards
- Introduction of main ideas (8 minutes)
  - Categories for objectives effectiveness
    - Getting others to do what you ask them to do.
    - Making refusals to unwanted requests stick.
    - Resolving interpersonal conflict.
    - Asking for your rights to be respected.
    - Getting your opinion taken seriously.
- Discussion: Objectives effectiveness—DEAR MAN (22 minutes)
  - Review of Handout 26.1. Interpersonal Effectiveness: Getting Someone to Do What You Want (10 minutes)
    - D: Describe
    - E: Express
    - A: Assert
    - R: Reinforce
    - M: (be) Mindful
    - A: Appear confident
    - N: Negotiate
  - Class exercise: Dyadic role plays and presentations (12 minutes)
- Lesson summary (3 minutes)
  - Review mnemonic by randomly calling on students.
- Homework assignment (2 minutes)
  - Homework 26.2. Interpersonal Effectiveness: Practicing DEAR MAN Skills
    - Write a DEAR MAN script and practice.
  - Diary cards

DETAILED LESSON PLAN

Mindfulness Exercise (5 minutes)

Participating: Singing "Row, Row, Row Your Boat" (3 minutes)

Welcome the class and state that today's mindfulness exercise will involve participating. Explain:

> *Today for mindfulness, we are going to sing "Row, Row, Row Your Boat." We are going to sing in rounds, so we will divide ourselves into three groups.*

Divide the students into three groups, so that when they stand and begin the practice, they will know which part they are to sing. Then continue:

> *Group 1 will begin singing the song. As soon as those of you in Group 1 have finished with the first line, "Row, row, row your boat," Group 2 will jump in singing the song from the beginning as Group 1 continues with the song, and then Group 3 will come in after Group 2 has sung the first line. We will sing the song for three rounds. Just as a reminder, here are the words to this song: "Row, row, row your boat, gently down the stream. Merrily, merrily, merrily, merrily, life is but a dream."*
>
> *Remember also that fully participating means throwing yourself in 100%. Let's have fun with this. Add in hand motions, and sing with zest! If you notice judgmental thoughts, just notice them, let them go and then bring yourself back to singing.*

It is important for you to model 100% participation by throwing yourself fully into the activity. (You may want to practice this ahead of time.) Then go on:

> *When I say 1, that's the signal to stand up next to your desk and push in any chairs around you. When I say 2, that's the signal to take a deep breath. When I say 3, that's the signal to begin the practice of fully participating one-mindfully and nonjudgmentally in the singing exercise. Group 1 will begin, and then Groups 2 and 3 will start at the appropriate points. I'll say, "Stop," to end the singing.*

Now start the practice by counting to 3.

> *1: Stand up and move the chairs in around you. 2: Take a deep breath. 3: Begin singing.*

Point to the students in Group 1 to start singing their part. Stop the exercise after 2 minutes.

Describing Observations of the Exercise (2 minutes)

After the third round of the song is finished, ask students to return to their seats, and have a few students share an observation. Provide feedback about observations as needed, ensuring that each statement consists of something a student can observe and describe nonjudgmentally (e.g., I noticed judgments about this exercise, I noticed I was able to participate 100%,

I noticed a thought about how this was different from last week, I noticed a thought . . . , I noticed the sensation . . . , I noticed my mind wandering to other thoughts. I had lots of thoughts about how this could be helpful to me, I noticed I liked last week's practice better, I noticed I was uncomfortable so had to move . . .).

Homework Review (10 minutes)

Homework 25.4. Interpersonal Effectiveness: Clarifying Priorities in Interpersonal Situations

SHARING WITH CLASS

Have students take out their completed copies of Homework 25.4. Ask:

> *Who completed the homework successfully and was able to identify priorities in an interpersonal situation? Who didn't do the homework or had difficulty determining priorities?*

As a method of reviewing last week's lesson, go through two examples of students who had difficulty and two examples of students who did not. As these students share their homework, ask whether other students had similar experiences, in order to normalize both those who completed the homework and those who had difficulty.

As usual, troubleshoot with any students who did not complete the homework what may have been in their way and how they will complete the homework this week.

Diary Cards

Ask all students to turn in their diary cards and homework sheets to be reviewed. If you are not able to review homework with each student each lesson, then be sure to get to each student over the course of several lessons. Comment on the amount of skill use you see marked on the diary cards for students. Encourage students who have low skill use to practice more, and remind them that only with practice will the skills become more helpful and automatic.

Introduction of Main Ideas (8 minutes)

Begin:

> *As a brief review from last class, remember that the first thing that you want to do in an interpersonal situation is to clarify your highest priority or most important goal. What are the three goals of interpersonal effectiveness?*

List them on the board:

- Meeting your objectives
- Maintaining and improving your relationships
- Maintaining and increasing your self-respect

Continue:

> *As we also discussed last week, there are three different sets of skills that you can use, depending on your goals. What are the three skills we will use to meet these goals?*

Write the corresponding skill next to each goal:

- Meeting your objectives: Objectives effectiveness
- Maintaining and improving relationships: Relationship effectiveness
- Maintaining and increasing your self-respect: Self-respect effectiveness

Now explain:

> *Today we are going to focus on learning and practicing the skills for objectives effectiveness. Objectives effectiveness is getting what you want out of an interpersonal situation or saying no to what you don't want. Today we are going to learn the skills to use when your top priority is this type of effectiveness.*

Have students refer back to their completed copies of Homework 25.4. If they did not complete the homework sheet, have them turn to the copies of Handout 25.2 that they filled out during Lesson 25. Instruct the students:

> *Please write down on a piece of scratch paper the objective that you listed when you completed the homework assignment or the objective that you wrote down in class last week. Then put this objective aside and save it for later in the class when you will use it in an exercise. Make sure that this is something you are willing to share with the class, and that it does not involve another student in this class.*

Next, ask:

> *What are some different times when you need to say no or when you need to ask for something that can be difficult? In general, most objectives effectiveness situations fall under five different categories.*

Write the following five categories on the board, and discuss each one as you go through them, using the examples provided below each one.

- *Getting others to do what you ask them to do.*
  - *Asking your parents to extend your curfew.*
  - *Asking a classmate whether you can copy his or her notes for a class since you were absent.*
  - *Asking a classmate for a ride home.*
- *Making your refusals to unwanted requests stick.*
  - *Telling your friends that you are not going to cut class any more with them.*
  - *Telling a friend that you aren't going to loan him or her any more lunch money.*

- *Resolving interpersonal conflict.*
  - ○ *Asking a friend or parent to listen to your side of a situation, and then asking this person to explain his or her side.*
- *Asking for your rights to be respected.*
  - ○ *Asking your locker neighbor not to put his or her backpack directly in front of your locker because it blocks you from being able to access your locker and you don't have time to wait for your neighbor to finish.*
- *Getting your opinion or point of view taken seriously.*
  - ○ *Being confident and direct when you are asking or saying no in any of the examples just given.*

Ask students to generate their own examples of times that they have had to ask for something or say no that has been difficult.

Now ask:

Are there situations in which you have no problem asking for things and other situations where you really struggle? Or are there some people you have no problem saying no to, and others you struggle with saying no to?

Again, gather examples. These examples may indicate that students already may have some of the skills they need; they just may not be able to use them in all different contexts or environments.

Discussion: Objectives Effectiveness—DEAR MAN (22 minutes)

Review of Handout 26.1. Interpersonal Effectiveness: Getting Someone to Do What You Want (10 minutes)

Have students turn to Handout 26.1. Explain:

DEAR MAN is a mnemonic (memory helper) for the skills to use for getting what you want or saying no. The DEAR stands for what you do, and the MAN stands for how you do it.

Write the mnemonic vertically on the board, filling in the word or words for each letter as you teach that letter. Continue:

We are going to learn and practice a strategy that will help us use our interpersonal effectiveness skills in situations or relationships that are personal to us. This is very important, so we are going to take our time and make sure each one of you is familiar with the strategy before practicing it in front of the group or trying it on your own. We are going to take each step of the strategy (in this case, each letter in DEAR MAN) one at a time and give examples for each different component. Remember, this exercise is to help us with our objectives effectiveness.

Below, three extended examples are provided to illustrate how the DEAR MAN skills are used in three different situations. You may use these examples to teach the DEAR MAN skills, or you may use your own example or a student's example in class. Choose one or two of the three examples to use in order to demonstrate how the skills all come together for one situation.

D: DESCRIBE

The D in DEAR MAN stands for Describe: Describe the current situation (if necessary). Stick to the facts, and avoid judgmental statements.

- *Example 1: You do not like your math teacher, and you are frustrated with the grade he or she gave you on the exam.*
  - *Describe (to the teacher): "My paper says that I got a C– on the test."*
- *Example 2: You are at a party with friends, and they are asking you to do ecstasy. You don't do drugs, but you are afraid they will not like you if you don't.*
  - *Describe (to your friends): "Thanks for offering to share the ecstasy with me."*
- *Example 3: You are at the fair, and your friends are all going on the rollercoaster. You are afraid of rollercoasters.*
  - *Describe (to your friends): "Thanks for asking me to go on the rollercoaster with you."*

E: EXPRESS

The E in DEAR MAN stands for Express: Express your feelings and opinions about the situation. Use "I" statements ("I feel . . . ," "I would like . . . ," etc.). Stay away from "you should."

- *Example 1: Express your feelings about the results of the exam—how you feel inside.*
  - *Express: "I am frustrated with my grade because I studied for 4 days for that test. I looked it over, and I think some of my answers are correct."*
- *Example 2: Express your feelings about not wanting to offend your friends.*
  - *Express: "I really appreciate you inviting me to the party and including me in the activities. I am worried that you will be mad at me."*
- *Example 3: Express your feelings about rollercoasters.*
  - *Express: "Rollercoasters are not any fun for me, and they kind of freak me out."*

A: ASSERT

The first A in DEAR MAN stands for Assert: Assert yourself by asking for what you want or saying no clearly. Be clear and concise.

- *Example 1: Ask your math teacher to go through the test with you.*
  - *Assert: "Would you please go through the problems I got wrong with me, so I can understand why my answers were not correct?"*

- *Example 2: Tell your friends clearly that you do not want to do drugs.*
  - *Assert: "No, thanks, I am not interested in doing any drugs."*
- *Example 3: Tell your friends clearly that you do not want to ride the rollercoaster.*
  - *Assert: "No, thanks, I don't want to go on the rollercoaster."*

R: REINFORCE

The R in DEAR MAN stands for Reinforce: Reinforce or reward the other person(s) ahead of time by explaining the consequences.

- *Example 1: Explain to your teacher why going through the exam with you will be good for you both.*
  - *Reinforce: "I would really appreciate you going through the exam with me, and it will be really helpful to me so I have a better understanding of the material."*
- *Example 2: Explain to your friends that you will still be their friend even if you choose not to do ecstasy.*
  - *Reinforce: "I appreciate your understanding, and I am really glad we can still hang out together."*
- *Example 3: Explain to your friends that you will still be their friend if you do not go on the rollercoaster, and that you can do something for them while you wait.*
  - *Reinforce: "Thanks for wanting me to go on the ride with you and for understanding. I will be happy to hold on to your bags and wait for you guys down here while you ride it."*

M: (BE) MINDFUL

The M in DEAR MAN stands for (be) Mindful: Stay mindful and keep your focus on your objectives. There are a couple of techniques for doing this.

1. *Repeating like a broken record: Keep asking, saying no, or expressing your opinion over and over again. You don't have to come up with a new way of saying it each time. You can continue to repeat the DEAR over and over again.*

2. *Ignoring: If another person attacks, threatens, or tries to change the subject, simply ignore the threats, comments, or attempts to divert you. Has anyone in here ever done any boxing or ever watched boxing? I think of this skill like the "bob and weave" move in boxing. You make your move and "bob" [make a light punching gesture], and then you "weave" your body [move your upper body from side to side after each "punch"] to avoid the other person's punch. So if the other person keeps throwing things at you, especially if they are things that are not immediately and directly related to the topic at hand, you are going to just bob and weave out of the way and allow the attacks to fly past you without reacting.*

A: APPEAR CONFIDENT

The second A in DEAR MAN stands for Appear confident. This means looking at the other person or persons when you are talking to them and using a confident voice tone.

Go up to a student and, without making eye contact, looking down, and with a meek voice, ask the student whether he or she would please stay after class to clean the desks and wipe board today. Afterward, ask students for their observations and feedback. This will generate a brief conversation about why it is important to make eye contact and appear confident.

N: NEGOTIATE

The N in DEAR MAN stands for Negotiate: Be willing to give to get. Offer and ask for alternative solutions to the problem. In addition, "turn the tables": That is, turn the problem over to the other person(s) and ask for alternative solutions.

It is also important to determine when we need to negotiate. Should we negotiate right away, when someone is not willing to accept our refusal or to do what we ask? The answer is no. If after two or three rounds there is no progress, you may decide to negotiate or ask the other person to come up with a solution. You might say, "Since you are not willing to accept my request/response, what solution do you think we should try?"

- *Example 1: Negotiate with the math teacher.*
  - *Negotiate: "I understand you are really busy, and I really need to go over my exam with you. What do you suggest we do so I can get some feedback on my exam?"*
- *Example 2: Negotiate with your friends at the party.*
  - *Negotiate: "I appreciate you want to include me in your fun, and I am not interested in doing drugs. I am happy to hang out with you, though. If I won't do drugs and you want to still hang out, what do you suggest we do?"*
- *Example 3: Negotiate with your friends at the fair.*
  - *Negotiate: "I know you want to go on the rollercoaster, and I don't want to. I am fine with waiting for you while you go on it. If you don't like that idea, what do you suggest we do? I am not going to go on the rollercoaster, and I still want you to have a good time."*

CLASS EXERCISE: DYADIC ROLE PLAYS AND PRESENTATIONS (12 MINUTES)

Have each student pair up with someone he or she has not worked with in a while. Explain:

You are going to use the objective from your homework in Lesson 25 that you wrote down on a piece of paper at the start of this lesson. (Remember, this objective should be something that you are open to sharing, and that does not involve someone else in the class.) You and your partner will take turns playing the role of the other person, and you can challenge each other, but only a moderate amount. Once one person has gone through it, switch roles. Practice enough to be prepared to show the group how you will implement the DEAR MAN strategy.

Ask the students to turn to Handout 26.2. Practice Cards for Learning the DEAR MAN Skills, or give each pair a set of DEAR MAN practice cards enlarged from the set in Handout 26.2. Explain:

You can use these cards as a means of remembering which letter you are focusing on while completing your DEAR MAN role plays. You can keep them on the desk in front of you while you are practicing at your desk, and bring them up front with you when we practice in front of the group.

You should walk around and assist pairs if they are having trouble with any of the components. After 5 minutes or so, bring all the pairs back together to their desks if they have moved around the classroom. Put a copy of Handout 26.2 (or an enlarged set of the DEAR MAN cards in this handout) out in the middle or front of the room to provide guidance. Randomly choose students in pairs (as time allows). to show the rest of the group their personal examples of implementing the DEAR MAN skills. Students may argue or change the subject, so that the students will have an opportunity to use repeating or ignoring. Ask the other students to coach the students doing each role play if one partner or the other should get stuck. Make sure that the group provides positive feedback for using the skills properly, as well as constructive criticism if an example does not fit the skills.

Allow as many students to give presentations as time allows. Students will be able to use the current practice examples in the following weeks as well.

Lesson Summary (3 minutes)

Briefly review the purpose of objectives effectiveness, as well as the DEAR MAN skills, with the class. Go around the classroom, randomly choosing students or having students call out the meaning of each letter in DEAR MAN.

Homework Assignment

Homework 26.3. Interpersonal Effectiveness: Practicing DEAR MAN Skills

Explain to students:

The DEAR MAN skills are really important skills to learn and will be useful on countless occasions in your daily lives. You are going to write out and practice a DEAR MAN situation for homework this week. Writing out your step-by-step DEAR MAN skills will make it easier for you to determine whether you are missing any steps. With practice over time, these skills will become more automatic. If you can't think of anything on your own, you can use some of the examples or ideas generated during this lesson and in Lesson 25. Furthermore, it is important that you write out each of the steps because next week we are going to spend considerable time during homework review going through your DEAR MAN situations.

Diary Cards

Hand out new skills diary cards to the students. Highlight that they have now learned the DEAR MAN skills, and that when they practice these skills for their homework, they are to circle the days and rate the skill use for the week on the diary card (along with the other skills that they have been taught).

Finally, do some troubleshooting: Ask students whether they have any questions about the homework or any obstacles to completing it. If so, answer the questions and address the obstacles. Obstacles may include, but are not limited to, the following: Students have no intention of doing the assignment, have too much other homework this week, are likely to forget, or don't understand the assignment. Help students to identify their obstacles, and work with them to make a plan to overcome them. Examples include encouraging a student to write down the assignment and set a reminder in a cell phone or calendar to complete it; discussing why a student has no intention of doing the homework, and working on increasing his or her motivation and the relevance of the assignment (e.g., grades); or clarifying any other points. Troubleshooting should be done each week after the homework is assigned.

Interpersonal Effectiveness
GIVE Skills

SUMMARY

Interpersonal effectiveness also involves building and maintaining healthy relationships. This is an important component of any interpersonal situation. We use the GIVE skills to focus on relationships—specifically, how to build and maintain relationships while obtaining our objectives. The amount of emphasis placed on these skills will be determined by how an individual prioritizes the goals of relationship effectiveness in relation to those of objectives effectiveness and self-respect effectiveness. GIVE stands for (be) Gentle, (act) Interested, Validate, and (use an) Easy manner. This lesson teaches students how to engage in each of these steps, with extra attention focused on how to validate another person. Validating another person is an important skill that will later translate into being able to validate oneself as well. Today's lesson includes opportunities for students to practice using their GIVE skills.

MAIN POINTS

1. If an important part of a person's goal is relationship effectiveness, then the GIVE skills ([be] Gentle, [act] Interested, Validate, [use an] Easy manner) are the skills to employ.
2. These skills work together with the other interpersonal effectiveness skills. The GIVE skills involve "how we say it."

MATERIALS

1. Handouts for this lesson:
   - Handout 27.1. Interpersonal Effectiveness: Building and Maintaining Positive Relationships
   - Homework 27.2. Interpersonal Effectiveness: Practicing GIVE Skills

303

2. Extra student skills binders, with pens or pencils, for students who attend class without materials.
3. Dry-erase markers or chalk for writing on the board.
4. Diary cards: Have new diary cards available to distribute at the end of class. If possible, highlight the "GIVE" skills.

PREPARATION

1. Review the lesson plan as well as handouts in student skills binder.
2. Arrange desks in the classroom, if possible, in order for students to be able to see each other.

LESSON OVERVIEW AND TIMELINE

- Mindfulness exercise (5 minutes)
  - Observing: Dropping into the pauses of the breath (3 minutes)
  - Describing observations of the exercise (2 minutes)
- Homework review (10 minutes)
  - Homework 26.3. Interpersonal Effectiveness: Practicing DEAR MAN Skills
    - Sharing with partners
    - Sharing with class
  - Diary cards
- Introduction of main ideas (5 minutes)
  - Goals of Relationship Effectiveness
    - Communicating your wants and needs in a manner that builds and maintains relationships.
    - How you want the other person to feel about you when interaction is over.
  - Important to clarify priority of relationship in each interaction.
- Discussion: Relationship effectiveness—GIVE (25 minutes)
  - Review of Handout 27.1. Interpersonal Effectiveness: Building and Maintaining Positive Relationships (15 minutes)
    - G: (be) <u>G</u>entle
    - I: (act) <u>I</u>nterested
    - V: <u>V</u>alidate
    - E: (use an) <u>E</u>asy manner
  - Class exercise: Dyadic role plays (10 minutes)
- Lesson summary (3 minutes)
  - Review mnemonic by randomly calling on students.
- Homework assignment (2 minutes)
  - Homework 27.2. Interpersonal Effectiveness: Practicing GIVE Skills
    - Identify two situations in which you used your GIVE skills.
  - Diary cards

DETAILED LESSON PLAN

Mindfulness Exercise (5 minutes)

Observing: Dropping into the Pauses of the Breath (3 minutes)

Welcome the class and state that today's mindfulness practice will involve observing. Explain:

> *Today for mindfulness, we are going to practice observing our breath. How often do you stop throughout the day to notice that you are about to engage in some behavior before you actually do it? Did you notice the urge to sit down in your chair just before you sat down? Or did you notice the urge to raise your hand just before it went up? Or did you notice the urge to yell at your mother, just before the words came flying out of your mouth? Of course, this can be difficult for many of us. As we practice observing, we will become more aware of these moments.*
>
> *So today we are going to do an exercise called "dropping into the pauses of the breath." Everybody take a breath in—pause—and now exhale. Pause. Now inhale. At the top and bottom of each breath, there is a natural pause between the inhale and exhale, and it may be very brief. As we focus on our breath today, we are going to drop into these pauses by noticing the space between each inhale and exhale.*

Continue:

> *When I say 1, that's the signal to sit in the mindful/wide-awake position we know well by now. This means keeping our feet flat on the floor, sitting up straight, and putting our hands in our laps. For this exercise, we will keep our eyes open with a soft gaze, looking forward and down, but at nothing in particular. If you notice any urges to move, other than blinking or swallowing, notice each urge without acting on it, and return to your breath. When I say 2, that's the signal to take a deep breath. When I say 3, that's the signal to begin the practice. I'll say, "Stop," to end it.*

Now start the practice by counting to 3.

> *1: Get yourself into the mindful/wide-awake position. 2: Take a deep breath. 3: Begin the practice.*

After 2 minutes, say, "Stop."

Describing Observations of the Exercise (2 minutes)

Have a few students share an observation in the moment. Provide feedback about observations as needed, ensuring that each statement consists of something a student can observe and describe nonjudgmentally (e.g., I noticed judgments about this exercise, I noticed I was able to participate 100%, I noticed a thought about how this was different from last week, I noticed a thought . . . , I noticed the sensation . . . , I noticed my mind wandering to other thoughts. I had lots of thoughts about how this could be helpful to me, I noticed I liked last week's practice better, I noticed I was uncomfortable so had to move . . .).

Homework Review

Homework 26.3. Interpersonal Effectiveness: Practicing DEAR MAN Skills

SHARING WITH PARTNERS

Ask the students to pair up. Explain:

> You are each going to share with your partner what you did as your DEAR MAN homework. I don't want you just to read the script to your partner; I want you to role-play how you did it. Pretend that your partner is the person with whom you did the DEAR MAN exercise. So instead of saying, "I said [blank]," say what you said, and how you said it, to your partner. Your partner should be prepared to tell you one aspect of the DEAR MAN exercise that was effective and also one area that could use improvement.
>
> After the first partner has finished and received his or her feedback, switch roles and have the other person share his or her DEAR MAN homework, also receiving feedback regarding one effective aspect, and one area that could be improved.

If a student reports that he or she did not complete the homework, tell him or her to use the example they practiced with their partner during the exercise last class.

SHARING WITH THE CLASS

Ask any students who completed a DEAR MAN exercise to share with the class. The example does not need to be one that was successful in achieving a student's objectives, because it is important for students to recognize that using the DEAR MAN skill only increases their likelihood of reaching their objectives.

Follow up with questions regarding whether the students were mindful, whether they had any attacks that needed ignoring, whether they employed repetition as a technique, if they employed broken record, or whether they had to turn the tables. Troubleshoot with any students who did not complete the homework what may have been in their way and how they will complete the homework this week.

Diary Cards

Ask all students to turn in their diary cards and homework sheets to be reviewed. If you are not able to review homework with each student each lesson, then be sure to get to each student over the course of several lessons. Comment on the amount of skill use you see marked on the diary cards for students. Encourage students who have low skill use to practice more, and continue to remind them that only with practice will the skills become more helpful and automatic.

Introduction of Main Ideas (5 minutes)

Ask the class to remind you of the goals of relationship effectiveness. List them on the board:

- Communicating your wants and needs in a way that builds and maintains the relationship.
- Thinking about how you want the other person to feel about you after the interaction is over.

Generate a discussion about the importance of focusing on relationships by asking the following questions:

How many friends do you think you would have if you constantly insisted on doing only what you want, talking only about yourself, and not acknowledging the other person's feelings at all?

How many of you pay attention to how you interact with your parents? Some teenagers don't pay much attention to their relationship with their parents, because they don't think that how they interact with their parents has any effect on the relationship. Do you think you would be more likely to get what you want from your parents if you actually attended to the relationship in a way that strengthens it?

What about relationships with friends or teachers? Do you think you could be more skillful in strengthening those relationships?

Today we are going to focus on learning the relationship effectiveness skills, called the GIVE skills. Notice how your level of emphasis on the relationship may change with different people.

Now explain:

There are different times when maintaining a relationship is more important than getting what you want or when maintaining your self-respect may be the most important goal. You will still try to get what you want in the interaction, only that may not be the most important thing to you. In addition, even when your objective is your highest priority, being mindful of the relationship and your self-respect are still important, so we have to use these skills as well as the DEAR MAN skills, even though they may not be your highest priority. Remember, these skills are not mutually exclusive and need to be used together. But we need to determine our priorities in each interaction to help us decide how much emphasis to give each goal of the interaction. Next week we will focus on the self-respect effectiveness skills.

Give this example:

You are going to a movie with a friend, and you each want to see a different movie. If seeing the movie that you want to see is your highest goal, then you are going to go heavy on the use of DEAR MAN skills to get your objective met of seeing the movie of your choice. If you are not so concerned about the movie, and maintaining the relationship with this friend is your most important goal, then you may go lighter on the DEAR MAN skills and put more emphasis on the use of GIVE skills to communicate that it is more important to you to have the company of your friend at the movie, although you are also hoping to see a different movie.

Ask students to provide their own examples of situations when they had to focus on building and maintaining a relationship.

Discussion: Relationship Effectiveness—GIVE (25 minutes)

Review of Handout 27.1. Interpersonal Effectiveness: Building and Maintaining Positive Relationships (15 minutes)

Have students turn to Handout 27.1. Write GIVE vertically on the board, filling in the word (or words) for each letter as you teach that letter. Explain:

GIVE is the mnemonic (memory helper) for the skills to use for building and maintaining a relationship. These are the skills that focus on how you interact with the other person, similar to the "how" skills in mindfulness.

G: (BE) <u>G</u>ENTLE

Have a student read the points on Handout 27.1 for the G in GIVE. Ask:

What is the difference between being assertive and being aggressive?

Allow students to generate responses. Then continue:

A person can be assertive without being aggressive by focusing on the G in GIVE.

"Being gentle" refers to being courteous, respectful, and pleasant in your approach to this person. Has anyone ever heard the phrase "You can catch more flies with honey than vinegar"? Using vinegar is the opposite of being gentle.

No attacks or threats: People do not like being attacked or threatened or having anger directed at them. Do not make threats such as "I'm going to fail my test if you don't do this for me," "Everybody is going to laugh at me if you don't buy me new clothes," or "I'm going to make your life miserable if you break up with me."

No judgments: Do not engage in name calling or make statements that are put-downs or have some element of judgment. No "shoulds" or guilt trips.

Voice tone: Be aware of your tone of voice. People often pay more attention to non-verbal behavior than to what is being said. So you can be using the kindest words and not attacking the other person at all, but if you are using a sarcastic or judgmental voice tone, the other person is likely only to hear that and to ignore your words. In other words, you have to be gentle all the way—with your words, thoughts, and tone of voice.

I: (ACT) U̲NTERESTED

Have a student read the points on Handout 27.1 for the I in GIVE. Then say:

> *Act interested in what the person is saying because you care about the relationship, even if you are not actually interested in the topic.*
>
> *Allow the person to finish his or her thoughts without being interrupted. Listen to the person's reason for saying no or for making a request of you or the person's responses to your request. Be patient with the person. In particular, do not try to talk over the person or make faces that indicate you don't agree with or care about what the person is saying. And maintain eye contact with the person.*

Ask:

> *Have any of you ever been in a conversation with another person, and while you were talking, the other person kept checking for text messages or Facebook updates? How did you feel during that experience? Did you think the other person cared about what you were saying? Again, our nonverbal behaviors can sometimes communicate more than our words.*

V: V̲ALIDATE

Have a student read the points on Handout 27.1 for the V in GIVE. Then go on:

> *Let's say that you tell a friend a story about a big blowout fight that you had with your parents, and the friend looks at you and says, "Well, of course you got mad, and I can see how that led to you yelling and swearing at them. Anybody would be pissed if their parents said that to them." And all of a sudden you feel better. Why? Because your friend gets it. You feel validated. Your friend may not agree with your swearing at your parents, and it may not have been effective, but you know your friend understands what you were experiencing. What if your friend responded by saying, "Wow, that was dumb. Seems like you blew up for no reason." Do you think you would feel better or worse? Probably worse. This is called invalidation.*
>
> *Our goal is to increase our validation. "Validation" is acknowledging the other person's feelings, behaviors, or opinions. We can validate <u>why</u> someone did something without validating <u>what</u> the person did.*
>
> *We can validate what the other person feels and, if needed, follow it up with what you didn't like about the situation. For example, if a friend hangs up on the phone with you, you can say, "I get it that you were so angry with me all you wanted to do was to hang up on me. And I don't think it's effective for us to break off our discussions like that when one of us is mad, because it will probably just make both of us more angry."*

Emphasize:

> <u>*Validation does not mean approval.*</u> *But we can always validate someone else's or our own emotions. It is invalidating to tell people they don't feel something that they feel.*

Ask:

> *Has anyone ever been told not to be sad, angry, guilty, or embarrassed about something? How did you feel when someone told you this?*

Allow students to generate answers. Then ask:

> *Did your emotion go up or down? Usually the intensity of an emotion goes up when we are invalidated by someone else or ourselves.*

Continue:

> *There are various ways to validate people. One is validation based on their past experiences—in other words, validating by stating that their reactions make sense given situations they have previously been in. For example, you could say, "Of course you were scared to tell your parents that you failed the chemistry test because the last time you failed a test, they grounded you for a month."*
>
> *Another type of validation is based on normalizing a person's reaction to his or her current situation. In other words, you can also validate someone based on the fact that many people would have a similar reaction in the same situation. For example, you could say, "I get that you are scared to tell your parents that you failed the chemistry test. Who wouldn't be? I know I would be too."*

Now ask students:

> *Now that you have a better understanding of what it means to validate or be validated, I want you to take a moment to think of a situation when you didn't feel validated by the other person. What was that like for you? Then think of a time when you did feel validated and understood by the other person. What was that like for you?*

Elicit responses.

E: (USE AN) <u>E</u>ASY MANNER

Have a student read the points on Handout 27.1 for the E in GIVE. Then say:

> *Smile, be easygoing, use humor, and use a light tone of voice. The idea is to minimize the person's defensiveness, which will help him or her hear your message.*

Have students practice nonthreatening and threatening body postures (e.g., relaxed and sitting back vs. standing in someone else's personal space, pointing fingers, and acting tense). Then ask:

> *Which body posture do you think is going to have a better effect on the relationship if you want to build and maintain it?*

Now have students practice saying, "Why didn't you call me last night?", using an attacking, harsh voice tone versus a soft, easy, light voice tone. Ask:

> *Which tone of voice do you think will cause less amount of defensiveness or anger in the other person? How would you react differently to the two statements?*

Allow students to generate responses.

Class Exercise: Dyadic Role Plays (10 minutes)

Have each student pair up with someone he or she has not worked with recently. Explain to students:

> *We are going to practice our GIVE skills right now, especially validation, and I want to see how this affects your relationships with your partners. First, I want the students in each pair to identify who will be the talker first and who will practice GIVE first. The talker will begin by thinking of something that happened to him or her today and that he or she would tell a friend. The person who is doing GIVE should practice being gentle with the talker, acting interested, using an easy manner, and validating the talker. Validation can include reflecting back what the talker says, acknowledging that things make sense given the situation, and being completely genuine with the talker.*

Have the dyads begin the role play. Bring the class back together as a group after about a minute or two. Now provide the students with a second set of instructions:

> *I want you to stay in your same roles, except that this time, I want the person in each pair who was practicing the GIVE skills to stop doing this. Don't pay attention to the other person; for instance, you can look around the room or look in your backpack. Also, don't validate, give up being gentle, and stop using an easy manner with the person. Talkers, continue with your story.*

Have the class begin again, and bring the class back together after a minute or two. Next, have students switch roles so that the other person in each pair has the opportunity to practice using his or her GIVE skills versus not using them.

Now, ask for observations about the exercise from several pairs of students. What was the experience of the storyteller in each pair when the listener stopped using the GIVE skills? Did the person continue talking? Did the volume in the room change? What was it like for the student practicing GIVE to be engaged versus not engaged?

After these role plays are finished, ask:

> *Who thinks these skills could help them strengthen their relationships?*

Elicit responses. Then ask:

> *Can you think of a time when, even though the relationship is not your top priority, it would be a good idea to use the GIVE skills?*

Again, allow for answers before continuing:

> *Even in a case when you don't care about the relationship, do you think it would be better to walk away from the other person with him or her thinking fondly of you rather than negatively? For example, if you break up with your girlfriend or boyfriend, do you want your ex hating and cursing you or wishing you well? What might your ex write about you on Facebook or Twitter if you do not use GIVE skills?*

Lesson Summary (3 minutes)

Briefly review the GIVE mnemonic by randomly choosing students around the room to define the abbreviations. Do this three or four times quickly to increase students' ability to generate the meanings of the letters.

Homework Assignment (2 minutes)

Homework 27.2. Interpersonal Effectiveness: Practicing GIVE Skills

Explain:

> *This is the homework for next week: You are to choose two situations over the next week where you will practice the GIVE skills. You are to report on your homework sheet the name of the person you engaged with, what the situation was, what the outcome was, and how you felt about the relationship afterward.*

Diary Cards

Hand out new diary cards to the students. Highlight that they have now learned the GIVE skills, and that when they practice these skills for their homework, they are to circle the days and rate the skill use for the week on the diary card (along with the other skills that they have been taught).

Finally, do some troubleshooting: Ask students whether they have any questions about the homework or any obstacles to completing it. If so, answer the questions and address the obstacles. Obstacles may include, but are not limited to, the following: Students have no intention of doing the assignment, have too much other homework this week, are likely to forget, or don't understand the assignment. Help students to identify their obstacles, and work with them to make a plan to overcome them. Examples include encouraging a student to write down the assignment and set a reminder in a cell phone or calendar to complete it; discussing why a student has no intention of doing the homework, and working on increasing his or her motivation and the relevance of the assignment (e.g., grades); or clarifying any other points. Troubleshooting should be done each week after the homework is assigned.

Interpersonal Effectiveness
FAST Skills

SUMMARY

Interpersonal effectiveness also involves keeping and maintaining your own self-respect. This lesson focuses on the FAST skills, aimed at the goal of self-respect effectiveness; specifically, it focuses on how to maintain self-respect while also obtaining objectives. Like the GIVE skills, the FAST skills are important to all social situations. The amount of emphasis placed on the FAST skills will be determined by how the individual prioritizes the goals of self-respect effectiveness in relation to those of objectives effectiveness and relationship effectiveness. FAST stands for (be) Fair, (no) Apologies, Stick to values, and (be) Truthful. This lesson teaches students how to engage in each of these steps in order to increase the probability that the students will like how they feel about themselves after a social interaction is over. Today's lesson includes opportunities for students to practice using all of their DEAR MAN, GIVE, and FAST skills.

MAIN POINTS

1. We are continuing to learn skills in the Interpersonal Effectiveness module. It is important to remember that the interpersonal effectiveness skills are not mutually exclusive, and we don't have to use only one at a time or always use them all together; the way in which we use these skills depends on the situation.
2. If the main goal of communication is self-respect effectiveness, then the FAST skills ([be] Fair, [no] Apologies, Stick to values, [be] Truthful) are the skills to employ.

MATERIALS

1. Handouts for this lesson:
    *   Handout 28.1. Interpersonal Effectiveness: Maintaining Your Self-Respect
    *   Homework 28.2. Interpersonal Effectiveness: Practicing FAST Skills

2. Extra student skills binders, with pens or pencils, for students who attend class without materials.

3. Dry-erase markers or chalk for writing on the board.

4. Diary cards: Have new diary cards available to distribute at the end of class. If possible, highlight the "FAST" skills.

PREPARATION

1. Review the lesson plan as well as handouts in student skills binder.

2. Arrange desks in the classroom, if possible, in order for students to be able to see each other.

LESSON OVERVIEW AND TIMELINE

- Mindfulness exercise (5 minutes)
  - Participating: Buzz (counting game) (3 minutes)
  - Describing observations of the exercise (2 minutes)
- Homework review (10 minutes)
  - Homework 27.2. Interpersonal Effectiveness: Practicing GIVE Skills
    - Sharing with partners
    - Sharing with class
  - Diary cards
- Introduction of main ideas (5 minutes)
  - Goals of self-respect effectiveness
  - Examples of impact when you violate your own values
- Discussion: Self-respect effectiveness—FAST (10 minutes)
  - Review of Handout 28.1. Interpersonal Effectiveness: Maintaining Your Self-Respect
    - F: (be) Fair
    - A: (no) Apologies
    - S: Stick to values
    - T: (be) Truthful
    - Balancing FAST skills with DEAR MAN and GIVE skills
- Class exercise: Dyadic role plays—putting skills all together (15 minutes)
  - Assign dyads priorities/goals.
    - Role-play DEAR MAN, GIVE, and FAST skills based on priority assigned.
    - Class guesses order of priorities/goals.
- Lesson summary (3 minutes)
  - Review skills associated with each interpersonal effectiveness skill (DEAR MAN, GIVE, FAST).
  - Review FAST mnemonic by randomly calling on students.
- Homework assignment (2 minutes)
  - Homework 28.2. Interpersonal Effectiveness: Practicing FAST Skills
    - Practice FAST skills in two different situations.
  - Diary cards

DETAILED LESSON PLAN

Mindfulness Exercise (5 minutes)

Participating: Buzz (Counting Game) (3 minutes)

Welcome the class and state that today's mindfulness practice will involve participating. Explain:

> *Today for mindfulness, we are going to focus on doing one thing in the moment nonjudgmentally. How often do you notice trying to think ahead and plan what you are going to do next? As a result of this, what may happen? You may end up missing the moment and making a mistake right now.*
>
> *So today we are going to play a game called Buzz. This is a counting game. When I say so, we are all going to stand up and move ourselves into a circle. [If there are more than 12 people in the class, then split the class into two circles.] In this game, one person is going to start off by counting 1; then the next person, to either the left or right, will count 2. However, the number with a 3 in it and any later number divisible by 3 will be a "Buzz" number; that is, instead of saying the number, you need to say, "Buzz." Then the next person will continue with the next number, and so on. For example, we would count: "1, 2, Buzz, 4, 5, Buzz, 7, 8, Buzz, 10, 11, Buzz, 13, 14, Buzz, 16 . . . "*
>
> *Let's see how high we can count. For the first minute, we will practice, and if someone makes a mistake, the next person should simply begin at 1 again. After the first minute, we will stop and then start again. This second time, if someone makes a mistake, that person should step outside the circle, and the next person will start at 1 again. Remember, the goal is to practice being present in this one moment and not thinking ahead to what number it may be at your turn. If you notice yourself doing that, notice it, and bring your attention back to the game and the person counting right now.*

An additional instruction you may give for more advanced groups if time allows or for future practice is to add in a "reverse" word. If the student says, "Buzz," the direction of the counting continues; however, if the student says "Bizz," the direction reverses.

Now continue:

> *When I say 1, that's the signal to stand up next to your desk and move into the circle [or one of the two circles]. When I say 2, that's the signal to take a deep breath. When I say 3, that's the signal to begin the practice of fully participating one-mindfully and nonjudgmentally and for one person to begin counting. I'll say, "Stop," to end the exercise.*

Now start the practice by counting to 3.

> *1: Stand up and move into a circle. 2: Take a deep breath. 3: Begin.*

Stop the exercise after 2 minutes.

Describing Observations of the Exercise (2 minutes)

After finishing the exercise, ask students to return to their seats, and ask some students to share one observation. Provide feedback about observations as needed, ensuring that each statement consists of something a student can observe and describe nonjudgmentally (e.g., I noticed judgments about this exercise, I noticed I was able to participate 100%, I noticed a thought about how this was different from last week, I noticed a thought . . . , I noticed the sensation . . . , I noticed my mind wandering to other thoughts. I had lots of thoughts about how this could be helpful to me, I noticed I liked last week's practice better, I noticed I was uncomfortable so had to move . . .).

Homework Review (10 minutes)

Homework 27.2. Interpersonal Effectiveness: Practicing GIVE Skills

SHARING WITH PARTNERS

Ask the students to pair up. Explain:

> *You are each going to share with your partner what you did as your GIVE homework. Pick one of the two situations that you wrote about on the homework sheet, and share this with your partner. Explain what you did for each letter of GIVE. Your partner is going to ask one question. If the outcome was effective, your partner can ask you what you think was done well. If the outcome was not as effective as hoped, your partner can ask you what you think could have been done differently, if anything, and can offer some suggestions to help. Then switch roles. Be sure that you both get a chance to tell about one situation for GIVE.*

SHARING WITH THE CLASS

Ask any students who completed their GIVE homework to share a situation with the class. As you review the homework scenarios, ask what was done for each letter of GIVE. Students may need further help understanding and explaining the V in GIVE, so drawing out any validation that was done is particularly important. Highlight an area where each student was especially effective and one area where further development seems needed.

Troubleshoot with any students who did not complete the homework what may have been in their way and how they will complete the homework this week.

Diary Cards

Ask all students to turn in their diary cards and homework sheets to be reviewed. If you are not able to review homework with each student each lesson, then be sure to get to each student over the course of several lessons. Comment on the amount of skill use you see marked on the diary cards for students. Encourage students who have low skill use to practice more, and keep reminding them that only with practice will the skills become more helpful and automatic.

Introduction of Main Ideas (5 minutes)

Explain:

> Today we are going to learn the skills to use when self-respect effectiveness is one of your priorities. We call these the FAST skills. We are going to discuss how to balance the seesaw of other people's needs and wants, and your own needs and wants.

Ask the class to remind you of the goals of self-respect effectiveness. List them on the board:

- Building and maintaining your self-respect during and after an interaction with someone else.
- Sticking to your beliefs and values. Giving up your beliefs for approval, or acting helpless when you are not, can hurt your self-respect.

Ask the following questions:

> How does it feel when you sacrifice your own needs to make a friend happy? Or how does it feel when you go against your own values to do something that somebody is pressuring you into doing?

Allow for answers. The goal is to have students generate answers indicating that when they go against their own values or principles, they may begin judging themselves and then feel worse about themselves. Then go on:

> Remember, even at times when your objective is your highest priority, being mindful of the relationship and your self-respect are still important, so you will need the GIVE and FAST skills as well as the DEAR MAN skills. These three sets of skills are not mutually exclusive, and we don't only use one at a time. We need to use our self-respect skills in every interaction.

Now ask:

> I want you to take a minute and think of examples in your life—ones that you are willing to share and ones that are appropriate for school—when maybe you didn't maintain your self-respect during an interaction with someone.

Elicit students' examples. Or use some of the following possible answers or themes:

- Feeling so angry that you screamed and yelled at someone to get them to do what you wanted.
- Bullying someone.
- Pressuring someone to do something the other person didn't really want to do (such as cheating at school, skipping class, drinking alcohol, taking drugs, smoking cigarettes, engaging in sexual behaviors, or the like.)

- Lying to your friends or family members.
- Crying so intensely that someone else did something you wanted because you were crying so much.

Then go on:

We have just discussed times when your self-respect went down or examples where it might have gone down. Now I want you to provide examples of situations when you did decide to focus on maintaining your own self-respect over the relationship or objective.

Again, allow students to share examples. Reinforce their participation and answers, especially when they include one of the FAST skills.

Discussion: Self-Respect Effectiveness—FAST (10 minutes)

Review of Handout 28.1. Interpersonal Effectiveness: Maintaining Your Self-Respect

Have students turn to Handout 28.1. Write FAST vertically on the board, filling in the words for each letter as you teach that letter. Explain:

The mnemonic (memory helper) for this skill is FAST. As we go through this, we can relate each skill to the examples we have previously discussed.

F: (BE) FAIR

Have a student read the points on Handout 28.1 for the F in FAST. Then ask:

What is fair to you? Are you always doing what the other person wants? And what is fair to the other person? If you were in that person's shoes, what would you want done? If you always do what you want, you may feel worse about yourself, and if you always do what the other person wants, you may also feel worse about yourself. Being fair means finding balance.

Draw a set of "seesaws" on the board like the ones in Figure L28.1. Say:

If you stand too far to one side or the other of the "seesaw," the relationship is out of balance. Being fair means balancing your needs with the other person's. Unbalanced relationships may lead you to feel negative about yourself and may decrease your self-respect.

A: (NO) APOLOGIES

Have a student read the points on Handout 28.1 for the A in FAST. Then say:

Apologizing when you do something that warrants an apology is of course OK. This is when it is important that you don't under-apologize. But when could over-apologizing to someone be a problem?

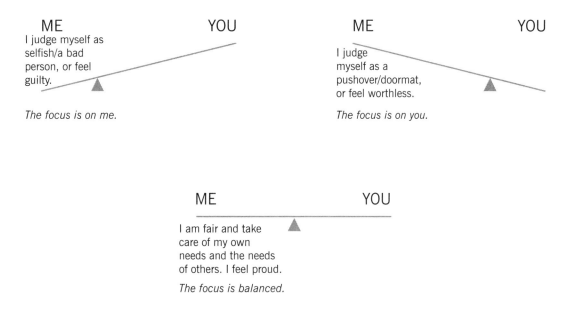

FIGURE L28.1. "Seesaws" illustrating imbalance and balance between one's own needs and those of another person.

Allow for multiple answers. Then go on:

> *Over-apologizing is a problem because it can imply that you did something egregiously wrong or made a huge mistake that you "should" feel bad about and keeps you from moving forward. When you over-apologize, it can also start to annoy other people as well. Sometimes people over-apologize because they are wanting the other person to tell them it's OK for whatever they did wrong or because they are trying to decrease their own guilt. This can make you feel worse about yourself over time because there is no way for you to let yourself move past the situation. Furthermore, you don't have to apologize for making a request from someone else or having an opinion.*

Ask for examples of when someone might have engaged in over-apologizing for something and how it affected his or her self-respect in the short term or long term. Or use this example:

> *Sally is in the lunchroom talking to Billy about their chemistry assignment. Sally's boyfriend, Mike, walks in and sees them talking, rolls his eyes at Sally, and walks out. Sally runs after Mike and starts apologizing multiple times for talking to Billy.*

Ask:

> *What do Sally's apologies imply? They imply that she was doing something wrong and that she should not have been working on her chemistry assignment. How do you think Sally feels about herself after multiple apologies?*

S: <u>S</u>TICK TO VALUES

Have a student read the points on Handout 28.1 for the S in FAST. Then instruct students:

> *Think about what your values are in regard to important issues in your life; honesty, money, stealing, sex, drugs, cheating, and so on. Write down some of your own values or moral beliefs. Remember, we reviewed values in the Emotion Regulation module, so if you need a quick review, you can flip back to Handout 19.5. Emotion Regulation: Wise Mind Values and Priorities List.*

> Now ask:

> *When might it be difficult to stick to your values?*

Allow students to generate examples, and then go on:

> *When your beliefs go against the beliefs of the group, you might struggle with being on the outside. What happens if you give up on your values repeatedly? You end up feeling worse about yourself over time and are likely to start judging yourself negatively.*

T: (BE) <u>T</u>RUTHFUL

Have a student read the points on Handout 28.1 for the T in FAST. Then ask:

> *What impact can lying have on your self-respect?*

Allow for responses, and then say:

> *Repeated lying can make you start to feel worse about yourself, and it can also erode relationships over time. Is acting helpless a form of not being truthful? Yes, it may increase the likelihood that someone does something for you, but over time it may also make you feel worse about yourself for "tricking" people into helping you—for example, crying in front of a teacher to get out of trouble or acting sicker than you are so someone will give up another activity to stay with you.*

Ask students for additional examples.

BALANCING FAST SKILLS WITH DEAR MAN AND GIVE SKILLS

Ask:

> *Are the FAST skills only needed when self-respect is the top priority in the interaction, or should they be used in all interactions?*

Allow students to answer that FAST skills are useful in most situations. Then ask:

Remember the example we used in Lesson 27 about going to the movies with a friend when you each want to see a different movie? If seeing the movie that you want to see is your goal, then you are going to use DEAR MAN skills to get your objective met of seeing the movie of your choice. If you are not as concerned about the movie as you are about maintaining the relationship with this friend, then you are going to increase the use of GIVE skills to communicate that you want to see a different movie or to agree to see the movie that your friend wants to see.

But what if this is a case where you always do what this friend wants, and you are starting to feel like a doormat? Then this is the time to increase your use of the FAST skills. What do you think the person should do in this situation?

Allow for input from students. Reinforce and praise responses that are effective and in line with the FAST skills. Then ask:

When might focusing too much on the FAST skills be problematic? Here's a hint: Think of your mindfulness skills. Focusing solely on your self-respect might be problematic if it is not effective, meaning that it is not in line with your long-term goals. The key is not to focus too little on them or too much on them, unless self-respect is your top priority.

Class Exercise: Dyadic Role Plays—Putting Skills All Together (15 minutes)

Divide students into pairs. Assign each pair a different order of priorities for (1) objectives effectiveness, (2) relationship effectiveness, and (3) self-respect effectiveness. Possible orders of priorities, using these numbers, are illustrated in Figure L28.2. (For classes with more than 12 students, there may be repeat pairs.) Only the pair should know what their order is. Later the class will have to guess the order. Instruct the students:

Now you and your partner are going to practice putting the DEAR MAN, GIVE, and FAST skills together, according to the priority order your pair has been assigned. Here is the situation: You are at lunch with a friend, standing in front of the cash register. You have just ordered your food. Your friend steps up, tells you that he or she doesn't have any money, and asks you to pay for his or her lunch. This friend has done this to you before and has never paid you back. This is a good friend, someone that you have worked hard to have as your friend. What is your goal here: not to pay, to keep the friend, or to maintain your self-respect? How will you use objectives, relationship, or self-respect effectiveness, depending on your assigned order of priorities? Each partner should take a turn responding to his or her friend. Again, I want you to practice using all three skill sets for interpersonal effectiveness: the DEAR MAN, GIVE, and FAST skills.

123	213	312
132	231	321

FIGURE L28.2. Possible orders of priorities for the class exercise.

Once the pairs have all finished practicing, have pairs come forward as time allows and practice their skills in front of the entire class, without telling the class how they ordered their priorities. The audience will guess the order of priorities.

Lesson Summary (3 minutes)

Congratulate the students for learning the new skills and for the great jobs they did role-playing. Then ask students to briefly review the three goals for interpersonal effectiveness, one at a time. Follow this by having other students identify the skills that go with each goal; that is, go quickly around the room and have students identify the words associated with each of the three mnemonics, with special emphasis on the FAST skills.

Homework Assignment (2 minutes)

Homework 28.2. Interpersonal Effectiveness: Practicing FAST Skills

Explain:

> *Use this sheet for the homework for next week: You are to choose two situations before the next lesson where you will practice the FAST skills. You are to report the relationship to the person you engaged with, what the situation was, what the outcome was, and how you felt about yourself afterward.*

Diary Cards

Distribute new diary cards to the students. Highlight that they have now learned the FAST skills, and that when they practice these skills for their homework, they are to circle the days and rate the skill use for the week on the diary card (along with the other skills that they have been taught).

Finally, do some troubleshooting: Ask students whether they have any questions about the homework or any obstacles to completing it. If so, answer the questions and address the obstacles. Obstacles may include, but are not limited to, the following: Students have no intention of doing the assignment, have too much other homework this week, are likely to forget, or don't understand the assignment. Help students to identify their obstacles, and work with them to make a plan to overcome them. Examples include encouraging a student to write down the assignment and set a reminder in a cell phone or calendar to complete it; discussing why a student has no intention of doing the homework, and working on increasing his or her motivation and the relevance of the assignment (e.g., grades); or clarifying any other points. Troubleshooting should be done each week after the homework is assigned.

Interpersonal Effectiveness

Evaluating Options for How Intensely to Ask or Say No

SUMMARY

Today's lesson focuses on helping students to determine how strongly they should make a request or say no to a request when they are using the DEAR MAN skills for objectives effectiveness. The lesson first introduces the 10 factors they should consider in determining this. Each student will then choose a situation in which to use the DEAR MAN skills. As the teacher, you will need to have an example as well. The class will walk through each of the factors, determining whether or not each factor is relevant to the situation and whether or not the intensity should be raised.

MAIN POINTS

1. There are different levels of intensity for asking for something or saying no in a situation.
2. Evaluating how intensely to ask for something or say no requires consideration of 10 factors: capability, priorities, self-respect, rights, authority, relationship, long-term versus short-term goals, give and take, homework, and timing.

MATERIALS

1. Handouts for this lesson:
   - Handout 29.1. Interpersonal Effectiveness: Evaluating Your Options
   - Handout 29.2. Interpersonal Effectiveness: Factors to Consider
   - Handout 29.3. Interpersonal Effectiveness: Figuring Out How Strongly to Ask or Say No
   - Homework 29.4. Interpersonal Effectiveness: Using Interpersonal Effectiveness Skills at the Same Time

2. Extra student skills binders, with pens or pencils, for students who attend class without materials.
3. Dry-erase markers or chalk for writing on the board.
4. Diary cards: Have new diary cards available to distribute at the end of class. If possible, highlight the "Evaluating options" skill.
5. A set of 10 dimes per student (paper clips can be used if dimes are not available).

PREPARATION

1. Review the lesson plan as well as handouts in student skills binder.
2. Arrange desks in the classroom, if possible, in order for students to be able to see each other.

LESSON OVERVIEW AND TIMELINE

- Mindfulness exercise (5 minutes)
  - Participating: Letter switch (3 minutes)
  - Describing observations of the exercise (2 minutes)
- Homework review (10 minutes)
  - Homework 28.2. Interpersonal Effectiveness: Practicing FAST Skills
    - Sharing with partners
    - Sharing with class
  - Diary cards
- Introduction of main ideas (10 minutes)
  - Review of Handout 29.1. Interpersonal Effectiveness: Evaluating Your Options
    - Deciding whether or not it is appropriate to ask for something or to say no.
    - Deciding how strongly you should ask or say no.
- Discussion: Factors to consider (20 minutes)
  - Review of Handout 29.2. Interpersonal Effectiveness: Factors to Consider
  - Review of Handout 29.3. Interpersonal Effectiveness: Figuring Out How Strongly to Ask or Say No
    - Capability
    - Priorities
    - Self-respect
    - Rights
    - Authority
    - Relationship
    - Long-term versus short-term goals
    - Give and take
    - Homework
    - Timing
- Lesson summary (3 minutes)
  - Briefly review 10 factors.
  - Have one or two students demonstrate differing levels of intensity when asking or saying no.

- Homework assignment (2 minutes)
  - Handout 29.3. Interpersonal Effectiveness: Figuring Out How Strongly to Ask or Say No
  - Homework 29.4. Interpersonal Effectiveness: Using Interpersonal Effectiveness Skills at the Same Time
    - Write a DEAR MAN, GIVE, and FAST script for the scenario practiced in class today while determining intensity of asking or saying no.
  - Diary cards

DETAILED LESSON PLAN

Mindfulness Exercise (5 minutes)

Participating: Letter Switch (3 minutes)

Welcome the class and state that today's mindfulness exercise will involve participating. Explain:

> As in all the other participating exercises we have practiced, our goal is to focus on engaging in the activity one-mindfully and nonjudgmentally. After I give you the instructions, we will stand up and get into a circle [if there are more than eight people in the class, form two circles]. For this exercise, I will begin by saying a three-letter word. The person to my right will change one letter in the word to form a new word. The next person will do the same thing. For example, "cat" becomes "pat" when the "c" is changed to a "p," and then "pat" becomes "put" when the "a" is changed to a "u," and then "put" becomes "cut" when the "p" is changed to a "c," and so on. We want to be fast and spontaneous, throwing ourselves completely into the exercise.
>
> If you notice yourself having any judgmental thoughts about the activity, your word, or about anything else, just notice the thoughts, let them go, and bring yourself back to the exercise. If someone makes a mistake, simply notice it, and then someone else in the circle just begins again. Remember, you can only change one letter in a word at a time!

Continue:

> When I say 1, that's the signal to stand up next to your desk and move into a circle [or one of two circles]. When I say 2, that's the signal to take a deep breath. When I say 3, that's the signal to begin the practice of fully participating one-mindfully and nonjudgmentally, and I will start with the first word. I'll say, "Stop," to end the exercise.

Now start the practice by counting to 3.

> 1: Stand up and move into a circle. 2: Take a deep breath. 3: Begin.

Give the first word and stop the exercise after 2 minutes.

Describing Observations of the Exercise
(2 minutes)

After finishing the exercise, ask all students to return to their seats, and ask a few students to share one observation. Provide feedback about observations as needed, ensuring that each statement consists of something a student can observe and describe nonjudgmentally (e.g., I noticed judgments about this exercise, I noticed I was able to participate 100%, I noticed a thought about how this was different from last week, I noticed a thought . . . , I noticed the sensation . . . , I noticed my mind wandering to other thoughts. I had lots of thoughts about how this could be helpful to me, I noticed I liked last week's practice better, I noticed I was uncomfortable so had to move . . .).

Homework Review (10 minutes)

Homework 28.4. Interpersonal Effectiveness:
Practicing FAST Skills

SHARING WITH PARTNERS

Divide the class into pairs. Explain:

> *You are each going to share with your partner what you did as your FAST homework. Choose one of the two situations that you wrote about, and share this with your partner. Explain what you did for each letter of FAST. Your partner is going to ask one question. If the outcome was effective, your partner can ask you what you think was done well. If the outcome was not as effective as intended, your partner can ask what you think could have been done differently and can offer some suggestions to help. Then switch roles. Be sure that you both get a chance to tell about one situation for FAST.*

SHARING WITH THE CLASS

Ask students to share with the class what their partners reported on. Students will explain what was done for each of the letters in FAST. Be sure to provide corrective feedback as needed, and reinforce students for sharing the homework and practicing the skill.

Troubleshoot with any students who did not complete the homework what may have been in their way and how they will complete the homework this week.

Diary Cards

Ask all students to turn in their diary cards and homework sheets to be reviewed. If you are not able to review homework with each student each lesson, then be sure to get to each student over the course of several lessons. Comment on the amount of skill use you see marked on the diary cards for students. Encourage students who have low skill use to practice more, and keep reminding them that only with practice will the skills become more helpful and automatic.

Introduction of Main Ideas (10 minutes)

Begin by asking:

Have you ever had a situation where you wanted something really badly but you asked for it too lightly, or quickly took no for an answer when you really, really wanted it and thought you deserved it? How about on the other side: Have you ever asked for something so strongly that the other person couldn't say no to you because you wouldn't accept no for an answer? In either case, how did that affect the relationship?

Elicit responses. Then explain:

In today's lesson, we will focus on two things. First, we will learn how to decide whether or not it is appropriate to ask for something or to say no right now. Second, we will focus on how strongly we should ask or say no in an interpersonal situation right now. Basically, we are going to focus on how strongly we should use our DEAR MAN, GIVE, and FAST skills before we put them all together.

A key component to being interpersonally effective is recognizing that these questions and situations do not always have black-and-white answers or solutions and that we need to consider different factors when asking for something or saying no. There are 10 factors that play important roles in these decisions because they affect the intensity with which we ask or say no.

Review of Handout 29.1. Interpersonal Effectiveness: Evaluating Your Options

Have students turn to Handout 29.1. Have one student read through the top part of the handout (the first two sentences).

Now draw a vertical line on the board and put a 1 at the top and a 10 at the bottom, with the remaining numbers spaced evenly in between. Highlight the different levels of intensity listed in the handout. Ask:

What would low-intensity behaviors for asking or saying no look like? What would high-intensity behaviors look like?

Have students discuss the difference between low-intensity behaviors (e.g., avoiding eye contact, low voice tone, hinting without being direct, giving in to the other person) and high-intensity behaviors (e.g., refusing to negotiate, louder voice tone, being firm). Then ask:

Where do you tend to fall on the continuum? Is it always different, or does your behavior tend to be more toward the top or the bottom? Where would you prefer to be?

Provide students a moment to think about their answers. A few may share if they desire. Then say:

Today we are going to learn 10 factors to consider in determining which level of intensity is appropriate for each situation. It is important to keep in mind that what works in one situation may not work in another. You can use a certain intensity to tell your younger sibling that you are not going to help him or her, but using that same intensity with your parents would probably get you in trouble. You may ask for money from one of your parents with a certain amount of intensity one day, but if that parent has just been fired, you would use a different intensity. Your behavior needs to be appropriate to the situation.

Discussion: Factors to Consider (20 minutes)

For this part of the lesson, you and the students are going to walk through the 10 factors, using their (and your) own examples. For each factor, have a student read the description on Handout 29.2, and then have all the students determine whether that is an important factor for them.

Review of Handout 29.2. Interpersonal Effectiveness: Factors to Consider
Review of Handout 29.3. Interpersonal Effectiveness: Figuring Out How Strongly to Ask or Say No

Ask all students to have viewable on their desks both Handout 29.2 and Handout 29.3. Explain:

In this part of the lesson, we are going to learn the 10 factors to take into account when we are deciding how firm or intense we want to be in asking or saying no. First, we all need to come up with an example of something we want to ask someone for or something we know we want to say no to. For this exercise, the examples need to be things that we are willing to share with the class and are appropriate for school discussion.

Give students a minute to generate a situation. As the teacher, you must come up with an example as well. Possible ideas for you include asking the principal for a raise, asking another teacher to cover your class so you can go to the gym, or asking a family member to clean his or her room. Possible examples for everyone include asking a partner or friend to go to a concert that the other person is unlikely to enjoy, saying no to giving someone a ride home after school, saying no to going to a concert with someone, or saying no to a good friend about getting "BFF" tattoos or piercings.

As the students are generating their examples and sharing them, go around and give each student 10 dimes (or paper clips, if you don't have dimes; if the class is large, you may also pass out the items before the class starts to save time). Once the students have their examples ready, go around the room and ask them to share briefly what they will be asking for or saying no to, in order to ensure that everyone has an example. Then explain:

We are going to walk through Handout 29.2 to determine how strongly to ask or say no, using our examples. Handout 29.3 is a practice worksheet for us to use. It lists all the factors and is an easy way for us to go through the factors quickly, once we learn them from Handout 29.2. Each time we go through one of the factors, for those of you trying to determine how strongly to ask for something, I want you to put a dime [or paper clip] in your bank by moving it to the top of your desk. On Handout 29.3, you can also circle the

10¢ symbol listed on the left side of the page each time your answer is yes for the specific factor. For those of you trying to determine how strongly to say no, I want you to put a dime [or paper clip] in your bank, or on Handout 29.3 circle the 10¢ symbol listed on the right side of the page, each time your answer is no for the specific factor. At the end, we will add up all of our dimes in the bank [or paper clips] and determine how strongly we should do our DEAR MAN skills.

Now walk the class through the exercise, using your own example as well as the students' examples. For illustrative purposes, the material below uses the example of asking a parent for permission to get a piercing; therefore, you will need to keep track of the yes responses for this request. As you go through each factor, have one student read the factor and description from Handout 29.2. Provide the further explanation as outlined below, and then determine together with the students whether that factor fits the scenario or not.

Depending on class size, you may not be able to have every student share his or her answer for each factor. Be sure to have all students share at least once, however. Also, be sure to ask whether any students are not sure of their answer, and have the class help those students decide. As the teacher, you will be also sharing your answer for each question with the class on the board. As you go through each factor, write the name of the factor on the board. Each time the factor fits for your example, place a check mark or write "10¢" next to it so the class can follow your model on the board.

CAPABILITY

Have a student read through the questions in Handout 29.2. Then say:

Is the person able to give you what you want? If the answer is yes, you put a dime [or a paper clip] in the bank. If the answer is no, then you keep your dime [or paper clip].

Example:

Let's look at our earlier example of asking your parents to allow you to get a piercing. In this case, the answer is yes: They are your legal guardians, so they are capable of giving permission. Therefore, you would put a dime in the bank and circle the 10¢ symbol on the left side of Handout 29.3.

Go around the room and ask students to identify whether or not the persons they are asking have the capability of giving them what they want. Or, if the students are being asked for something, do the students have the capability? Ask clarifying questions as needed. In addition, use your own example as needed to provide further clarification and practice.

PRIORITIES

Have a student read through the questions on Handout 29.2. Then say:

Next, you have to decide what your priority is. Is your objective a higher priority than the relationship? If the objective is a higher priority, then your answer is yes, and you put a dime [or paper clip] in the bank. If the relationship is a higher priority, then your answer is no, and you keep your dime [or paper clip].

Example:

So let's look to our example of asking your parents to allow you to get a piercing. Do you care more about what you want than about keeping the relationship? No, you may want that piercing really badly, but it is probably not worth destroying your relationship with your parents. For this example, then, you would keep your money.

Go around the room and ask students to state briefly state what their priority is and to share it with the class. Ask clarifying questions as needed, and use your own example as needed.

SELF-RESPECT

Have a student read through the questions on Handout 29.2. Then say:

How will you feel about yourself after you ask? Do you typically ask for many things, or do you usually do things on your own? Can you ask without acting helpless?

Example:

Let's assume in this case that you don't ask your parents for things like this all the time. Let's also assume that you will retain your self-respect by asking directly without whining or yelling, even if they say no. So the answer to this question is yes: You can increase your intensity of asking, and therefore you would put a dime [or paper clip] in the bank.

Go around the room and ask students to identify whether or not making the request or saying no to a request will have an impact on their self-respect. If the students are not acting helpless and usually do things for themselves, then the answer to making a request is yes, and the dime (or paper clip) goes in the bank. If saying no to a request doesn't make the students feel worse about themselves, then the answer is no, and they put the dime (or paper clip) in the bank. Ask clarifying questions as needed, and use your own example as needed.

RIGHTS

Have a student read through the questions on Handout 29.2. Then say:

Is the person required by law or moral code to give you what you want?

Example:

In the piercing example, no, there is no law that says you have to get a piercing, so you would keep your dime. But if your parents were required by law to say yes to the piercing, then the answer to the question about rights would be yes, and you would add a dime [or paper clip] to the bank and increase your intensity of asking.

Go around the room and ask students to identify whether or not either they or the persons making the request of them are required by law or moral code to make the request. Ask clarifying questions as needed, and use your own example as needed.

AUTHORITY

Have a student read through the questions on Handout 29.2. Then say:

Are you responsible for directing the person or telling the person what to do?

Example:

In the piercing example, no, actually, it is the opposite. So you would keep your dime [or paper clip]. If a person making a request of you does not have authority over you, then your answer would be no, and you would put a dime [or paper clip] in the bank. This would increase your intensity of saying no to the request.

Go around the room and ask students to identify whether or not either they or the person making the request has the authority to make the request. Ask clarifying questions as needed, and use your own example as needed. (With the piercing example, a student may argue that the student who wants the piercing has authority over his or her own body. Although this is true, the student needs the parents' written permission to get the piercing; therefore, the parents have authority over the student.)

RELATIONSHIP

Have a student read through the questions on Handout 29.2. Then say:

Is asking appropriate to the current relationship?

Example:

In the piercing example, yes, since you are a minor, you need your parents' written permission in order to get the piercing from a reputable place. So you would add a dime [or paper clip] to your bank. Let's assume for a moment, however, that you are asking your 22-year-old brother's permission (and that he is not your legal guardian). Would that be appropriate to the relationship? In this case, no, it would not be. So your answer for this factor in this case would be no, and you would not put a dime [or paper clip] in your bank.

Go around the room and ask students to identify whether or not either the request they are making or the request being made of them is appropriate to the relationship. Ask clarifying questions as needed, and use your own example as needed.

LONG-TERM VERSUS SHORT-TERM GOALS

Have a student read through the questions on Handout 29.2. Then say:

How will asking now affect the relationship in the long run?

Example:

In the piercing example, will not asking for the piercing now maintain the peace in the short term, but be likely to cause more frustration later? The answer is no: If you don't ask now, it won't cause more problems later. So you would keep your dime [or paper clip], and your intensity of asking would not increase.

Ask for examples of situations where a person may give in to keep the short-term peace, although it may cause frustration or resentment later. Or you can use these examples:

- *A friend, Linh, asks you to let her copy your homework for geometry at least once or twice a week. She asks you again today. Although you are frustrated with her copying your work, you know she will start saying bad things about you to your friends if you don't give in.*
- *You really want to go to the football game on Friday night with your friends, but your mom usually has you babysit on Friday nights because that is your parents' date night. You think that if you ask her to give up her date night with your father, she will get angry or complain that she never gets time for herself. However, you know if you miss out on another Friday night event with your friends, you are going to be really angry at your parents for a long time (and probably will not be very nice to your younger siblings).*

Go around the room and ask students to identify whether or not making the request or saying no to a request is likely to keep the peace in the short term, but to create problems later. Ask clarifying questions as needed, and use your own example as needed.

GIVE AND TAKE

Have a student read through the questions on Handout 29.2. Then say:

In your relationship with this person, do you give as much as you are asking for?

Example:

In the piercing example, let's say that you clean the table and do the dishes after dinner each night, and you babysit your younger siblings on the weekends when your parents ask you to. So your answer would be yes, and you would add a dime [or paper clip] to your bank.

Go around the room and ask students to identify whether or not they have reciprocal relationships with the other persons, meaning, "Do I do as much for them when they ask me as I ask of them?" Ask clarifying questions as needed, and use your own example as needed.

HOMEWORK

Have a student read through the questions on Handout 29.2. Then say:

> *When you are making a request, "doing your homework" includes having all the necessary information needed to make the request and making both your request and goals clear to the person you are asking. If you have done all your homework and your request is clear, then your answer is yes, and you would put a dime [or paper clip] in your bank. If you are saying no to someone, then you want to ask yourself whether the request being made of you is clear, so that you know exactly what is being asked of you. If the request is not clear, your answer to this question is no, and you would put a dime [or paper clip] in the bank.*

Example:

> *In the piercing example, do you know all the facts you need to know to support your request? Let's assume that you have looked into different places, that you have checked prices, and that you have obtained all the information about keeping a piercing safe and healthy and avoiding infection. Let's also assume that the piercing you want is a small gold ball on the left side of your nose. You will provide a picture of the type of piercing you are requesting.*

Go around the room and ask students to identify whether or not either they or the persons making the request have done all their homework and whether the request is clear. Ask clarifying questions as needed. (For example, if the piercing example does not include information about the type of piercing and where the student wants it, the parents will not know what they were being asked. The parents may assume that the student wants an ear or tongue piercing, and may have a different reaction based on this assumption.)

TIMING

Have a student read through the questions on Handout 29.2. Then say:

> *Is this a good time to ask?*

Example:

> *In the piercing example, let's assume that you just got good grades on the latest progress report, so your parents are happy with you and are in a good mood right now. But when do you think might not be a good time to ask for something or say no?*

Allow students to generate multiple examples of good times and bad times to ask for something or to say no to something. In the piercing example, the parents may be happy with the student for getting good grades, but if the parents have just finished having an argument or are experiencing increased stress right now because they are cleaning the house for a party, then it might not be a good time.

Once all 10 factors have been reviewed with the students, have everyone add up all of the yes or no responses for the example used. For instance, for the piercing example, there are six yes responses. Turn back to Handout 29.1 and read the intensity for the corresponding number. For an intensity level of 6, the student who wants the piercing should "ask confidently; take no." Have students count their dimes (or paper clips) in the bank and determine the intensity of how strongly they should ask or say no to a request.

Now ask:

Do you think it is always as simple as this to determine how to ask a question? Do you think that some factors sometimes outweigh other factors?

Allow students to answer, and then continue:

Sometimes we need to make a wise mind adjustment by going up or down in intensity, depending on the weight of some factors. For instance, in the piercing example, you may want to go back and see whether any of the factors should be weighed more than the others. For timing, yes, it may be a good time to ask because we have assumed that you have good grades and that your parents are in a good mood. However, you may also be aware that your father has just learned he has to spend money on getting the car fixed, so money may be an issue. Once you know that, you may weigh timing a little higher than the other factors and decrease your intensity. So now your intensity rating may be a 5, which says I should "Ask gracefully [rather than confidently], but take no."

Ask the students whether they have any questions about this. Then have the students go through their own examples and make wise mind adjustments as needed. Allow some students to share any adjustments they have made. Remind all students about the importance of listening to wise mind when doing this activity.

Lesson Summary (3 minutes)

State:

Being interpersonally effective requires thinking through whether it is appropriate to ask for something or to say no to a request. The 10 factors we have learned in this lesson give us a way to approach the question of how strongly to ask for something or to say no.

Briefly review the 10 factors as needed. If time allows, have one or two students model the intensity of how they will ask or say no, based on the results of the exercise.

Homework Assignment (2 minutes)

Handout 29.3. Interpersonal Effectiveness: Figuring Out How Strongly to Ask or Say No

Explain:

> *Use Handout 29.3 to review the 10 factors we have learned today and determine your intensity again. You can also go through this handout again if another situation occurs this week.*

Homework 29.4. Interpersonal Effectiveness: Using Interpersonal Effectiveness Skills at the Same Time

Explain:

> *The second part of your homework assignment is to practice the DEAR MAN, GIVE, and FAST skills with the example you used today in class or the one you use for Handout 29.3 if another situation occurs, and to report back to us next week on how it went. Write down the scenario and what you said and did for each skill.*
>
> *Finally, remember that the Interpersonal Effectiveness Test is also next week, so review all the skills in this module in addition to the mindfulness skills.*

Diary Cards

Distribute new diary cards to the students. Highlight that they have now learned the skill of evaluating options, and that when they practice this skill for their homework, they are to circle the days and rate the skill use for the week on the diary card (along with the other skills that they have been taught).

Finally, do some troubleshooting: Ask students whether they have any questions about the homework or any obstacles to completing it. If so, answer the questions and address the obstacles. Obstacles may include, but are not limited to, the following: Students have no intention of doing the assignment, have too much other homework this week, are likely to forget, or don't understand the assignment. Help students to identify their obstacles, and work with them to make a plan to overcome them. Examples include encouraging a student to write down the assignment and set a reminder in a cell phone or calendar to complete it; discussing why a student has no intention of doing the homework, and working on increasing his or her motivation and the relevance of the assignment (e.g., grades); or clarifying any other points. Troubleshooting should be done each week after the homework is assigned.

Interpersonal Effectiveness
Interpersonal Effectiveness Test

SUMMARY

The purpose of this final lesson is for students to demonstrate what they have learned in the Interpersonal Effectiveness module and to assess for areas of weakness that may need review.

MATERIALS

1. Interpersonal Effectiveness Test (make enough copies for the whole class).
2. Diary cards: Have blank diary cards available to distribute at the end of class.
3. Pens and/or pencils for the students.

PREPARATION

1. Arrange desks as usual for taking exams.
2. Review the Interpersonal Effectiveness Test in order to be able to answer any questions students may have.

LESSON OVERVIEW AND TIMELINE

- Mindfulness exercise (5 minutes)
    - Observing/wise mind: Breathing in "Wise," breathing out "Mind" (3 minutes)
    - Describing observations of the exercise (2 minutes)
- Homework review (10 minutes)
    - Handout 29.3. Interpersonal Effectiveness: Figuring Out How Strongly to Ask or Say No

- Homework 29.4. Interpersonal Effectiveness: Using Interpersonal Effectiveness Skills at the Same Time
  - Sharing in small groups
  - Sharing with class
- Diary cards
- Module and test review (5 minutes)
- Administration of test (28 minutes)
- Distribution of diary cards (2 minutes)

DETAILED LESSON PLAN

Mindfulness Exercise (5 minutes)

Observing/Wise Mind: Breathing in "Wise," Breathing out "Mind" (3 minutes)

Welcome the class. Explain:

> *Because today is a test day, for mindfulness we are going to do an exercise we have done before to observe our breath and access wise mind. We are going to try to find that still point within us, focusing on the present moment while we breathe in the word "Wise" and breathe out the word "Mind." As we inhale, we are going to say the word "Wise" to ourselves, and as we exhale, we are going to say the word "Mind" to ourselves. This is a practice we can use whenever we need to access wise mind. Since our breath is always with us, we can use this practice anywhere as well. You may find yourself practicing this today either before or during this test or any test on any day. Skill in accessing wise mind comes with regular practice. Again, if thoughts or judgments come up, notice them and then just let them go, returning to your wise mind breathing.*

Continue:

> *When I say 1, that's the signal to sit in the mindful/wide-awake position we are familiar with by now. This means keeping our feet flat on the floor, sitting up straight, and putting our hands in our laps. For this exercise, we will keep our eyes open with a soft gaze, looking forward and down, but at nothing in particular. If you notice any urge to move, other than blinking or swallowing, notice it without acting on it, and return to your breath. When I say 2, that's the signal to take a deep breath. When I say 3, that's the signal to begin the practice. I'll say, "Stop," to end it.*

Now start the practice by counting to 3.

> *1: Get yourself into the mindful/wide-awake position. 2: Take a deep breath. 3: Begin the practice.*

After 2 minutes, say, "Stop."

Describing Observations of the Exercise (2 minutes)

Have students share an observation in the moment. Provide feedback about observations as needed, ensuring that each statement consists of something a student can observe and describe nonjudgmentally (e.g., I noticed the urge to move my body, I noticed I held my breath between inhaling and exhaling, I noticed a thought about how this was different from last week, I noticed a thought . . . , I noticed the sensation . . . , I noticed my mind wandering to other thoughts. I had lots of thoughts about how this could be helpful to me, I noticed I liked last week's practice better, I noticed I was uncomfortable so had to move . . .).

Homework Review (10 minutes)

Handout 29.3. Interpersonal Effectiveness: Figuring Out How Strongly to Ask or Say No
Homework 29.4. Interpersonal Effectiveness: Using Interpersonal Effectiveness Skills at the Same Time

SHARING IN SMALL GROUPS

Have students divide into small groups of three. Explain:

> *Each of you is first going to report on the practice of using the 10 factors to determine the intensity of asking for or saying no to someone. Second, each of you is to report on your use of the DEAR MAN, GIVE, and FAST skills for either last week's example or the one used in the 10 factors and describe the intensity you used to ask or say no. How did it go?*

Walk around and listen to the groups, offering feedback and answering questions as needed.

SHARING WITH THE CLASS

Ask two or three students to share their homework with the whole class. Choose at least one person who completed the homework, as well as at least one student who reported not completing the homework or struggling with the assignment. Provide feedback and coaching to the student(s) who had difficulty on how to improve the skill practice.

Troubleshoot with any students who did not complete the homework what may have been in their way and how they will complete the homework this week.

Diary Cards

Ask all students to turn in their diary cards and homework sheets to be reviewed. This is the last of the lessons; thus comment on the amount of skill use you have seen, especially compared to skill use at the beginning of the curriculum.

Module and Test Review (5 minutes)

Answer students' questions about the material presented in the Interpersonal Effectiveness module (and remind them that the test will also include a few questions about the Mindfulness module) before you distribute the test.

Administration of Test (28 minutes)

Administer the Interpersonal Effectiveness Test.

Distribution of Diary Cards (2 minutes)

Distribute new diary cards to students after they have turned in their tests. Say to them:

> *Congratulations! You have completed the entire DBT STEPS-A curriculum! Although completing diary cards is no longer required, I want to encourage all of you to continue completing these cards in order to remind yourself regularly of all the skills you have learned in this class. I also hope that you continue to use your skills and refer to your handouts and homework sheets for help with the skills. Remember, these are skills that we all need to use every day of our lives in order to be effective!*

Distress Tolerance Test

Name: _____

Note: Although the test mainly covers the distress tolerance skills, it also includes some questions on mindfulness skills.

1. Fill in the three states of mind:

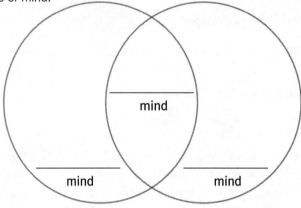

2. Name the "what" skills and explain how you would use them.

3. Name "how" skills and explain how you use them.

(continued)

4. Distress tolerance skills are: (circle one)

    a. Skills for interacting effectively with other people.

    b. Skills for getting through a difficult situation without making it worse.

    c. Skills for finding your wise mind.

    d. Skills for accepting and tolerating urges to act on your emotions in distressing situations.

5. Name the two types of distress tolerance skills.

    a. _____

    b. _____

Mnemonic Quiz

6. TIP your body chemistry:

    T_____

    I_____

    P_____

7. IMPROVE the moment:

    I_____

    M_____

    P_____

    R_____

    O_____

    V_____

    E_____

8. Describe the purpose of the self-soothing skills, and give an example of each.

    Purpose: _____

    _____

    _____

    _____

    a. _____

    _____

    b. _____

    _____

    c. _____

    _____

(continued)

d. _____

_____

e. _____

_____

f. _____

_____

9. What system is activated when we use the TIP skills to change the intensity of our emotions?

_____

10. What are the five key components to maximizing the effectiveness of managing extreme emotions by using temperature?

a. _____

b. _____

c. _____

d. _____

e. _____

11. Situation: You are walking down the hall at school, heading to take an exam that is worth 90% of your grade for a class you need to graduate, and you get a call from your mom that your dog has just been hit by a car and died. You want to leave school and skip your exam. Using your distress tolerance skills other than pros and cons, what would you do?

(continued)

12. Complete the pros-and-cons table below, based on the scenario in question 11. Decision 1 is staying in class and taking the exam; Decision 2 is leaving school and skipping the exam.

	Pros	Cons
Decision 1: Avoiding Impulsive Behavior		
Decision 2: Engaging in Impulsive Behavior		

Distress Tolerance Test Answer Key

1. Fill in the three states of mind:

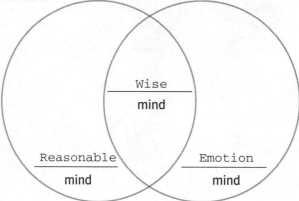

2. Name the "what" skills and explain how you would use them.

   The "what" skills are observing, describing, and participating. The description of how to use them needs to include that each of these skills has to be used one at a time.

3. Name "how" skills and explain how you use them.

   The "how" skills are nonjudgmentally, one-mindfully, and effectively. The description of how to use them needs to include that they can be used simultaneously.

4. Distress tolerance skills are: (circle one)
   a. Skills for interacting effectively with other people.
   b. Skills for getting through a difficult situation without making it worse.
   c. Skills for finding your wise mind.
   d. Skills for accepting and tolerating urges to act on your emotions in distressing situations.

5. Name the two types of distress tolerance skills.

   a. Crisis survival skills

   b. Reality acceptance skills

(continued)

Mnemonic Quiz

6. TIP your body chemistry:

Temperature

Intense exercise

Paced breathing

7. IMPROVE the moment:

Imagery

Meaning

Prayer

Relaxation

One thing in the moment

Vacation

Encouragement

8. Describe the purpose of the self-soothing skills, and give an example of each.

Purpose: To engage in behaviors that one would consider loving, soothing, and enjoyable during times of emotional distress.

a. Seeing

b. Hearing

c. Tasting

d. Touching

e. Smelling

f. Movement

Refer to Handout 7.1 for examples of skills.

9. What system is activated when we use the TIP skills to change the intensity of our emotions?

Parasympathetic nervous system (PNS)

(continued)

10. What are the five key components to maximizing the effectiveness of managing extreme emotions by using temperature?

   a. <u>Cold</u>

   b. <u>Wet</u>

   c. <u>Face</u>

   d. <u>Bend over</u>

   e. <u>Hold breath</u>

11. Situation: You are walking down the hall at school, heading to take an exam that is worth 90% of your grade for a class you need to graduate, and you get a call from your mom that your dog has just been hit by a car and died. You want to leave school and skip your exam. Using your distress tolerance skills, what would you do?

   ```
   Answer may include the use of various crisis survival skills in
   order to tolerate the urge to leave school and skip the exam; and/
   or the use of radical acceptance of the facts that there is nothing
   that the student can do right now to help the dog, and that he or
   she won't be able to retake the exam.
   ```

12. Complete the pros-and-cons table below, based on the scenario in question 11. Decision 1 is staying in class and taking the exam; Decision 2 is leaving school and skipping the exam.

   ```
   Answers should include both short-term and long-term consequences,
   and should also include the impact on emotions. Below is only an
   example of possible answers.
   ```

	Pros	**Cons**
Decision 1: Avoiding Impulsive Behavior	• Won't fail exam. • Keeps me in line for graduation. • Won't have to see my dog in injured state.	• Won't be able to see my dog. • Others may see me crying. • Too hard to focus on the exam. • Have to experience my sadness. • Won't be able to concentrate on the test.
Decision 2: Engaging in Impulsive Behavior	• Others won't see me crying. • Get to see my dog. • Don't have to focus on the exam while I am distracted by my dog dying.	• Will miss the exam. • Won't graduate on time. • My mother will be angry at me for skipping the exam. • My teacher may be angry at me for skipping the exam. • I might not be able to retake the exam. • I will feel shame for skipping the exam.

Emotion Regulation Test

Name: _____

Note: Although the test mainly covers the emotion regulation skills, it also includes some questions on mindfulness skills.

1. What are the three "what" skills? (circle one)
   a. Observing, describing, effectively
   b. Observing, one-mindfully, nonjudgmentally
   c. Participating, describing, observing
   d. Nonjudgmentally, one-mindfully, effectively

2. Wordless watching is part of which skill? (circle one)
   a. Describing
   b. Nonjudgmentally
   c. Observing
   d. Wise mind

3. Focusing on what works is part of which skill? (circle one)
   a. Participating
   b. Wise mind
   c. Nonjudgmentally
   d. Effectively

(continued)

4. Fill in the labels for the model of emotions: Model of Emotions

Inside the Body

Outside the Body

(continued)

5. Pick and circle an emotion (joy, love, sadness, anger, fear, shame). Then fill in the blanks:

   a. A prompting event for this emotion could be _____.

   b. An interpretation of this could be _____.

   c. The experience of this emotion is _____.

   d. The expression of this emotion is _____.

   e. The aftereffects of this emotion are _____.

6. List the three functions of emotions.

   a. _____

   b. _____

   c. _____

7. Challenging black-and-white thinking or catastrophic thoughts is a step in which skill?

   _____

   _____

8. If you are going to focus on Accumulating positive experiences, you will: (circle one)

   a. Identify at least one pleasurable activity to enjoy daily.

   b. Identify your values.

   c. Engage in behaviors that increase your confidence in yourself and make you think you are competent.

   d. All of the above.

   e. Only a or b.

9. What is the most important thing to identify when using the skill of Coping ahead? (circle one)

   a. The prompting event.

   b. The best possible outcome.

   c. The most likely outcome.

   d. The threat.

   e. None of the above.

10. List and describe the skills for reducing vulnerability to emotion mind by taking care of your body.

    _____

    _____

    _____

    _____

    _____

    _____

    _____

(continued)

11. What are the action urge and opposite action for each of the following emotions when the emotion *does not* fit the facts?

Emotion	Action urge	Opposite action
1. Fear		
2. Guilt		
3. Sadness		
4. Anger		

12. In general, when is it the appropriate time to use problem-solving skills?

_____

_____

_____

13. In the Distress Tolerance module, we learned that sometimes it is important to distract from our emotions. In the Emotion Regulation module, we learned that sometimes it is important to sit with and experience our emotions. Name the emotion regulation skill we would use to sit with our emotion, and describe when we should use the emotion regulation skill of experiencing the emotion over the distress tolerance skill of distracting from it.

_____

_____

_____

_____

_____

_____

_____

_____

_____

_____

Emotion Regulation Test Answer Key

1. What are the three "what" skills? (circle one)

    a. Observing, describing, effectively

    b. Observing, one-mindfully, nonjudgmentally

    c. Participating, describing, observing

    d. Nonjudgmentally, one-mindfully, effectively

2. Wordless watching is part of which skill? (circle one)

    a. Describing

    b. Nonjudgmentally

    c. Observing

    d. Wise mind

3. Focusing on what works is part of which skill? (circle one)

    a. Participating

    b. Wise mind

    c. Nonjudgmentally

    d. Effectively

4. Fill in the labels for the model of emotions:

    Refer to Handout 16.1 for the labels to the model of emotions.

5. Pick and circle an emotion (joy, love, sadness, anger, fear, shame). Then fill in the blanks:

    Refer to Handout 16.2 for ways to describe emotions.

6. List the three functions of emotions.

    a. Emotions motivate and prepare us for action.

    b. Emotions communicate to and influence others.

    c. Emotions communicate and provide information to ourselves.

7. Challenging black-and-white thinking or catastrophic thoughts is a step in which skill?

    Checking the facts

(continued)

8. If you are going to focus on <u>A</u>ccumulating positive experiences, you will: (circle one)
   a. Identify at least one pleasurable activity to enjoy daily.
   b. Identify your values.
   c. Engage in behaviors that increase your confidence in yourself and make you think you are competent.
   d. All of the above.
   e. Only a or b.

9. What is the most important thing to identify when using the skill of Coping ahead? (circle one)
   a. The prompting event.
   b. The best possible outcome.
   c. The most likely outcome.
   d. The threat.
   e. None of the above.

10. List and describe the skills for reducing vulnerability to emotion mind by taking care of your body.

    PL: Treat <u>P</u>hysica<u>L</u> Illness—if you are sick, get treatment.

    E: Balance <u>E</u>ating—not too much or too little.

    A: <u>A</u>void mood-altering drugs—don't use drugs or alcohol.

    S: Balance <u>S</u>leep—not too much or too little.

    E: Get <u>E</u>xercise—get at least 20 minutes per day.

11. What are the action urge and opposite action for each of the following emotions when the emotion *does not* fit the facts?

Emotion	Action urge	Opposite action
1. Fear	Escape or avoiding	Approach
2. Guilt	Overpromise not to do it again; disclaim all responsibility; hide; beg forgiveness	Don't apologize or try to make up for it; change body posture; do the behavior repeatedly
3. Sadness	Withdraw; become passive; isolate	Get active
4. Anger	Attack	Gently avoid Be a little nicer to person. Put yourself in the other person's shoes.

(continued)

12. In general, when is it the appropriate time to use problem-solving skills?

    When the emotion fits the facts (or is justified).

13. In the Distress Tolerance module, we learned that sometimes it is important to distract from our emotions. In the Emotion Regulation module, we learned that sometimes it is important to sit with and experience our emotions. Name the emotion regulation skill we would use to sit with our emotion, and describe when we should use the emotion regulation skill of experiencing the emotion over the distress tolerance skill of distracting from it.

    Mindfulness to current emotions (the wave skill): It is effective
    to distract from our emotions and their action urges when we need
    to get through a difficult situation without making it worse. For
    example, we might need to distract from emotions when we are about
    to take a test. It is also important to allow ourselves to
    experience emotions by using mindfulness to current emotions—
    that is, mindfully observing an emotion and the physical sensations
    associated with the emotion. We must learn to experience our
    emotions, so we learn that emotions are not catastrophic and that
    they can be tolerated.

Interpersonal Effectiveness Test

Name: _____

Although the test mainly covers the interpersonal effectiveness skills, it also includes some questions on mindfulness skills.

Mnemonic Quiz

1. DEAR

    D_____.

    E_____.

    A_____.

    R_____.

2. MAN:

    M_____.

    A_____.

    N_____.

3. GIVE:

    G_____.

    I_____.

    V_____.

    E_____.

4. FAST:

    F_____.

    A_____.

    S_____.

    T_____.

(continued)

5. The DEAR MAN skills focus on what priority? _____, which entails _____ and _____.

6. The FAST skills focus on what priority? _____.

7. List and describe 7 of the 10 factors to consider when determining the intensity of your DEAR MAN skills.

   a. _____ _____

   b. _____ _____

   c. _____ _____

   d. _____ _____

   e. _____ _____

   f. _____ _____

   g. _____ _____

8. Situation: Your friend borrowed your favorite DVD and then returned it with a scratch so deep that it skips. You feel that your friend should buy you a replacement DVD, only you are nervous about his or her reaction if you bring it up. You have the money to replace it yourself, but then you can't afford to go to the movie that you wanted to see this weekend if you do that. Using your wise mind, rank your interpersonal effectiveness priorities. Then describe how you will skillfully address the situation by using your interpersonal skills and what you will say to your friend, keeping in mind your goals. Also name the skills that you would use.

   Priorities:

   a. _____
   _____

   b. _____
   _____

   c. _____
   _____

   Description and skills used:

   _____

   _____

   _____

   _____

   _____

   _____

   _____

   _____

   _____

   _____

(continued)

9. Situation: It is the day of a big test at school. Your friend wants you to ditch class to go to the mall. This is a new friend, so you are really trying to make sure that this person likes you—but you also know that this is a big test in your class, and that you need to do well on it to keep from failing the class. Using your wise mind, describe how you are going to handle this situation by using your interpersonal effectiveness skills and what you will say to your friend, keeping in mind your goals. Also name the skills that you would use.

_____

_____

_____

_____

_____

_____

_____

_____

_____

_____

_____

10. Situation: You just received your homework assignment back from your teacher and were given a failing grade. You know that you didn't do your best on the assignment, but you are thinking, "What a jerk this teacher is," and "I am the worst student in the world." Now the teacher is handing out a pop quiz. Using your mindfulness "how" skills, describe how you are going to participate fully in the quiz.

_____

_____

_____

_____

_____

_____

_____

_____

_____

_____

_____

Interpersonal Effectiveness Test Answer Key

Mnemonic Quiz

1. DEAR:

   <u>D</u>escribe

   <u>E</u>xpress

   <u>A</u>ssert

   <u>R</u>einforce

2. MAN:

   <u>M</u>indful

   <u>A</u>ppear confident

   <u>N</u>egotiate

3. GIVE:

   (be) <u>G</u>entle

   (act) <u>I</u>nterested

   <u>V</u>alidate

   (use an) <u>E</u>asy (manner)

4. FAST:

   (be) <u>F</u>air

   (no) <u>A</u>pologies

   <u>S</u>tick to values

   (be) <u>T</u>ruthful

5. The DEAR MAN skills focus on what priority? <u>Objectives effectiveness</u>, which entails <u>asking for what you want</u> and <u>saying no to things you don't want</u>.

6. The FAST skills focus on what priority?: <u>Self-respect effectiveness</u>.

7. List and describe the 7 of the 10 factors to consider when determining the intensity of your DEAR MAN skills.

   See Handout 29.2 for the names and desscriptions of all 10 factors.

(continued)

8. Situation: Your friend borrowed your favorite DVD and then returned it with a scratch so deep that it skips. You feel that your friend should buy you a replacement DVD, only you are nervous about his or her reaction if you bring it up. You have the money to replace it yourself, but then you can't afford to go to the movie that you wanted to see this weekend if you do that. Using your wise mind, rank your interpersonal effectiveness priorities. Then describe how you will skillfully address the situation by using your interpersonal skills and what you will say to your friend, keeping in mind your goals. Also name the skills that you would use.

   Priorities:

   > Priorities will vary, depending on the student's reading of the situation.

   Description and skills used:

   > A correct answer will employ the GIVE, FAST, and/or DEAR MAN skills and should match the priorities the student has listed above.

9. Situation: It is the day of a big test at school. Your friend wants you to ditch class to go to the mall. This is a new friend, so you are really trying to make sure that this person likes you—but you also know that this is a big test in your class, and that you need to do well on it to keep from failing the class. Using your wise mind, describe how you are going to handle this situation by using your interpersonal effectiveness skills and what you will say to your friend, keeping in mind your goals. Also name the skills that you would use.

   > The answers will vary; a wise mind decision should use the DEAR MAN skills, although some students may choose to answer using GIVE.

10. Situation: You just received your homework assignment back from your teacher and were given a failing grade. You know that you didn't do your best on the assignment, but you are thinking, "What a jerk this teacher is," and "I am the worst student in the world." Now the teacher is handing out a pop quiz. Using your mindfulness "how" skills, describe how you are going to participate fully in the quiz.

    > A correct answer will describe being one-mindful, letting go of judgments toward the self and the teacher and focusing on what works.

STUDENT HANDOUTS

Part III consists of handouts for the students participating in a DBT STEPS-A class. There are two different types of student handouts. The ones with the word "Handout" in their numbers are informational or work activity sheets corresponding to the designated lessons (e.g., Handouts 1.1 and 1.2 are the first two handouts in Lesson 1). The handouts with the word "Homework" in their numbers are designed for students to complete on their own outside of class (e.g., Homework 2.3 is the homework sheet for Lesson 2, to be reviewed early in Lesson 3). There may be several occasions where students begin to complete their homework sheets in class, but the majority of the homework sheets are designed for practicing the skills beyond the DBT STEPS-A classroom. Also included at the beginning of Part III is the student diary card, which lists all the skills that will be taught throughout the DBT STEPS-A curriculum.

DBT STEPS-A Skills Daily Diary Card

Name: _____ Date started: _____

Scale for determining effectiveness of the skills used:

0 = Not thought about or used	4 = Tried, could do it/them, but they didn't help
1 = Thought about, not used, didn't want to	5 = Tried, could use it/them, helped
2 = Thought about, not used, wanted to	6 = Didn't think about it, used it/them, didn't help
3 = Tried but couldn't use it/them	7 = Didn't think about it, used it/ them, helped

NS = Have not learned the skill

Circle Days Practiced	DBT STEPS-A Skills	Weekly Skills Use Rating/Comments
	MINDFULNESS	
M T W Th F Sa Su	1. Wise mind (balance between emotion mind and reasonable mind)	
M T W Th F Sa Su	2. Observe (just noticing the experience)—one of the "what" skills	
M T W Th F Sa Su	3. Describe (put words to the experience)—one of the "what" skills	
M T W Th F Sa Su	4. Participate (throwing yourself completely into it)—one of the "what" skills	
M T W Th F Sa Su	5. Nonjudgmentally (seeing but not evaluating; just the facts)—one of the "how" skills	
M T W Th F Sa Su	6. One-mindfully (being completely present)—one of the "how" skills	
M T W Th F Sa Su	7. Effectively (focusing on what works)—one of the "how" skills	
	DISTRESS TOLERANCE	
M T W Th F Sa Su	8. ACCEPTS (Activities, Contributing, Comparisons, Emotions, Pushing away, Thoughts, Sensations)	
M T W Th F Sa Su	9. IMPROVE (Imagery, Meaning, Prayer, Relaxation, One thing in the moment, Vacation, Encouragement)	
M T W Th F Sa Su	10. Self-Soothe (with five senses, plus movement)	
M T W Th F Sa Su	11. TIP (Temperature, Intense exercise, Paced breathing)	
M T W Th F Sa Su	12. Pros and cons	
M T W Th F Sa Su	13. Radical acceptance (freedom from suffering requires acceptance) ≠ approval	
M T W Th F Sa Su	14. Turning the mind (to the acceptance road); willingness (doing just what is needed)	
M T W Th F Sa Su	15. Mindfulness of current thoughts	

(continued)

363

DBT STEPS-A Skills Daily Diary Card *(page 2 of 2)*

Circle Days Practiced	DBT STEPS-A Skills	Weekly Skills Use Rating/Comments
	EMOTION REGULATION	
M T W Th F Sa Su	16. Describing emotions	
M T W Th F Sa Su	17. Check the facts	
M T W Th F Sa Su	18. Opposite action (acting opposite to your current emotion action urge)	
M T W Th F Sa Su	19. Problem solving	
M T W Th F Sa Su	20. Accumulate positives in the short term (daily pleasant events) and long term (values)	
M T W Th F Sa Su	21. Build mastery (doing things that make you feel competent and effective)	
M T W Th F Sa Su	22. Cope ahead (rehearsing a plan ahead of time so you are prepared to cope skillfully)	
M T W Th F Sa Su	23. *PLEASE* (reduce PhysicaL illness, balance Eating, Avoid mood-altering drugs, balance Sleep, Exercise daily)	
M T W Th F Sa Su	24. *Wave skill* (riding the wave of emotion—mindfulness of current emotion)	
	INTERPERSONAL EFFECTIVENESS	
M T W Th F Sa Su	25. Ranking priorities (objectives, relationship, self-respect)	
M T W Th F Sa Su	26. *DEAR MAN* (Describe, Express, Assert, Reinforce) (Mindful, Appear confident, Negotiate)	
M T W Th F Sa Su	27. *GIVE* (be Gentle, act Interested, Validate, use an Easy manner)	
M T W Th F Sa Su	28. *FAST* (be Fair, no Apologies, Stick to values, be Truthful)	
M T W Th F Sa Su	29. Evaluating options (low or high intensity for asking or saying no)	

General Guidelines

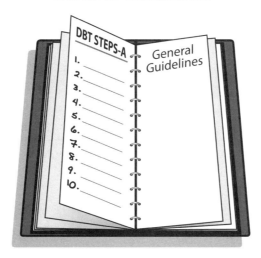

General school rules apply, including but not limited to the following:

1. Attend each class. Arrive on time.

2. Your binder includes all of the handouts and homework assignments for this course. You are expected to bring your binder to each class, with your homework completed.

3. Be nonjudgmental: No put-downs. Abusive language or behavior will not be tolerated.

4. What is discussed in the class stays in the class. Information about other people in the class may be private and should be respected.

5. We will identify target behaviors for each of us that you are willing to work on increasing or decreasing in class. We will refer to these identified behaviors as "target behaviors" in class, rather than naming the specific behaviors themselves.

Goals of DBT STEPS-A

Problems		Skills	
Behaviors to Decrease		**Behaviors to Increase**	
1. **Difficulty managing emotions** (fast, intense mood changes with little control, or a steady negative emotional state; your emotions control your actions)		1. **Emotion regulation skills**	
2. **Confusion: reduced awareness and focus (distraction)** (you are not always aware of what you are feeling, why you get upset, or what your goals are; and/or you have trouble staying focused)		2. **Mindfulness skills**	
3. **Impulsiveness** (acting without thinking it all through; escaping or avoiding emotions)		3. **Distress tolerance skills**	
4. **Relationship problems** (pattern of difficulty keeping relationships, getting what you want, keeping self-respect; loneliness)		4. **Interpersonal effectiveness skills**	

Goals for DBT STEPS-A: What are your goals?	
Behaviors to Decrease	**Behaviors to Increase**
1.	1.
2.	2.
3.	3.
4.	4.
5.	5.

(continued)

Where do you fall on each continuum of problems?

Place an X on each continuum for where you think you are. Sometimes people think that they fall on both sides of a continuum and rarely in the middle. If that is true for you, you can place two X's on the continuum.

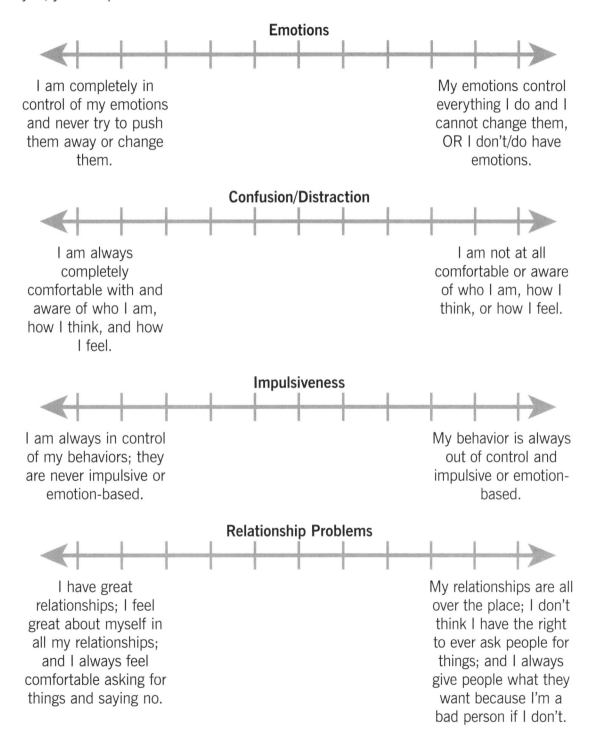

Emotions

I am completely in control of my emotions and never try to push them away or change them.

My emotions control everything I do and I cannot change them, OR I don't/do have emotions.

Confusion/Distraction

I am always completely comfortable with and aware of who I am, how I think, and how I feel.

I am not at all comfortable or aware of who I am, how I think, or how I feel.

Impulsiveness

I am always in control of my behaviors; they are never impulsive or emotion-based.

My behavior is always out of control and impulsive or emotion-based.

Relationship Problems

I have great relationships; I feel great about myself in all my relationships; and I always feel comfortable asking for things and saying no.

My relationships are all over the place; I don't think I have the right to ever ask people for things; and I always give people what they want because I'm a bad person if I don't.

Options for Solving Any Problem

When life presents you with problems, what are your options?

1. **Solve the Problem**

   Change the situation . . . OR avoid, leave, or get out of the situation for good.

2. **Feel Better about the Problem**

   Change (or regulate) your feelings about the problem.

3. **Tolerate the Problem**

   Accept and tolerate both the problem and your response to the problem.

4. **Stay Miserable**

   Or possibly make it worse!

DBT STEPS-A Skills to Use

1. *To Solve the Problem:*

   Use interpersonal effectiveness skills.

   Be dialectical.

   Use problem-solving skills (from emotion regulation skills).

2. *To Feel Better about the Problem:*

   Use emotion regulation skills.

3. *To Tolerate the Problem:*

   Use distress tolerance and mindfulness skills.

4. *To Stay Miserable:*

   Use NO skills.

Class Schedule

Lesson 1	Orientation
Lesson 2	Dialectics
Lesson 3	Mindfulness: Wise Mind
Lesson 4	Mindfulness: "What" Skills
Lesson 5	Mindfulness: "How" Skills
Lesson 6	Distress Tolerance: Introduction to Crisis Survival, and ACCEPTS
Lesson 7	Distress Tolerance: Self-Soothe and IMPROVE the Moment
Lesson 8	Distress Tolerance: TIP Skills for Managing Extreme Emotions
Lesson 9	Distress Tolerance: Pros and Cons
Lesson 10	Distress Tolerance: Introduction to Reality Acceptance Skills, and Radical Acceptance
Lesson 11	Distress Tolerance: Turning the Mind and Willingness
Lesson 12	Distress Tolerance: Mindfulness of Current Thoughts (and Distress Tolerance Test)
Lesson 13	Mindfulness: Wise Mind
Lesson 14	Mindfulness: "What" and "How" Skills
Lesson 15	Emotion Regulation: Goals of Emotion Regulation and Functions of Emotions
Lesson 16	Emotion Regulation: Describing Emotions
Lesson 17	Emotion Regulation: Check the Facts and Opposite Action
Lesson 18	Emotion Regulation: Problem Solving
Lesson 19	Emotion Regulation: The A of ABC PLEASE
Lesson 20	Emotion Regulation: The BC PLEASE of ABC PLEASE
Lesson 21	Emotion Regulation: The Wave Skill—Mindfulness of Current Emotions
Lesson 22	Emotion Regulation: Emotion Regulation Test
Lesson 23	Mindfulness: Wise Mind Review
Lesson 24	Mindfulness: "What" and "How" Skills Review
Lesson 25	Interpersonal Effectiveness: Goals and Overview
Lesson 26	Interpersonal Effectiveness: DEAR MAN Skills
Lesson 27	Interpersonal Effectiveness: GIVE Skills
Lesson 28	Interpersonal Effectiveness: FAST Skills
Lesson 29	Interpersonal Effectiveness: Evaluating Options for How Intensely to Ask or Say No
Lesson 30	Interpersonal Effectiveness: Interpersonal Effectiveness Test

Dialectics: What Is It? What's the Big Deal?

Dialectics teach us:

- There is always more than one way to see a situation and more than one way to solve a problem.
- All people have unique qualities and different points of view.
- Change is the only constant.
- Two things that seem like (or are) opposites can both be true.
- Trying to **honor the truth** on both sides of a conflict is the best approach. This does not mean giving up your values or selling out. Avoid seeing the world in "black-or-white," "all-or-nothing" ways. Trying to honor the truth on both sides does not mean compromise.

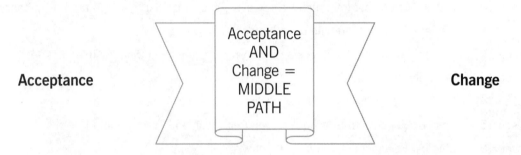

Acceptance

Acceptance
AND
Change =
MIDDLE
PATH

Change

Examples:

I am doing the best I can, **AND** I need to do better, try harder, and be more effective and more motivated to change.

I can do this, **AND** it's going to be hard.

My mom is strict, **AND** she really cares about me.

You are tough, **AND** you are gentle.

This perspective helps pave the way toward the middle path by helping you:

- Expand your thoughts and ways of considering life situations.
- "Unstick" standoffs and conflicts.
- Be more flexible and approachable.
- Avoid assumptions and blaming.

Adapted with permission from Rathus and Miller (2015). Copyright © The Guilford Press.

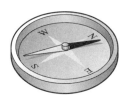

Dialectical Thinking: "How To" Guide

Hints for thinking and acting dialectically:

1. Move to "both–and" thinking and away from "either–or" thinking. Avoid extreme words, such as "always," "never," and "you make me." Be descriptive.
   a. Example: Instead of saying, "Everyone always treats me unfairly," say, "Sometimes I get treated fairly, AND at other times I am treated unfairly."

2. Practice looking at all sides of a situation and all points of view. Be generous and dig deep. Find the kernel of truth in every side by asking, "What is being left out?"
   a. Example: "Why does Mom want me to be home at 10 P.M.? Why do I want to stay out until midnight?

3. Remember: **no one** has the absolute truth. Be open to alternatives.

4. Use "I feel . . ." statements, instead of "You are . . .", "You should . . .", or "That's just the way it is" statements.
   a. Example: Say, "I feel angry when you say I can't stay out later just because you said so," instead of "You never listen, and you are always unfair to me."

5. Accept that different opinions can be valid, even if you do not agree with them: "I can see your point of view, even though I do not agree with it."

6. Check your assumptions. Do not assume that you know what others are thinking. "What did you mean when you said . . . ?"

7. Do not expect others to know what you are thinking: "What I am trying to say is . . ."

PRACTICE:

Circle the dialectical statements:
1. a. "It is hopeless. I just cannot do it."
   b. "This is easy . . . I got no problems."
   c. "This is really hard for me, and I am going to keep trying."
2. a. "I know I am right about this."
   b. "You are totally wrong about that, and I am right."
   c. "I can understand why you feel this way, and I feel differently."

Practice in Thinking and Acting Dialectically

Name: _____ Date: _____

Identify times this week when you did NOT think or act dialectically.

Situation 1: Briefly describe the situation (who, what, when): _____

_____

_____

_____

How did you think or act in this situation? _____

_____

_____

Describe both sides of the dialectic:

Side A   **Side B**

_____

_____

_____

_____

_____

_____

How can you honor both sides of the dialectic? _____

_____

_____

What was the outcome? _____

_____

_____

(continued)

Situation 2: Briefly describe the situation (who, what, when): _____

_____

_____

_____

How did you think or act in this situation? _____

_____

_____

Describe both sides of the dialectic:

Side A   **Side B**

_____

_____

_____

_____

_____

How can you honor both sides of the dialectic? _____

_____

_____

What was the outcome? _____

_____

_____

Mindfulness: Taking Hold of Your Mind

From: **To:**

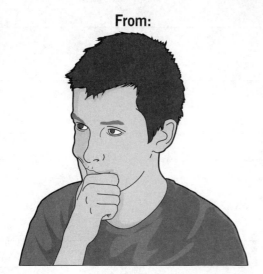

Mindfulness: Being in control of your mind, rather than letting your mind be in control of you.

1. **Full Awareness (Opened Mind):** Being aware of the present moment (i.e., thoughts, feelings, and physical sensations) without judgment and without trying to change it.

2. **Attentional Control (Focused Mind):** Staying focused on one thing at a time.

Practice, practice, practice!

Adapted with permission from Rathus and Miller (2015). Copyright © The Guilford Press.

Mindfulness: Why Bother?

Being mindful can:

1. Give you more choices and more control over your behavior.

2. Reduce your emotional suffering and increase your pleasure.

3. Help you make important decisions.

4. Help focus your attention and make you more effective and productive.

5. Increase your compassion for yourself and others.

6. Lessen your pain, tension, and stress, and even improve your health.

Practice, practice, practice!

Mindfulness: Three States of Mind

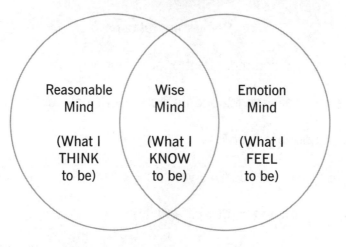

Emotion mind is "hot"—ruled by your feelings and urges.

Emotion mind is: _____

When I am in emotion mind, I . . . (please describe what you do or think): _____

_____

_____

Reasonable mind is "cool"—ruled by facts, reason, and logic.

Reasonable mind is: _____

When I am in reasonable mind, I . . . (please describe what you do or think): _____

_____

_____

Wise mind includes both reason and emotion—the wisdom within each person. It is the state of mind to access when you want to make an important decision.

Wise mind is: _____

When I am in wise mind, I . . . (please describe what you do or think): _____

_____

_____

Adapted with permission from Rathus and Miller (2015). Copyright © The Guilford Press.

_____

HANDOUT 3.4

Practicing Wise Mind

Mindfulness skills often require a lot of practice. Like any new skill, it is important to practice first when you don't need the skill. If you practice in easier situations, the skill will become automatic, and you will have it when you need it. Practice with your eyes closed and with your eyes open.

1. ☐ **Stone flake on the lake.** Imagine that you are by a clear blue lake on a beautiful sunny day. Then imagine that you are a small flake of stone, flat and light. Imagine that you have been tossed out onto the lake and are now gently, slowly, floating through the calm, clear blue water to the lake's smooth, sandy bottom.
   - Notice what you see, what you feel as you float down, perhaps in slow circles, floating toward the bottom. As you reach the bottom of the lake, settle your attention there within yourself.

2. ☐ **Walking down the spiral stairs.** Imagine that within you is a spiral staircase, winding down to your very center. Starting at the top, walk very slowly down the staircase, going deeper and deeper within yourself.
   - Notice the sensations. Rest by sitting on a step, or turn on lights on the way down if you wish. Do not force yourself further than you want to go. Notice the quiet. As you reach the center of yourself, settle your attention there—perhaps in your gut or your abdomen.

3. ☐ **Breathing "Wise" in, "Mind" out.** Breathing in, say to yourself, "Wise"; breathing out, say, "Mind."
   - Focus your entire attention on the word "Wise," then focus it again entirely on the word "Mind."
   - Continue until you sense that you have settled into wise mind.

4. ☐ **Asking: Is this wise mind?** Breathing in, ask yourself, "Is this [action, thought, plan, etc.] wise mind?"
   - Breathing out, listen for the answer.
   - Listen, but do not give yourself the answer. Do not tell yourself the answer; listen for it.
   - Continue asking during each inhale. If no answer comes, try again another time.

(continued)

Adapted with permission from Linehan (2015b). Copyright © Marsha M. Linehan.

From *DBT Skills in Schools: Skills Training for Emotional Problem Solving for Adolescents (DBT STEPS-A)* by James J. Mazza, Elizabeth T. Dexter-Mazza, Alec L. Miller, Jill H. Rathus, and Heather E. Murphy. Copyright © 2016 The Guilford Press. Permission to photocopy this material is granted to purchasers of this book for personal use or use with individual students (see copyright page for details). Purchasers can download additional copies of this material (see the box at the end of the table of contents).

377

5. ☐ **Expanding awareness.** Breathing in, focus your awareness on your center.
   - Breathing out, stay aware of your center, but expand awareness to the space you are in now.
   - Continue in the moment.

6. ☐ **Dropping into the pauses between inhaling and exhaling.**
   - Breathing in, notice the pause after inhaling (top of breath).
   - Breathing out, notice the pause after exhaling (bottom of breath).
   - At each pause, let yourself "fall into" the center space within the pause.

7. ☐ **Other wise mind practice ideas:** _____

_____

_____

_____

_____

_____

_____

_____

_____

_____

_____

_____

_____

Practice Observing Yourself in the Three States of Mind

Name: _____

Due Date: _____

Emotion mind

One example of emotion mind this week was (please describe your emotion[s], thoughts, behaviors): _____

_____

_____

Reasonable mind

One example of reasonable mind this week was (please describe your emotion[s], thoughts, behaviors): _____

_____

_____

Wise mind

One example of wise mind this week was (please describe your emotion[s], thoughts, behaviors): _____

_____

_____

_____

Mindfulness: "What Skills"

Observe

- Engage in wordless watching: Just notice the experience in the present moment.

- Watch your thoughts and feelings come and go, as if they are on a conveyor belt.

- Observe both inside and outside yourself, using all of your five senses.

- Have a "Teflon mind," letting experiences come into your mind and slip right out (not holding on).

- Don't push away your thoughts and feelings. Just let them happen, even when they are painful.

- *Note:* We cannot observe another's inner experience (e.g., "He's upset")—only external features (e.g., a tear rolling down a cheek) or our thoughts about another's experience ("I observed the thought, 'He's upset'").

Describe

- Put words on the experience. Label what you observe with words. Some examples are: "I feel sad," or "My face feels hot," or "I feel my heart racing."

- Describe only what you observe *without* interpretations. Stick to the facts! Instead of "That person has an attitude," you could describe that person as "rolling his [or her] eyes and speaking with a loud voice."

Participate

- Throw yourself into the present moment fully (e.g., dancing, cleaning, taking a test, feeling sad in the moment). Try not to worry about tomorrow or focus on yesterday.

- Become one with whatever you're doing: Get "into the zone."

- Fully experience your feelings without being self-conscious.

- Experience even negative emotions fully to help your wise mind make a decision about what to do (instead of acting impulsively).

Adapted with permission from Rathus and Miller (2015). Copyright © The Guilford Press.

Mindfulness: Observing Practice

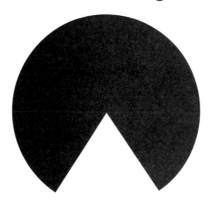

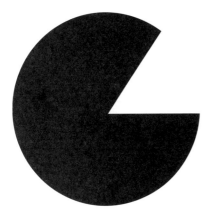
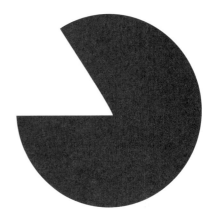

Reprinted with permission from Linehan (2015a). Copyright © Marsha M. Linehan.

Mindfulness: Practicing "What" Skills

Name: _____

Due Date: _____

Check off one "what" skill that you practiced during the week:

_____ Observe

_____ Describe   R W E

_____ Participate

Briefly describe your experience of using the skill during the week (include when and where you used it):

_____

_____

_____

_____

Briefly describe whether the skill affected your thoughts, feelings, or behaviors. If so, how?

_____

_____

_____

_____

If you did not complete this practice exercise, please explain why not/what interfered:

_____

_____

_____

_____

Adapted with permission from Rathus and Miller (2015). Copyright © The Guilford Press.

_____

Mindfulness: "How Skills"

Nonjudgmentally

- Notice, but don't evaluate or judge. Stick to the observable facts.
- Acknowledge the harmful and the helpful, but don't judge it. For example, replace "He's a jerk" with "He walked away while we were talking."
- You can't go through life without making judgments; your goal is to catch them so you have more control over your emotions.
- When you find yourself judging, don't judge your judging.

- Discriminating/differentiating judgments: _____

- Evaluating judgments: _____

- Three steps to being nonjudgmental:
  1. _____
  2. _____
  3. _____

One-Mindfully

- Stay focused: Focus your attention on *only* one thing in this moment. Slow yourself down to accomplish this.
- Stop doing two things at once (the opposite of multitasking).
- Concentrate your mind: Let go of distractions, and refocus your attention when it drifts, again and again.
- Stay focused so that the past, future, and current distractions don't get in your way.

Effectively

- Be effective: Focus on what works to achieve your goal.
- Don't let emotions control your behavior, cutting the cord between feeling and doing.
- Play by the rules (which may vary at home, school, work).
- Act as skillfully as you can to achieve your goals.
- Let go of negative feelings (e.g., vengeance and useless anger) and "shoulds" (e.g., "My teacher should have . . .") that can hurt you and make things worse.

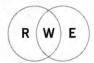

Mindfulness: Practicing "How" Skills

Name: _____

Due Date: _____

Check off one "how" skill that you practiced during the week:

_____ Nonjudgmentally

_____ One-mindfully

_____ Effectively

Briefly describe your experience of using the skill during the week (include when and where you used it):

_____

_____

_____

_____

Briefly describe whether the skill affected your thoughts, feelings, or behaviors. If so, how?

_____

_____

_____

_____

If you did not complete this practice exercise, please explain why not/what interfered:

_____

_____

_____

_____

Distress Tolerance:
Why Bother Coping with Painful Feelings and Urges?

Because . . .

1. Pain is part of life and can't always be avoided.

2. If you can't deal with your pain, you may act impulsively.

3. When you act impulsively, you may end up hurting yourself, hurting someone else, and not getting what you want.

Two Types of Distress Tolerance Skills

Crisis survival skills are for: _____

_____

_____

_____

Reality acceptance skills are for: _____

_____

_____

_____

Distress Tolerance: When to Use Crisis Survival Skills

YOU ARE IN A CRISIS when the situation is:

- Highly stressful.

- Short term (that is, it won't last a long time).

- Creating intense pressure to resolve the crisis *now.*

USE CRISIS SURVIVAL SKILLS when:

1. You have intense pain that cannot be helped quickly.

2. You want to act on your emotions, but it will only make things worse.

3. Emotion mind threatens to overwhelm you, and you need to stay skillful.

4. You are overwhelmed, yet demands must be met.

5. Your arousal is extreme, but your problems can't be solved immediately.

DON'T USE CRISIS SURVIVAL SKILLS for:

- Everyday problems.

- Solving all your life problems.

- Making your life worth living.

Adapted with permission from Linehan (2015b). Copyright © Marsha M. Linehan.

Distress Tolerance: Crisis Survival Skills

Skills for tolerating painful events and emotions when you cannot make things better right away and you don't want to make things worse!

DISTRACT with Wise Mind ACCEPTS

<u>A</u>ctivities
<u>C</u>ontributing
<u>C</u>omparisons
<u>E</u>motions
<u>P</u>ushing Away
<u>T</u>houghts
<u>S</u>ensations

SELF-SOOTHE with the Five Senses (plus Movement)

Vision
Hearing
Smell
Taste
Touch
Movement

IMPROVE the Moment

<u>I</u>magery
<u>M</u>eaning
<u>P</u>rayer
<u>R</u>elaxation
Do <u>O</u>ne thing at a time
take a <u>V</u>acation
provide <u>E</u>ncouragement

TIP Your Body Chemistry

<u>T</u>emperature
<u>I</u>ntense exercise
<u>P</u>aced breathing

Pros and Cons

Adapted with permission from Rathus and Miller (2015). Copyright © The Guilford Press.

Distress Tolerance:
Distract with Wise Mind ACCEPTS

Distract yourself with . . .

Activities   ***Do something.*** Call, email, or visit a friend; watch a favorite movie or TV show; play video games; write in a journal; clean your room; go for a walk or run; exercise intensely; read a book; listen to music, go online and download music or apps; play a game with yourself or others.

Contributing   ***Contribute to (or do something nice) for someone.*** Help a friend or sibling with homework; make something nice for someone else; give away things you don't need; surprise someone with a big hug, a note, or a favor; volunteer.

Comparisons   ***Compare yourself to those less fortunate.*** Compare how you are feeling now to a time when you were doing worse. Think about others who are coping the same as or less well than you.

Emotions   ***Create different emotions.*** Watch a funny TV show or emotional movie; listen to something soothing or to upbeat music; get active when you are sad; go to a store and read funny greeting cards or joke books.

Pushing away   ***Push the painful situation out of your mind temporarily.*** Leave the situation mentally by moving your attention and thoughts away; build an imaginary wall between you and the situation; put the pain in a box and on a shelf for a while.

Thoughts   ***Replace your thoughts.*** Read; do word or number puzzles; count numbers, colors in a poster, tiles on a wall, or anything else; repeat words to a song in your mind.

Sensations   ***Intensify <u>other</u> sensations.*** Hold or chew ice; listen to loud music; take a warm or cold shower; squeeze a stress ball; do sit-ups or push-ups; pet your dog or cat.

Adapted with permission from Rathus and Miller (2015). Copyright © The Guilford Press.

Distress Tolerance: Practicing Wise Mind ACCEPTS

Name: _____

Due Date: _____

Write down at least two specific ACCEPTS skills to practice during the week when you are experiencing a crisis or urge to act on an emotion (e.g., for Activities, play video games or the guitar; for Contributing, baking cookies for a neighbor).

Activities _____

Contributing _____

Comparisons _____

Emotions _____

Pushing away _____

Thoughts _____

Sensations _____

Briefly describe the stressful situation(s) you were in when you chose to practice your skills: _____

_____

_____

Did using the skills help you to (1) cope with uncomfortable feelings and urges and/or (2) avoid conflict of any kind? Circle   Yes   or   No.

If yes, please describe how it helped: _____

_____

If no, please describe why you believe it did not help: _____

_____

(continued)

_____

Write down your level of distress (emotional pain) before and after using your skill: 100 = No tolerance, life is a nightmare, high urges to act impulsively. 0 = Lots of tolerance, life is manageable, much lower urges.

Before: _____

After: _____

If you did not practice this skill, please explain why: _____

_____

_____

_____

_____

_____

_____

_____

_____

_____

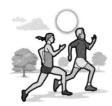

Distress Tolerance: Self-Soothe Skills

A good way to remember these skills is to think of soothing your five senses, plus movement:

Vision	**Hearing**
Smell	**Taste**
Touch	**Movement**

Vision   Go to your favorite place and take in all the sights; look at a photo album; "zone out" to a poster/picture; watch people; notice colors in a sunset.

Hearing   Listen to your favorite music and play it over and over again; pay attention to sounds in nature (birds, rain, thunder, traffic); play an instrument or sing; listen to a sound machine.

Smell   Put on your favorite lotion; light a scented candle; make cookies or popcorn; smell fresh-brewed coffee; go to the park and smell the roses.

Taste   Eat some of your favorite foods; drink your favorite nonalcoholic beverage; have your favorite flavor of ice cream; really notice the food you eat; eat one thing mindfully; don't overdo it!

Touch   Take a long bath or shower; pet your dog or cat; get a massage; brush your hair; hug or be hugged; put a cold cloth on your head; change into your most comfortable clothes.

Movement   Rock yourself gently; stretch; go for a run; do yoga or pilates; dance!

Adapted with permission from Rathus and Miller (2015). Copyright © The Guilford Press.

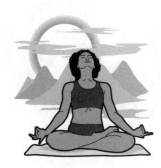

Distress Tolerance:

IMPROVE the Moment

"IMPROVE" the Moment with . . .

Imagery
Imagine a very relaxing scene. Imagine a calming, safe place. Imagine things going well; imagine coping well. Imagine painful emotions draining out of you like water out of a pipe.

Meaning
Find or create some purpose, meaning, or value in the pain. Make lemonade out of lemons!

Prayer
Open your heart to a supreme being, greater wisdom, or your own wise mind. Ask for strength to bear the pain in this moment.

Relaxation
Try muscle relaxing by tensing and relaxing each large muscle group, starting with the top of your head and then working down. Download a relaxation audio or video; stretch; take a bath; get a massage.

One thing at a time
Focus your entire attention on what you are doing right now. Keep your mind in the present moment. Be aware of body movements or sensations while you're walking, cleaning, eating.

Vacation
Give yourself a brief vacation. Get outside; take a short walk; go get your favorite coffee drink or smoothie; read a magazine or newspaper; surf the web; take a 1-hour breather from hard work that must be done. Unplug from all electronic devices.

Encouragement
Cheerlead yourself. Repeat over and over: "I can stand it," "It won't last forever," "I will make it through this," I am doing the best I can."

Distress Tolerance: Practicing IMPROVE the Moment

Name: _____

Due Date: _____

Write down ideas for practicing at least two specific IMPROVE skills during the week when you feel upset (e.g., Encouragement, Vacation).

Imagery _____

Meaning _____

Prayer _____

Relaxation _____

One thing at a time _____

Vacation _____

Encouragement _____

Briefly describe the stressful situation(s) you were in when you chose to practice your skills: _____

_____

_____

_____

Did using the skills help you to (1) cope with uncomfortable feelings and urges and/or (2) avoid conflict of any kind? Circle Yes or No.

If yes, please describe how it helped: _____

_____

_____

If no, please describe why you believe it did not help: _____

_____

_____

(continued)

Distress Tolerance: Practicing IMPROVE the Moment *(page 2 of 2)*

Write down your level of distress (emotional pain) before and after using your skill: 100 = No tolerance, life is a nightmare, high urges to act impulsively. 0 = Lots of tolerance, life is manageable, lower urges.

Before: _____

After: _____

If you did not practice this skill, please explain why: _____

_____

_____

_____

_____

_____

_____

_____

_____

_____

Distress Tolerance: Creating Your Crisis Survival Kit

Name: _____

Due Date: _____

List below 10 "tools" to go into your home crisis survival kit. Choose from your ACCEPTS skills, your self-soothe skills, and your IMPROVE skills. Take a shoebox, sturdy bag, or basket, and place the relevant items inside—for example, your iPod, a stress ball, your favorite scented lotion, perfume, or cologne, a picture of your favorite vacation spot, a favorite magazine, a crossword book, herbal tea bags, a favorite piece of candy, a relaxation CD or DVD.

1. _____

2. _____

3. _____

4. _____

5. _____

6. _____

7. _____

8. _____

9. _____

10. _____

Create a smaller version of your kit for school or work—one that fits in a pencil case or lunch box. Consider items that can be used at your desk—for example, multicolored rubber bands to stretch; paper and pens for doodling; a mini-pack of Play-Doh; a squeeze ball; Silly Putty; a list of visual stimuli in your class or office that can distract or soothe you; snacks to self-soothe; a list of friends, teachers, or counselors you can approach when you have a break.

1. _____

2. _____

3. _____

4. _____

Distress Tolerance: TIP Skills for Managing Extreme Emotions

Use these skills when emotional arousal is very high!

- You are completely caught in emotion mind.
- Your brain is not processing information.
- You are emotionally overwhelmed.

TIP your body chemistry to reduce extreme emotion mind quickly with:

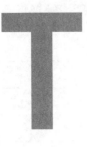

TEMPERATURE

Tip the temperature of your face with cold water to calm down fast.
Holding your breath, put your face in a bowl of cold water; keep water above 50°F. Or hold a cold pack or zipper-lock bag with ice water* on your eyes and cheeks, or splash cold water on your face. Hold for 30 seconds.

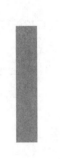

INTENSE EXERCISE

To calm down your body when it is revved up by emotion.
Engage in intense aerobic exercise, if only for a short while. Expend your body's stored-up physical energy by running, walking fast, jumping rope or jumping jacks, playing basketball, weightlifting, or putting on music and dance. Don't overdo it!

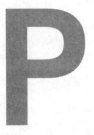

PACED BREATHING

Slow your pace of breathing way down (to about 5–7 in- and out-breaths per minute). Breathe deeply from the abdomen. Breathe out more slowly than you breathe in (e.g., 4 seconds in and 6 seconds out). Do this for 1–2 minutes to bring down your arousal.

*Ice water decreases your heart rate rapidly. Intense exercise will increase heart rate. If you have a heart or medical condition, have a lower base heart rate due to medications, take a beta blocker, or have an eating disorder, consult your health care provider before using these skills. Avoid ice water if you are allergic to the cold.

Adapted with permission from Rathus and Miller (2015). Copyright © The Guilford Press.

Distress Tolerance:
Using TIP Skills for Managing Extreme Emotions

Name: _____

Due Date: _____

Practice each TIP skill at least one time. Prepare yourself to use this skill when emotional arousal gets very high.

Rate your emotional arousal before you use the skill: 1–100: ____

Describe the situation you were in when you chose to practice the skill.

T

TEMPERATURE
Used ice or something cold to change emotions
Arousal: Before (0–100) ____   After (0–100) ____
Distress tolerance: After (0 = can't stand it; 5 = I can definitely survive) _____
What I did (describe) _____
_____

I

INTENSE EXERCISE
Arousal: Before (0–100) ____   After (0–100) ____
Distress tolerance: After (0 = can't stand it; 5 = I can definitely survive) _____
What I did (describe) _____
_____

P

PACED BREATHING
Arousal: Before (0–100) ____   After (0–100) ____
Distress tolerance: After (0 = can't stand it; 5 = I can definitely survive) _____
What I did (describe) _____
_____

Adapted with permission from Rathus and Miller (2015). Copyright © The Guilford Press.

Distress Tolerance: Pros and Cons

Select one crisis (emotionally upsetting situation) where you found it *really* hard to tolerate your distress, avoid destructive behavior, and/or not act impulsively.

Crisis I am faced with: _____

Crisis urges: _____

	Pros	Cons
Acting on crisis urges	Pros of acting on impulsive urges:	Cons of acting on impulsive urges:
Resisting crisis urges	Pros of resisting impulsive urges:	Cons of resisting impulsive urges:

1. **Consider short-term and long-term pros and cons.**
2. Before an overwhelming urge hits:
   a. Write out your pros and cons, and carry them with you.
3. When an overwhelming urge hits:
   a. Review your pros and cons.
   b. Imagine the positive consequences of resisting the urge.
   c. Imagine (and remember past) negative consequences of giving in to the urges.

Adapted with permission from Rathus and Miller (2015). Copyright © The Guilford Press.

Distress Tolerance: Practice with Pros and Cons

Name: _____

Due Date: _____

Select one crisis (emotionally upsetting situation) where you found it *really* hard to tolerate your distress, avoid destructive behavior, and/or not act on your urges.

Crisis I am faced with: _____

Crisis urges: _____

Directions:

1. Make a list for acting on crisis urges.
2. Make a second list for resisting crisis urges.
3. Weigh which side is "heavier"—the pros or cons—and act accordingly.
4. Think about how writing the pros and cons helped you to get into wise mind.
5. Remember to consider how the behavior affects you in the short term and long term.

	Pros	Cons
Acting on crisis urges	Pros of acting on impulsive urges:	Cons of acting on impulsive urges:
Resisting crisis urges	Pros of resisting impulsive urges:	Cons of resisting impulsive urges:

(continued)

Adapted with permission from Rathus and Miller (2015). Copyright © The Guilford Press.

1. **Consider short-term and long-term pros and cons.**
2. Before an overwhelming urge hits:
   a. Write out your pros and cons and carry them with you
3. When an overwhelming urge hits:
   a. Review your pros and cons.
   b. Imagine the positive consequences of resisting the urge.
   c. Imagine (and remember past) negative consequences of giving in to the urges.

Distress Tolerance: Overview of Reality Acceptance Skills

How to live a life that is not the life you want

Radical Acceptance

Turning the Mind

Willingness

Mindfulness of Current Thoughts

Adapted with permission from Linehan (2015b). Copyright © Marsha M. Linehan.

Distress Tolerance: Accepting Reality

*Many of our skills focus on changing your behavior in order to change the situation.
But when there is **no way** to change the situation . . .*

Accepting Reality: Choices We Can Make

Four things to do when a serious problem comes into your life:

1. Figure out how to solve the problem.
2. Change how you feel about the problem.
3. Accept it.
4. Stay miserable—or make things worse (by acting on your impulsive urges).

*When you can't solve the problem or change your emotions about the problem, try
acceptance as a way to reduce your suffering.*

Why Bother Accepting Reality?

✓ Rejecting reality does not change reality.
✓ Changing reality requires first accepting reality.
✓ Rejecting reality turns pain into suffering.
✓ Refusing to accept reality can keep you stuck in unhappiness, anger, shame,
   sadness, bitterness, or other painful emotions.

Radical Acceptance

✓ RADICAL ACCEPTANCE is the skill of accepting the things you cannot change.
✓ "RADICAL" = complete and total accepting in mind, heart, and body.
✓ "ACCEPTANCE" = seeing reality for what it is, even if you don't like it.
✓ Acceptance means to acknowledge, recognize, endure—not give up or give in.
✓ It is when you stop fighting reality, stop throwing tantrums about reality, and let go
   of bitterness. It is the opposite of "Why me?" It *is* "Things are as they are."
✓ Life can be worth living, even with painful events in it.

List one important thing that you need to accept in your life now: _____

_____

List one less important thing you need to accept this week: _____

_____

Distress Tolerance: Radical Acceptance, Step by Step

1. Observe that you are questioning or fighting reality ("It shouldn't be this way").

2. Remind yourself that the unpleasant reality is just as it is and cannot be changed ("This is what happened").

3. Remind yourself that there are causes for the reality. Acknowledge that some sort of history led up to this moment. Notice that given these causes and the history that led up to this moment, this reality had to occur just this way ("This is how things happened that made them this way").

4. Practice accepting with the whole self (mind, body, and spirit). Be creative in finding ways to involve your whole self. Use accepting self-talk, but also consider using relaxation, mindfulness of your breath, going to a place that helps bring you to acceptance, or imagery.

5. Practice opposite action. List all the behaviors you would do if you did accept the facts. Then act as if you have already accepted the facts. Engage in the behaviors that you would do if you really had accepted.

6. Cope ahead with events that seem unacceptable. Imagine (in your mind's eye) believing what you don't want to accept. Rehearse in your mind what you would do if you accepted what seems unacceptable.

7. Attend to your body sensations as you think about what you need to accept.

8. Allow disappointment, sadness, or grief to arise within you.

9. Acknowledge that life can be worth living, even when there's pain.

10. Do pros and cons if you find yourself resisting practicing acceptance.

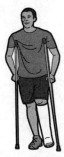

Distress Tolerance: Choosing Things
for Radical Acceptance Practice

Name: _____

Due Date: _____

Figure out what you need to radically accept.

1. Make a list of two **very important** things in your life right now that you need to radically accept.

    Then put a number indicating how much you accept this part of yourself or your life:

    0 = No acceptance (I am in complete denial)

    5 = Complete acceptance (I am at peace with this; it doesn't bother me any more)

    What I need to accept: (Acceptance, 0–5)

    a. _____ (_____)

    b. _____ (_____)

2. Make a list of two **less important** things in your life you are having trouble accepting **this week**.

    What I need to accept: (Acceptance, 0–5)

    a. _____ (_____)

    b. _____ (_____)

Refine your list

3. Review your two lists above:

    - **Check the facts**— is this my interpretation and/or opinions?
    - **Check for judgments**—avoid "good," "bad," and judgmental language.
    - **Rewrite list (if necessary)**—to be factual and nonjudgmental.

    (continued)

Adapted with permission from Linehan (2015b). Copyright © Marsha M. Linehan.

Practice radical acceptance

4. Choose one item from the very important list and one from the less important list to practice on:

a. _____

b. _____

5. Focus your mind on each of these facts or events separately, allowing your wise mind to radically accept that these *are* facts of your life. *Check off* any of the following exercises that you did.

☐ Observed that I was questioning/ fighting reality.	☐ Considered the causes of the reality, and nonjudgmentally accepted that causes exist.
☐ Reminded myself that reality is what it is.	☐ Practiced accepting all the way with my whole spirit (mind, body, spirit).
☐ Practiced opposite action.	☐ Did pros and cons of acceptance versus denial and rejection.
☐ Imagined coping with problems that could arise if I accept.	☐ Attended to my body sensations as I thought about what I need to accept.
☐ Noticed that life can be worth living even with pain in my life.	☐ Allowed myself to experience disappointment, sadness, or grief.

6. Rate your degree of acceptance after practicing radical acceptance (0–5): _____

Distress Tolerance: Turning the Mind

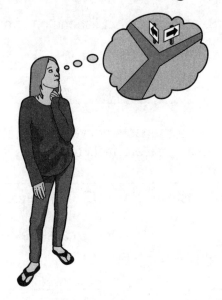

Turning the Mind

✓ ACCEPTANCE is a choice. It is like coming to a "fork in the road." You may have to turn your mind toward the "ACCEPTANCE Road" and away from the REJECTING "Reality Road."

- **Step 1:** Notice when you are not accepting (anger, bitterness, "Why me?").
- **Step 2:** Make an inner commitment to accept.
- **Step 3:** You may have to turn your mind over and over and over again.

Factors That Interfere with Acceptance

✓ Beliefs get in the way: You believe that if you accept your painful situation, you will become weak and just give up (or give in), approve of reality, or accept a life of pain.
✓ Emotions get in the way: Intense anger at the person or group that caused the painful event; unbearable sadness; guilt about your own behavior; shame regarding something about you; rage about the injustice of the world.

REMEMBER: ACCEPTANCE DOES NOT MEAN APPROVAL!

Distress Tolerance: Willingness

WILLFULNESS

- Willfulness is refusing to tolerate a situation or giving up.
- Willfulness is trying to change a situation that cannot be changed, or refusing to change something that must be changed.
- Willfulness is the "terrible twos": "No . . . no . . . no . . ."
- Willfulness is the opposite of "DOING WHAT WORKS."

REPLACE WILLFULNESS WITH WILLINGNESS

- Willingness is allowing the world to be what it is and participating in it fully.
- Willingness is doing just what is needed—no more, no less. It is being effective.
- Willingness is listening carefully to your wise mind and deciding what to do.
- When willfulness doesn't budge, ask: "What is the threat?"

How can you feel the difference between when you are **willing** and when you are **willful**? (Some clues that you are being willful: extreme thoughts like "No way!", muscles tightening.)

Describe a situation when you noticed **willingness and willfulness.**

Where were you willful? _____

How were you willful (e.g., thoughts, feelings, body sensations)? _____

_____

What happened? _____

_____

Where were you willing? _____

How were you willing (e.g., thoughts, feelings, body sensations)? _____

_____

What happened? _____

_____

Adapted with permission from Rathus and Miller (2015). Copyright © The Guilford Press.

Distress Tolerance:
Practice with Turning the Mind and Willingness

Name: _____

Due Date: _____

Practice each skill and rate your level of acceptance of reality as it is before and after as follows: 0 = "no acceptance at all" to 5 = "I'm at peace with this." List what you tried specifically under the rating.

TURNING THE MIND: Acceptance   Before _____   After _____

OBSERVE not accepting. What did you observe? What were you having trouble accepting?
MAKE AN INNER COMMITMENT to accept what feels unacceptable. How did you do this?
Describe your **PLAN FOR CATCHING YOURSELF** the next time you drift from acceptance.

WILLINGNESS: Acceptance   Before _____   After _____

Describe **EFFECTIVE BEHAVIOR** you did to move forward toward a goal.
NOTICE WILLFULNESS. Describe how you are not participating effectively in the world as it is, or how you are not doing something you know needs to be done to move toward a goal:
MAKE AN INNER COMMITMENT to accept what feels unacceptable. How did you do this?
Describe what you did that was **WILLING.**

Adapted with permission from Linehan (2015b). Copyright © Marsha M. Linehan.

Distress Tolerance: Mindfulness of Current Thoughts, Step by Step

1. OBSERVE YOUR THOUGHTS.

- Observe them as waves, coming and going.
- Do not suppress thoughts.
- Do not judge thoughts.
- Acknowledge their presence.
- Do not keep thoughts around.
- Do not analyze thoughts.
- Practice willingness.
- Step back and observe your thoughts.

2. ADOPT A CURIOUS MIND.

- Ask: Where do my thoughts come from?
- Notice that every thought that comes also goes out of your mind.
- Observe but do not evaluate your thoughts. Let go of judgments.

3. REMEMBER: YOU ARE NOT YOUR THOUGHTS.

- Do not necessarily *act* on your thoughts.
- Remember times when you have had very different thoughts.
- Remind yourself that crisis thinking is "emotion mind."
- Remember how you think when you are not feeling such intense suffering and pain.

4. DON'T BLOCK OR SUPPRESS THOUGHTS.

- Ask: What sensations are these thoughts trying to avoid? Turn your mind to the sensations. Then come back to the thoughts. Repeat this several times.
- Step back, and allow your thoughts to come and go.
- Play with your thoughts: Repeat them out loud over and over as fast as you can. Sing them. Imagine the thought as the words of a clown or as a cute animal you can cuddle up to.
- Try *loving* your thoughts.

Adapted with permission from Linehan (2015b). Copyright © Marsha M. Linehan.

Distress Tolerance:
Ways to Practice Mindfulness of Current Thoughts

PRACTICE MINDFULNESS OF CURRENT THOUGHTS BY USING WORDS AND VOICE TONE.

☐ 1. Say a thought or belief out loud, using a nonjudgmental tone, over and over and over . . .

    ☐ as *fast* as you can until it makes no sense.

    ☐ very, very *slowly*—one syllable or word per breath.

    ☐ in a *different voice* from yours (higher or lower pitch).

    ☐ as a *dialogue* on a TV comedy show ("You'll never believe what thought went through my mind. I was thinking, 'I'm a jerk.' Can you believe that?").

    ☐ as a *song*, singing it wholeheartedly and dramatically, in a tune that fits the thoughts.

PRACTICE MINDFULNESS OF CURRENT THOUGHTS WITH OPPOSITE ACTION.

☐ 2. Relax your face and body while imagining accepting your thoughts as only thoughts, or sensations of the brain.

☐ 3. Imagine things you would do if you stopped believing everything you think.

☐ 4. Practice loving your thoughts as they go through your mind.

Thoughts that get in my way: _____

_____

_____

PRACTICE MINDFULNESS OF CURRENT THOUGHTS BY OBSERVING THEM.

☐ 5. Notice thoughts as they come into your mind. As a thought comes into your mind, say, "A thought has entered my mind." Label the thought as a thought, saying, "The thought [describe thought] came into my mind."

☐ 6. As you notice thoughts in your mind, ask, "Where did the thought come from?"

☐ 7. Step back from your mind, as if you are on top of a mountain and your mind is just a rock down below. Gaze at your mind, watching what thoughts come up.

(continued)

PRACTICE MINDFULNESS OF CURRENT THOUGHTS BY IMAGINING THAT YOUR MIND IS:

☐ 8. *A conveyor belt,* and that thoughts and feelings are coming down the belt. Put each thought or feeling in a box labeled with the type of thought that it is (e.g., "worry thoughts," "thoughts about my past," "thoughts about my mother," "thoughts about planning what to do"). Just keep observing and sorting thoughts into the labeled boxes.

☐ 9. *A river,* and that thoughts and feelings are boats going down the river. Imagine sitting on the grass, watching the boats go by. Try not to jump on any of the boats.

☐ 10. *A railroad track,* and that thoughts and feelings are train cars going by. Try not to jump on the train.

☐ 11. *A leaf that has dropped* into a beautiful creek flowing by you as you sit on the grass. Each time a thought or image comes into your mind, imagine that it is written or pictured on the leaf floating by. Let each leaf go by, watching as it goes out of sight.

☐ 12. *The sky, and thoughts are clouds*. Notice each thought-cloud as it drifts by, letting each drift out of your mind.

Distress Tolerance:
Practicing Mindfulness of Current Thoughts

Name: _____

Due Date: _____

Describe your efforts to observe your thoughts in the past week. Practice observing thoughts each day at least once. Don't focus just on thoughts that are painful; also focus on observing pleasant and neutral thoughts. For each thought, first practice saying, "The thought [describe thought] went through my mind." Then practice one or more strategies to observe and let go of thoughts.

Check off any of the following exercises that you did:

☐ 1. Used words and voice tones to say a thought over and over, as fast as I could, very, very slowly, in a voice different from mine, as a dialogue on a TV comedy show, or as a song.

☐ 2. Relaxed my face and body imagining accepting my thoughts as sensations of my brain.

☐ 3. Rehearsed in my mind what I would do if I did not view my thoughts as facts.

☐ 4. Practiced loving my thoughts as they went through my mind.

☐ 5. Allowed my thoughts to come and go as I focused on observing my breath coming in and out.

☐ 6. Asked, "Where did the thought come from?"

☐ 7. Stepped back from my mind, as if I was on top of a mountain.

☐ 8. Imagined that in my mind thoughts were coming down a conveyor belt, were boats on a river, were train cars on a railroad track, were written on leaves flowing down a river, or were clouds floating in the sky. (Underline the image you used.)

☐ 9. Other: _____

(continued)

Describe thoughts you were mindful of during the week. State each thought as it went through your mind.

1. Thought: "_____"

   List the strategies you used (or give the numbers from above): _____

   _____

   Circle how effective this was at helping you be more mindful and less reactive to your thoughts.

1	2	3	4	5
Not effective		Somewhat effective		Very effective

2. Thought: "_____"

   List the strategies you used (or give the numbers from above): _____

   _____

   Circle how effective this was at helping you be more mindful and less reactive to your thoughts.

1	2	3	4	5
Not effective		Somewhat effective		Very effective

3. Thought: "_____"

   List the strategies you used (or give the numbers from above): _____

   _____

   Circle how effective this was at helping you be more mindful and less reactive to your thoughts.

1	2	3	4	5
Not effective		Somewhat effective		Very effective

Mindfulness: Solutions Using Three States of Mind

Name: _____

Due Date: _____

```
     Reasonable    Wise    Emotion
        Mind       Mind      Mind
```

Situation 1:

_____

_____

Solutions:

Reasonable mind	Wise mind	Emotion mind

Situation 2:

_____

_____

Solutions:

Reasonable mind	Wise mind	Emotion mind

Mindfulness: Practicing "What" and "How" Skills

Name: _____

Due Date: _____

Check off one "what" and one "how" skill that you practiced during the week.

"What" Skills	**"How" Skills**
_____ Observe	_____ Nonjudgmentally
_____ Describe	_____ One-mindfully
_____ Participate	_____ Effectively

Briefly describe your experience using the skill during the week (include when and where you used it):

_____

_____

_____

_____

Briefly describe whether the skill affected your thoughts, feelings, or behaviors. If so, how?

_____

_____

_____

_____

If you did not complete this practice exercise, please explain why not/what interfered:

_____

_____

_____

_____

Emotion Regulation: Goals of Emotion Regulation

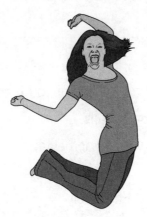

1. **Understand emotions you experience.**
   - Identify (observe and describe) emotions.
     - Use your mindfulness!
   - Know what your emotions do for you. (Are your emotions working for or against you in this moment?)

2. **Reduce emotional vulnerability.**
   Stop unwanted emotions from starting in the first place.
   - Increase your positive emotions.
   - Decrease your vulnerability to emotion mind.

3. **Decrease the frequency of unwanted emotions.**

4. **Decrease emotional suffering.**
   Stop or reduce suffering from unwanted emotions once they start.
   - Let go of your painful emotions, using mindfulness.
   - Change your emotions through opposite action.

Emotion Regulation: Short List of Emotions

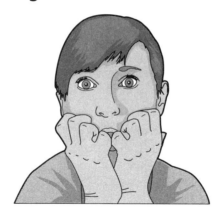

LOVE   HATE   FEAR   JOY   shame   Guilt   ANXIETY
loneliness

ANGER Excited FRUSTRATION sadness   shyness   envy
BOREDOM SURPRISE! embarrassed

CONFUSED   CURIOUS   PRIDE SUSPICIOUS   HAPPY

Rage INTEREST   DEPRESSED WORRY   IRRITABLE PANIC

Jealous   optimistic   hopeless   Disgust   hurt
sympathy   DISAPPOINTED   Content   Calm

Other names for emotions _____   _____
I frequently have:
_____   _____

_____   _____

_____   _____

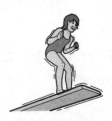

What Good Are Emotions?

Emotions give us information.

- Emotions provide us with a signal that something is happening (e.g., "I feel very nervous standing alone in this dark alley").
- Sometimes our emotions are communicated by "gut feelings" or intuition.
- However, it can be a problem when we treat emotions as if they are facts about the world—for example, "If I am afraid, there must be a threat," or "I love him, so he must be good for me."
- We need to be mindful that emotions are *not* facts. Therefore, it is important to check the facts about each situation.

Emotions communicate to and influence others.

- Facial expressions, body posture, and voice tone say a lot about how you're feeling. They communicate emotions to others (e.g., your sad face may cause someone to ask you if you are OK and give you some support).
- Whether you realize it or not, your emotions—expressed by your words, face, or body language—influence how other people respond to you.

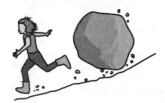

Emotions motivate and prepare us for action.

- The action urge connected to specific emotions is often "hard-wired." For example, when we hear a loud horn beep suddenly, we are startled.
- Emotions save time in getting us to act in important situations. Our nervous systems activate us (e.g., we instantly jump out of the way of an oncoming car). We don't have to think everything through.
- Strong emotions can help us overcome obstacles—in our minds and in the environment.

Adapted with permission from Rathus and Miller (2015). Copyright © The Guilford Press.

Emotion Regulation: Myths about Emotions

Name: _____

Due Date: _____

For each myth, write down a challenge that makes sense to you. Although the one already written may make a lot of sense, try to come up with another one or rewrite the one here in your own words.

1. There is a right way to feel in every situation.

   Challenge: **Every person responds differently to a situation. There is no correct or right way.**

   My Challenge: _____

2. Letting others know that I am feeling bad is a weakness.

   Challenge: **Letting others know that I am feeling bad is a healthy form of communication.**

   My Challenge: _____

3. Negative feelings are bad and destructive.

   Challenge: **Negative feelings are natural responses. They help me to create a better understanding of the situation.**

   My Challenge: _____

4. Being emotional means being out of control.

   Challenge: **Being emotional means being a normal human being.**

   My Challenge: _____

5. Some emotions are stupid.

   Challenge: **Every emotion indicates how I am feeling in a certain situation. All emotions are useful to help me understand what I am experiencing.**

   My Challenge: _____

(continued)

6. Drama is cool.

   Challenge: ***I can be dramatic and regulate my emotions.***

   My Challenge: _____

7. If others don't approve of my feelings, I obviously shouldn't feel the way I do.

   Challenge: ***I have every right to feel the way, I do regardless of what other people think.***

   My Challenge: _____

8. Other people are the best judge of how I am feeling.

   Challenge: ***I am the best judge of how I feel. Other people can only guess how I feel.***

   My Challenge: _____

Emotion Regulation: Emotion Diary

Name: _____   Due Date: _____

Record emotions (either the strongest emotion of the day, the longest-lasting one, or the one that was the most painful or gave you the most trouble).

EMOTIONS	MOTIVATE	COMMUNICATE TO OTHERS		COMMUNICATE TO ME	
Emotion name	What did my emotion motivate me to do (i.e., what goal did my emotion serve)?	How was my emotion expressed to others (my body language, my words, my actions)?	What message did my emotion express to others?	What was the effect of my emotion on others?	What was my emotion saying to me?	How did I check the facts?

Adapted with permission from Linehan (2015b). Copyright © Marsha M. Linehan.

Emotion Regulation: Model of Emotions

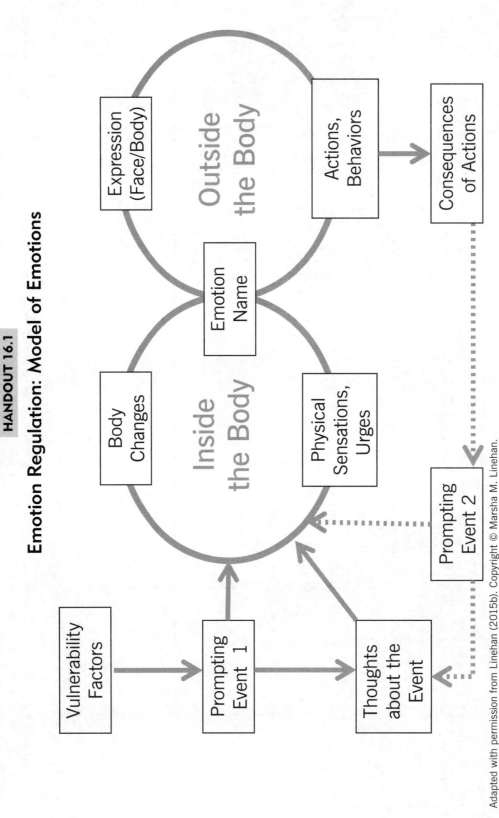

Adapted with permission from Linehan (2015b). Copyright © Marsha M. Linehan.

Emotion Regulation: Ways to Describe Emotions (Anger)

ANGER WORDS

anger	exasperation	grumpiness	outrage
aggravation	frustration	hostility	rage
agitation	fury	irritation	vengefulness
annoyance	grouchiness	bitterness	wrath

Prompting Events for Feeling Anger

• Having an important goal blocked or prevented. • You or someone you care about being attacked or threatened by others. • Losing power, status, or respect	• Not having things turn out as expected. • Physical or emotional pain. • Other: _____

Thoughts about the Events That Prompt Feelings of Anger

• Believing that you have been treated unfairly. • Blaming. • Believing that important goals are being blocked or stopped. • Believing that things "should" be different than they are.	• Rigidly thinking, "I'm right." • Judging that the situation is wrong or unfair. • Ruminating about the event that set off the anger in the first place. • Other: _____

Inside the Body: Body Changes and Sensations

• Muscles tightening. • Teeth clamping together. • Hands clenching. • Feeling your face flush or get hot. • Feeling as if you are going to explode.	• Being unable to stop tears. • Wanting to hit, bang the wall, throw something, blow up. • Wanting to hurt someone. • Other: _____

Outside the Body: Expressions and Action

• Physically or verbally attacking. • Making aggressive or threatening gestures. • Pounding, throwing things, breaking things. • Walking heavily, stomping, slamming doors. • Walking out. • Using a loud, quarrelsome, or sarcastic voice. • Using obscenities or swearing.	• Criticizing or complaining. • Clenching your hands or fists. • Frowning, not smiling, or mean expression. • Brooding or withdrawing from others. • Crying. • Grinning. • A red or flushed face. • Other: _____

Consequences of Anger

• Narrowing of attention. • Attending only to the situation that is making you angry. • Thinking about the situation making you angry (or another situation in the past), and not being able to think of anything else.	• Imagining future situations that will make you angry. • Numbness. • Checking out. • Other: _____

Adapted with permission from Linehan (2015b). Copyright © Marsha M. Linehan.

Emotion Regulation: Ways to Describe Emotions (Fear)

FEAR WORDS

fear	fright	feeling overwhelmed	uneasiness
anxiety	horror	panic	worry
apprehension	hysteria	shock	
dread	jumpiness	tenseness	
edginess	nervousness	terror	

Prompting Events for Feeling Fear

• Having your life, your health, or your well-being threatened. • Being in a similar or the same situation where you have been threatened or gotten hurt in the past or where painful things have happened. • Flashbacks.	• Silence. • Being in situations where you have seen others threatened or be hurt. • Being in a new or unfamiliar situation. • Being alone (e.g., walking alone, being home alone, living alone). • Being in the dark.	• Being in crowds. • Leaving your home. • Having to perform in front of others (e.g., school, work). • Pursuing your dreams. • Other: _____

Thoughts about the Events That Prompt Feelings of Fear

Believing that: • You might die, or you are going to die. • You might be hurt or harmed. • You might lose something valuable. • Someone might reject you, criticize, or dislike you. • You will embarrass yourself. • Failure is possible; expecting to fail.	Believing that: • You will not get help you or need. • You might lose help you already have. • You might lose someone important. • You lose something important. • You are helpless or are losing a sense of control. • Other: _____

Inside the Body: Body Changes and Sensations

• Breathlessness. • Fast heartbeat. • Choking sensation, lump in throat. • Muscles tensing, cramping.	• Clenching teeth. • Feeling as if you will vomit. • Getting cold, feeling clammy. • Wanting to scream or call out.	• Feeling of "butterflies" in stomach. • Wanting to run away or avoid things. • Other: _____

Outside the Body: Expressions and Actions

• Fleeing, running away. • Running or walking fast. • Hiding from or avoiding what you fear. • Engaging in nervous, fearful talk. • Pleading or crying for help. • Talking less or becoming speechless.	• Screaming or yelling. • Darting eyes or quickly looking around. • Frozen stare. • Talking yourself out of doing what you fear. • Freezing, trying not to move. • Crying or whimpering.	• Shaking, quivering, or trembling. • A shaky or trembling voice. • Sweating or perspiring. • Diarrhea, vomiting. • Other: _____

Consequences of Fear

• Narrowing of attention. • Being on high alert to threat. • Losing your ability to focus. • Being dazed.	• Losing control. • Imagining the possibility of more loss or failure. • Isolating yourself.	• Remembering other threatening times. • Other: _____

Adapted with permission from Linehan (2015b). Copyright © Marsha M. Linehan.

Emotion Regulation: Ways to Describe Emotions (Happiness)

HAPPINESS WORDS

happiness	satisfaction	delight	zeal
joy	bliss	enthusiasm	gladness
enjoyment	cheerfulness	thrill	pride
relief	triumph	jolly	elation
amusement	excitement	eagerness	glee
hope	jubilation	pleasure	optimism

Prompting Events for Feeling Happiness

• Receiving a wonderful surprise.	• Receiving love, liking, or affection.
• Reality exceeding your expectations.	• Being accepted by others.
• Getting what you want.	• Belonging somewhere or with someone or a group.
• Getting something you have worked hard for or worried about.	• Being with or in contact with people who love or like you.
• Being successful at a task.	• Other: _____
• Achieving a desirable outcome.	
• Receiving esteem, respect, or praise.	

Thoughts about the Events That Prompt Feelings of Happiness

• Thinking about the joyful event just as it is, without adding or subtracting.	• Other: _____

Inside the Body: Body Changes and Sensations

• Feeling excited.	• Feeling open or expansive.
• Feeling physically energetic, active.	• Feeling calm.
• Feeling like giggling or laughing.	• Urge to keep doing what is making you happy.
• Feeling your face flush.	• Other: _____
• Feeling at peace.	

Outside the Body: Expressions and Action

• Smiling.	• Hugging people.
• Having a bright, glowing face.	• Jumping up and down.
• Being bouncy or bubbly.	• Saying positive things.
• Communicating your good feelings.	• Using an enthusiastic or excited voice.
• Sharing the feeling.	• Being talkative or talking a lot.
• Silliness.	• Other: _____

Consequences of Happiness

• Being courteous or friendly to others.	• Remembering and imagining other times you have felt happy.
• Doing nice things for other people.	• Expecting to feel happy in the future.
• Having a positive outlook; seeing the bright side.	• Other: _____
• Having a high threshold for worry or annoyance.	

Adapted with permission from Linehan (2015b). Copyright © Marsha M. Linehan.

Emotion Regulation: Ways to Describe Emotions (Jealousy)

JEALOUSY WORDS

jealous cautious clinging	defensive fear of losing someone/ something	mistrustful possessive suspicious	self-protective wary watchful

Prompting Events for Feeling Jealous

• An important relationship is threatened or in danger of being lost.
• A potential competitor pays attention to someone you love.
• Someone:
  ■ Is threatening to take away important things in your life.
  ■ Goes out with the person you like.
  ■ Ignores you while talking to a friend of yours.
  ■ Is more attractive, outgoing, or self-confident than you.
	• A person you are romantically involved with looks at someone else.
	• Your boyfriend or girlfriend appears to flirt with someone else.
	• You are treated as unimportant by a person you want to be close to.
	• Your boyfriend or girlfriend tells you that he or she desires more time alone.
	• You find out that your boyfriend or girlfriend is cheating on you.
	• Other: _____

Thoughts about the Events That Prompt Feelings of Jealousy

Believing that: • Your boyfriend or girlfriend does not care for you anymore. • You are nothing to him or her. • He or she is going to leave you. • He or she is behaving inappropriately.	Believing that: • You don't measure up to your peers. • You were cheated. • No one cares about you anymore. • Other: _____

Inside the Body: Body Changes and Sensations

• Breathlessness. • Fast heartbeat. • Choking sensation, lump in throat. • Muscles tensing. • Clenching teeth. • Becoming suspicious of others. • Having injured pride.	• Feelings of rejection. • Needing to be in control. • Feeling helpless. • Wanting to grasp or keep hold of what you have. • Wanting to push away or eliminate your rival. • Other: _____

Outside the Body: Expressions and Actions

• Violent behavior or threats of violence toward the person threatening to take something away. • Attempting to control the freedom of the person or thing that you are afraid of losing. • Verbal accusations of disloyalty or unfaithfulness. • Spying on the person.	• Questioning the person, demanding an accounting of his or her time or activities. • Collecting evidence of wrongdoings. • Clinging, enhanced dependency. • Increased or excessive demonstrations of love. • Other: _____

Consequences of Jealousy

• Narrowing of attention. • Being mistrustful of everyone. • Being on high alert for threats to your relationships.	• Becoming isolated or withdrawn. • Seeing the worst in others. • Other: _____

Adapted with permission from Linehan (2015b). Copyright © Marsha M. Linehan.

Emotion Regulation: Ways to Describe Emotions (Love)

LOVE WORDS

love	caring	infatuation	sympathy
adoration	charmed	kindness	tenderness
affection	compassion	liking	warmth
arousal	desire	longing	
attraction	fondness	passion	

Prompting Events for Feeling Love

• A person:
  ▪ Offers or gives you something you want, need, or desire.
  ▪ Does things you want or need the person to do.
  ▪ Does things you particularly value or admire.
• You feel physically attracted to someone.
	• You spend a lot of time with a person.
	• You share a special experience together with a person.
	• You have exceptionally good communication with a person.
	• You are with someone you have fun with.
	• Other: _____

Thoughts about the Events That Prompt Feelings of Love

• Believing that a person loves, needs, or appreciates you. • Thinking that a person is physically attractive. • Judging a person's personality as wonderful, pleasing, or attractive.	• Believing that a person can be counted on or will always be there for you. • Other: _____

Inside the Body: Body Changes and Sensations

• When you are with or thinking about someone:
  ▪ Feeling excited and full of energy.
  ▪ Fast heartbeat.
  ▪ Feeling self-confident.
  ▪ Feeling invulnerable.
  ▪ Feeling happy, joyful, or exuberant.
  ▪ Feeling warm, trusting, and secure.
  ▪ Feeling relaxed and calm.
	▪ Wanting the best for a person.
	▪ Wanting to give things to a person.
	▪ Wanting to see and spend time with a person.
	▪ Wanting to spend your life with a person.
	▪ Wanting physical closeness or intimacy.
	▪ Wanting emotional closeness.
	▪ Other: _____

Outside the Body: Expressions and Actions

• Saying, "I love you." • Expressing positive feelings to a person. • Eye contact, mutual gaze. • Touching, hugging, holding, cuddling. • Smiling.	• Sharing time and experiences with someone. • Doing things that the other person wants or needs that you are comfortable doing. • Other: _____

Consequences of Love

• Only being able to see a person's positive side. • Feeling forgetful or distracted; daydreaming. • Feeling openness and trust. • Feeling "alive," capable. • Remembering other people you have loved.	• Remembering other people who have loved you. • Remembering and imagining other positive events. • Believing in yourself; believing you are wonderful, capable, competent. • Other: _____

Adapted with permission from Linehan (2015b). Copyright © Marsha M. Linehan.

Emotion Regulation: Ways to Describe Emotions (Sadness)

SADNESS WORDS

sadness	disappointment	feeling crushed	sorrow	loneliness
despair	pity	homesickness	defeat	unhappy
grief	dismay	neglect	disconnected	depression
misery	hurt	displeasure	suffering	glum
agony	rejection	insecurity	gloom	alone

Prompting Events for Feeling Sadness

• Losing something or someone that you cannot get back. • Things are not the way you expected or wanted. • The death of someone you love. • Being separated from someone you care for. • Being rejected, disapproved of, or excluded. • Not getting what you believe you need in life.	• Discovering that you are powerless or helpless. • Being with someone else who is sad or in pain. • Reading or hearing about other people's problems or troubles in the world. • Being alone, isolated, or an outsider. • Thinking about your losses. • Thinking about missing someone. • Other: _____

Thoughts about the Events That Prompt Feelings of Sadness

• Believing that a separation from someone will last for a long time or will never end. • Believing that you will not get what you want or need in your life.	• Seeing things or your life as hopeless. • Believing that you are worthless or not valuable. • Other: _____

Inside the Body: Body Changes and Sensations

• Feeling tired, run-down, or low in energy. • Feeling slow, wanting to stay in bed all day. • Feeling as if nothing is pleasurable any more. • Pain or hollowness in your chest or gut. • Feeling empty.	• Feeling as if you can't stop crying, or as if you ever start crying you will never be able to stop. • Difficulty swallowing. • Breathlessness. • Other: _____

Outside the Body: Expressions and Actions

• Avoiding things. • Acting helpless, staying in bed, being inactive. • Moping, brooding, or acting moody. • Making slow, shuffling movements. • Withdrawing from social contact. • Avoiding activities that used to bring pleasure. • Saying sad things.	• Giving up and no longer trying to improve. • Talking little or not at all. • Using a quiet, slow, or monotonous voice. • Frowning, not smiling. • Posture slumping. • Sobbing, crying, whimpering. • Other: _____

Consequences of Sadness

• Not being able to remember happy things. • Feeling irritable, touchy, or grouchy. • Yearning and searching for the thing lost. • Having a negative outlook.	• Blaming or criticizing yourself. • Thinking about sad events in the past. • Insomnia. • Appetite disturbance, indigestion. • Other: _____

Adapted with permission from Linehan (2015b). Copyright © Marsha M. Linehan.

Emotion Regulation: Ways to Describe Emotions (Shame)

SHAME WORDS

shame	embarrassment humiliation	self-conscious shyness

Prompting Events for Feeling Shame

• Being rejected by people you care about. • Having others find out that you have done something wrong. • Doing (or feeling or thinking) something that people you admire believe is wrong or immoral. • Comparing some aspect of yourself or your behavior to a standard and feeling like you do not live up to that standard. • Being laughed at or made fun of. • Being criticized in public or remembering public criticism.	• Being reminded of something wrong, immoral, or "shameful" you did in the past. • Being rejected or criticized for something you expected praise for. • Exposure of a very private aspect of yourself or your life. • Exposure of a physical characteristic you dislike. • Failing at something you feel you are (or should be) competent to do. • Other: _____

Thoughts about the Events That Prompt Feelings of Shame

• Believing that others will reject you (or have rejected you). • Judging yourself to be inferior, not "good enough," not as good as others, or a "loser." • Believing yourself unlovable. • Thinking that you are defective. • Thinking that you are a bad person or a failure.	• Believing that your body (or a body part) is too big, too small, or ugly. • Thinking that you have not lived up to others' expectations of you. • Thinking that your behavior, thoughts, or feelings are silly or stupid. • Other: _____

Inside the Body: Body Changes and Sensations

• Pain in the pit of the stomach. • Sense of dread.	• Wanting to shrink down and/or disappear. • Wanting to hide or cover your face and body. • Other: _____

Outside the Body: Expressions and Actions

• Hiding the behavior or characteristic you are ashamed of from other people. • Avoiding the person you have harmed. • Avoiding people who have criticized you. • Avoiding yourself (distracting, ignoring). • Withdrawing, covering the face. • Bowing your head, groveling.	• Making amends; saying you are sorry over and over and over. • Looking down and away from others. • Sinking back; slumped and rigid posture. • Halting speech, lower speech volume. • Other: _____

Consequences of Shame

• Avoiding thinking about what you did wrong; shutting down, blocking all emotions. • Engaging in distracting, impulsive behaviors to divert your mind or attention. • High amount of "self-focus"; preoccupation with yourself.	• Attacking or blaming others. • Conflicts with other people. • Feelings of isolation, alienation. • Difficulty in problem solving. • Other: _____

Adapted with permission from Linehan (2015b). Copyright © Marsha M. Linehan.

Emotion Regulation: Ways to Describe Emotions (Guilt)

GUILT WORDS

guilt being apologetic	regret remorse	being sorry

Prompting Events for Feeling Guilt

• Doing or thinking something you believe is wrong. • Doing or thinking something that violates your personal values. • Not doing something you said that you would do.	• Causing harm/damage to another person or object. • Causing harm/damage to yourself. • Being reminded of something wrong you did in the past. • Other: _____

Thoughts about the Events That Prompt Feelings of Guilt

• Thinking that your actions are to blame for something. • Thinking that you behaved badly.	• Thinking "if only you had done something differently . . ." • Other: _____

Inside the Body: Body Changes and Sensations

• Hot, red face. • Jitteriness, nervousness.	• Feeling as if you are suffocating. • Other: _____

Outside the Body: Expressions and Actions

• Trying to repair the harm, make amends for the wrongdoing, fix the damage, or change the outcome. • Asking for forgiveness; apologizing, confessing.	• Giving gifts/making sacrifices to try to make up for the wrongdoing. • Bowing your head, kneeling before the person. • Other: _____

Consequences of Guilt

• Making resolutions to change. • Making changes in behavior.	• Joining self-help programs. • Other: _____

Adapted with permission from Linehan (2015b). Copyright © Marsha M. Linehan.

Emotion Regulation: Practice with the Model of Emotions

Name: _____   Due Date: _____

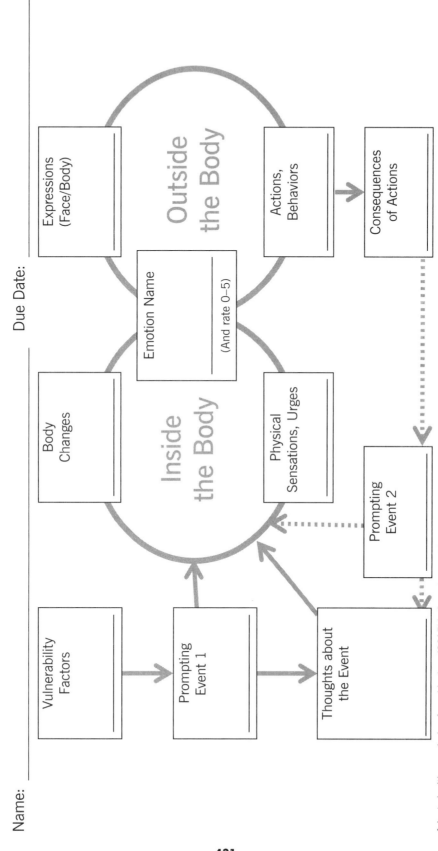

Adapted with permission from Linehan (2015b). Copyright © Marsha M. Linehan.

Emotion Regulation:
Overview of Skills for Changing Emotional Responses

CHECK THE FACTS

1. Check out whether your reactions fit the facts of the situation.

2. Changing your interpretation if it does not fit the facts can help you change your emotional reactions.

OPPOSITE ACTION

1. Acting opposite to your emotions that don't fit the facts can also change your emotions.

PROBLEM SOLVING

1. When the emotions do fit the facts, then move to problem solving, which will reduce the frequency of negative emotions.

Emotion Regulation: Check the Facts

Here Are the FACTS

Many emotions and actions are set off by our thoughts and interpretations of events, not by the events themselves.

Event → Thoughts → Emotion

Our emotions can also have a big effect on our thoughts about events.

Event → Emotion → Thoughts

Examining our thoughts and *checking the facts* can help us change our emotions.

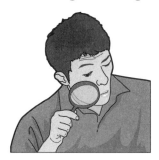

Three Steps to Check the Facts

1. Ask: "What is the emotion I want to change?"

2. Ask: "What is the event prompting my emotion?"

   Challenge judgments, extremes, and black-and-white thinking.
   Describe the facts that you observed through your senses.

3. Ask: "Am I interpreting the situation correctly?"

   Are there other possible interpretations?

Additional Questions That May or May Not Fit Each Situation:

a. "Am I thinking in extremes (all-or-nothing thoughts, catastrophic thinking)?"
   If so, think of as many other possible outcomes as you can.

b. "What is the likelihood of the worst thing happening"?

c. "Even if the worst were to happen, can I imagine coping well with it?"
   Imagine saying, "So what?"

Emotion Regulation: Examples of Emotions That Fit the Facts

Fear
- There is a threat to your life or that of someone you care about.
- There is a threat to your health or that of someone you care about
- There is a threat to your well-being or that of someone you care about.

Anger
- An important goal is blocked or prevented.
- You or someone you care about is attacked or hurt by others.
- Losing power, status, or respect.

Jealousy
- An important relationship is being threatened and in danger of being lost.
- Someone is threatening to take a valued relationship or object away from you.

Love
- A person, animal, or object gives you something you want, need, or desire.
- A person, animal, or object improves quality of life for you or for those you care about.

Sadness
- You have lost something or someone you care about.
- Things are not the way you wanted or hoped them to be.

Shame
- You are being rejected by a person or group you care about over an issue that publicly involves your behavior or characteristics.

Guilt
- You are doing something you believe is wrong.
- You are doing something that violates your own personal values or long-term goals.

Intensity and duration of an emotion are justified by:
1. How likely it is that the expected outcomes will occur?
2. How great and/or important the outcomes are?
3. How effective the emotion is in your life now?

Adapted with permission from Linehan (2015b). Copyright © Marsha M. Linehan.

Emotion Regulation: Opposite Action to Change Emotions

Emotions come with specific action urges that push us to act in certain ways. Often we escape the pain of the emotion in harmful ways.

These are the common urges associated with a sample of emotions:

Fear → Escaping or avoiding

Anger → Attacking

Sadness → Withdrawing, becoming passive, isolating

Shame → Hiding, avoiding, withdrawing, saving face by attacking others

Guilt → Overpromising that you will not commit the offense again, disclaiming all responsibility, hiding, lowering head, begging forgiveness

Jealousy → Verbal accusations, attempts to control, acting suspicious

Love → Saying, "I love you," making efforts to spend time with the person, doing what the other person wants and needs, giving affection

Acting Opposite = acting opposite to the action urge when the emotion is doing more harm than good.

EMOTION → **OPPOSITE ACTION**

Fear/anxiety → **Approach**
- Approach events, places, tasks, activities, or people you are afraid of, over and over. Confront.
- Do things to increase a sense of control and mastery over fears.

Anger → **Gently avoid**
- Gently avoid the person you are angry with (rather than attacking).
- Take time out and breathe in and out deeply and slowly.
- Be kind rather than mean or attacking (Try to have sympathy or empathy for the other person).

Sadness → **Get active**
- Approach, don't avoid.
- Build mastery and increase pleasant activities.

Shame → **Face the music** (when your behavior violates your moral values, or something shameful has been revealed about you, and the shame fits the facts):
- Apologize and repair the harm when possible.
- Try to avoid making the same mistake in the future and accept consequences.
- Forgive yourself and let it go.

   Go public (when your behavior *does not* violate your moral values, and the shame *does not* fit the facts):
- You continue to participate fully in social interactions, hold your head high, keep your voice steady, and make eye contact.

(continued)

- **Go public** with your personal characteristics or your behavior (with people who won't reject you).
- Repeat the behavior that sets off shame over and over (without hiding it from those who won't reject you).

Guilt   → **Face the music** (when your behavior violates your moral values, or it hurts feelings of significant others, and the guilt fits the facts).
- Experience the guilt.
- Ask but don't beg for forgiveness, and accept the consequences.
- Repair the transgression and work to prevent it from happening again.

            Don't apologize or try to make up for it (when your behavior *does not* violate your moral values and the guilt *does not* fit the facts).
- Change your body posture: Look innocent and proud, hold your head up, puff up your chest, and maintain eye contact. Keep your voice steady and clear.

Jealousy   → **Let go of controlling others' actions** (when it *does not* fit the facts or *is not* effective).
- Stop spying or snooping.
- Relax your face and body.

Love   → **Stop expressing love** (when it *does not* fit the facts or *is not* effective (e.g., the relationship is truly over, not accessible, or abusive).
- Avoid the person, and distract yourself from thoughts of the person.
- Remind yourself of why love does not fit the facts, and rehearse the "cons" of loving this person.
- Avoid contact with things that remind you of the person (e.g., pictures).

Opposite Action Works Best When:
1. The emotion **DOES NOT fit the facts.**
   a. An emotion DOES NOT fit thev facts when:
      - The emotion *does not* fit the facts of the actual situation (e.g., terror in response to speaking in public), *or*
      - The emotion, its intensity, or its duration is not effective for your goals in the situation (e.g., you feel angry at your math teacher, but three periods later you're still fuming and can't focus on science).
2. It is done **ALL THE WAY.**
   - Opposite behavior.
   - Opposite words and thinking.
   - Opposite facial expressions, voice tone, and posture.

Opposite Action Requires These Seven Steps:
1. Figure out the emotion you are feeling.
2. What is the action urge that goes with the emotion?
3. Ask yourself: "Does the emotion fit the facts in this situation? If yes, will acting on the emotion's urge be effective?"
4. Ask yourself: "Do I want to change the emotion?"
5. If yes, figure out the *opposite action*.
6. Do the opposite action—all the way.
7. Repeat acting opposite until the emotion goes down enough for you to notice.

Emotion Regulation: Practice with Check the Facts

Name: _____

Due Date: _____

It is hard to problem-solve emotional situations if you don't have your facts straight. It is important to know what the problem is before you can solve it. This worksheet can help you figure out whether it is the event that occurred that is causing your emotion, your interpretation of the event, or both. Before you can figure out what to change, you have to figure out what really happened. You have to use your mindfulness skills of observing and describing. You have to **check the facts** and then describe the facts you observed.

Emotion Name: _____ **Intensity (0–5) Before:** _____ **After** _____

Step 1: What is the emotion I want to change?

Step 2: Describe the prompting event: Who did what to whom? What led up to what? What is it about this event that is a problem for me?

Step 3: Am I interpreting the situation correctly? Are there other possible interpretations?

Additional questions you may need to ask:
1. Am I thinking in extremes (all-or-nothing thoughts, catastrophic thinking)?

2. What is the likelihood of the worst thing happening? And if the worst thing happens, can I imagine myself coping well with it? (Describe in detail the worst outcome I can reasonably expect and ways to cope if the worst thing does happen.)

Do my emotion and its intensity fit the facts? (0 = not at all, 5 = I am certain): Describe what you did to check the facts.

Emotion Regulation:
Practice with Changing Emotions by Opposite Action

Name: _____

Due Date: _____

Ask yourself the following questions as a guide to OPPOSITE ACTION:

Observe and **describe** the emotion: What is the current emotion you are having?
What is your action urge?
Do opposite action **ALL THE WAY.**
How did you feel after acting opposite to your emotion?

Adapted with permission from Linehan (2015b). Copyright © Marsha M. Linehan.

Emotion Regulation: Problem Solving

START PROBLEM SOLVING.

First, ask yourself: Can the problem be solved?

If yes, try problem solving!

If no, use your radical acceptance and mindfulness skills to manage the problem and your emotional reaction to it.

Steps for Problem Solving

1. **DESCRIBE** the problem situation.

2. **CHECK THE FACTS.**
   a. Am I interpreting the situation correctly?
   b. Am I thinking in extremes (all-or-nothing thoughts, catastrophic thinking)?
   c. What is the probability of the worst thing happening?
   d. Even if the worst thing happened, could you imagine coping well?
   e. If you are still faced with a big problem, then continue the steps below.

3. **IDENTIFY YOUR GOAL(S)** in solving the problem.
   a. Identify what needs to happen or change for you to feel OK.
   b. Keep it simple; keep it something that can actually happen.

4. **BRAINSTORM** lots of solutions.
   a. Think of as many solutions as you can. Ask for suggestions from people you trust.
   b. Don't be critical of any ideas at first (wait for Step 5 to evaluate ideas).

5. **CHOOSE at leastvv one solution** that is likely to work.
   a. If you are unsure, choose two or three solutions that look good.
   b. Do pros and cons to compare the solutions. Choose the best to try first.

6. Put the solution(s) into **ACTION.**
   a. ACT: try out the solution(s).
   b. Take the first step, and then the second . . .

7. **EVALUATE** each outcome.
   a. Did it work? Yeah! Reward yourself!
   b. It didn't work? Validate yourself for trying, and don't give up!
   c. Try a new solution.

Adapted with permission from Rathus and Miller (2015). Copyright © The Guilford Press.

Emotion Regulation:
Putting Opposite Action and Problem Solving Together

	Events that fit the facts	Act opposite to emotion urge	Act on emotion, avoid or problem-solve
Fear	1. Your life is in danger. 2. Your health is in danger. 3. Your well-being is in danger.	1. Approach what you are afraid of doing . . . over and over. 2. Do what gives you a sense of control and mastery.	1. Remove the threatening event. 2. Do what gives you a sense of control and mastery. 3. Avoid the threatening event.
Anger	A. An important goal is blocked or prevented. B. You or someone you care about is attacked or hurt by others. C. You are losing power, status, or respect.	1. Gently avoid. 2. Take a time out and breathe in and out deeply. 3. Be kind rather than mean or attacking. 4. Have sympathy or empathy for the other person.	1. Overcome obstacles to your goals. 2. Stop further attacks, insults, and threats. 3. Avoid or walk out on people who are threatening.
Jealousy	A. An important relationship is being threatened and in danger of being lost. B. Someone is threatening to take a valued object away from you.	1. Let go of trying to control others. 2. Stop spying and snooping. 3. Relax your face and body.	1. Protect what you have. 2. Work at being more desirable to the person you want to be in a relationship with (i.e., fight for the relationship). 3. Leave the relationship.
Love	A. A person, animal, or object gives you something you want, need, or desire. B. A person, animal, or object improves the quality of life for you or those you care about.	1. Stop expressing love. 2. Distract yourself from thoughts of the person. 3. Avoid contact with things that remind you of the person. 4. Remind yourself of why love does not fit the facts.	1. Be with the person, animal, or thing that you love. 2. Touch, hold, etc., the beloved. 3. Avoid separations when possible. If the beloved is lost: 4. Work to get the beloved back (if it is possible).

(continued)

Adapted with permission from Linehan (2015b). Copyright © Marsha M. Linehan.

	Events that fit the facts	Act opposite to emotion urge	Act on emotion, avoid or problem-solve
Sadness	A. You have lost something or someone you care about. B. Things are not the way you wanted or hoped them to be.	1. Get active. 2. Approach, don't avoid. 3. Build mastery; do things that make you feel competent and self-confident. 4. Increase pleasant events.	1. Grieve; process the loss or disappointment. 2. Plan how to rebuild your life without the person or thing you have lost. 3. Replace what is lost (if possible). 4. Ask for help. 5. Accept help when offered.
Shame	A. You are being rejected by a person or group you care about over an issue that publicly involves your behavior or characteristics.	1. Go public. 2. Participate fully in social interactions (hold your head high). 3. Repeat the behavior without hiding from people who won't reject you.	1. Hide what will get you rejected. 2. Apologize and repair the harm when possible. 3. Change your behavior or personal characteristics to fit in. 4. Avoid groups that disapprove of you. 5. Find a new group that fits your values or that likes your personal characteristics. 6. Work to change society's or a person's values.
Guilt	A. You are doing something you believe is wrong. B. You are doing something that violates your own personal values or long-term goals.	1. Don't apologize or try to make up for it. 2. Do what makes you feel guilty over and over and over. 3. Change your body posture (look innocent and proud).	1. Ask but don't beg for forgiveness. 2. Repair the harm and work to prevent it from happening again. 3. Accept the consequences gracefully.

Emotion Regulation:
Practice with Problem Solving to Change Emotions

Name: _____

Due Date: _____

Select a prompting event that triggers a painful emotion. Select an event that can be changed. Turn the event into a problem to be solved. Follow the steps below and describe what happened.

Emotion Name: _____

Intensity (0–5)   Before: _____   **After:** _____

1. **DESCRIBE THE PROBLEM SITUATION.** Describe exactly what makes this situation a problem.

   _____

   _____

2. **CHECK THE FACTS.** (Check all the facts; sort them out from interpretations—see Handout 17.2.)

   _____

   _____

3. **IDENTIFY YOUR GOAL(S)** in solving the problem:

   _____

   _____

4. **BRAINSTORM SOLUTIONS:** List as many solutions and coping strategies as you can think of. Don't evaluate!

   a. _____   d. _____

   b. _____   e. _____

   c. _____   f. _____

(continued)

5. CHOOSE at least one solution that is likely to work. Do pros and cons to compare solutions.

a. _____

b. _____

	Pros	Cons
Using this solution	1.	1.
	2.	2.
	3.	3.
Not using this solution	1.	1.
	2.	2.
	3.	3.

6. Put the solution(s) into **ACTION**. You might need to try out more than one!

a. _____

b. _____

7. EVALUATE each outcome. Did it work? Yeah! Reward yourself. If it didn't work, try a new solution. **Don't give up!**

_____

_____

Emotion Regulation: Overview of ABC PLEASE

How to **increase** positive emotions
and
reduce vulnerability to emotion mind:

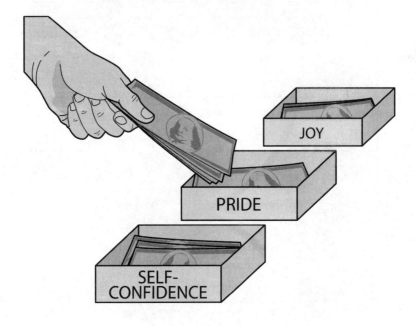

Accumulate positive experiences

Build mastery

Cope ahead of time with emotional situations

Treat **P**hysica**L** illness

Balance **E**ating

Avoid mood-altering drugs

Balance **S**leep

Get **E**xercise

Adapted with permission from Rathus and Miller (2015). Copyright © The Guilford Press.

Emotion Regulation:
Accumulating Positive Experiences in the Short Term

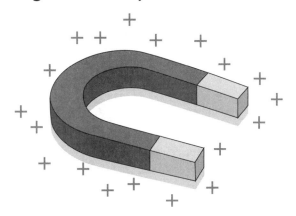

In the Short Term:

Do pleasant things that are possible right now.

- Increase pleasant activities that lead to positive emotions.
- Do one thing each day from the Pleasant Activities List (Handout 19.3).

Be Mindful of Positive Experiences:

- Focus your attention on positive events while they are happening.
- Refocus your attention when your mind wanders to the negative.
- Participate fully in the experience.

Be Unmindful of Worries:

- Don't destroy positive experiences by thinking about when they will end.
- Don't worry about whether you deserve this positive experience.
- Don't worry about how much more might be expected of you now.

Emotion Regulation: Pleasant Activities List

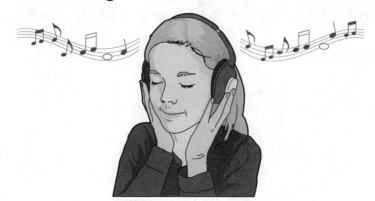

1. Soaking in the bathtub
2. Thinking about school holidays or vacations
3. Going out with friends
4. Relaxing
5. Going to a movie
6. Going running
7. Listening to music
8. Lying in the sun (with sunscreen)
9. Reading magazines or books
10. Saving money
11. Planning the future
12. Dancing
13. Fixing or cleaning things around the house
14. Having a quiet night
15. Cooking good food
16. Taking care of your pets
17. Going swimming
18. Writing
19. Drawing or doodling
20. Playing sports (list: _____)
21. Going to a party
22. Talking with friends
23. Working out
24. Singing
25. Roller skating or in-line skating
26. Going to a beach
27. Playing a musical instrument
28. Traveling
29. Making a gift for someone
30. Downloading music or new apps
31. Watching sports on TV
32. Going out to dinner
33. Baking
34. Planning a party for someone
35. Buying clothes
36. Getting a haircut or styling your hair
37. Enjoying an early cup of hot chocolate, coffee, or tea
38. Kissing

(continued)

39. Going to hear live music
40. Getting a manicure or pedicure
41. Spending some time with little kids
42. Going for a bike ride
43. Going sledding in a snowstorm
44. Getting a massage
45. Emailing or texting friends
46. Writing in a diary or journal
47. Looking at photos
48. Dressing up however you like
49. Playing video games
50. Walking around where you live
51. Noticing birds or trees (something in nature)
52. Surfing the Internet
53. Surprising someone with a favor
54. Completing something you will feel great about
55. Shooting pool or playing ping-pong
56. Contacting a relative you have been out of touch with
57. Tweeting, posting online
58. Thinking about taking lessons (sports, dance, music, martial arts)
59. Bowling
60. Fantasizing about life getting better
61. Saying, "I love you"
62. Writing a poem, song, or rap
63. Thinking about a friend's good qualities
64. Putting on makeup
65. Making a smoothie and drinking it slowly
66. Putting on your favorite piece of clothing
67. Playing a game
68. Writing a story

69. Instant-messaging someone
70. Watching reruns on TV
71. Making a card and giving it to someone you care about
72. Figuring out your favorite scent
73. Buying yourself a treat
74. Noticing a storm coming
75. Building furniture or carpentry

Add your own:

76. _____
77. _____
78. _____
79. _____
80. _____

Emotion Regulation:
Accumulating Positive Experiences in the Long Term

In the Long Term:

Make changes in your life so that positive events will occur more often. Build a life worth living.

Work toward Goals Based on Your Values:
- Identify one goal (e.g., graduate from high school).
- List small steps toward goals/value (e.g., get out of bed, go to first class).
- Take first step (e.g., buy an alarm clock or set cell phone alarm).

Pay Attention to Relationships:
- Repair old, create new, and work on current relationships.
- Avoid avoiding, and **avoid giving up!**

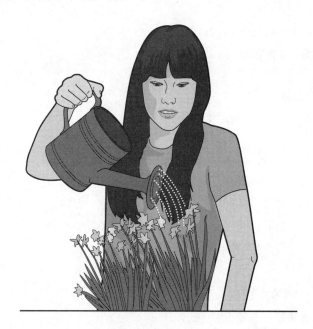

Adapted with permission from Rathus and Miller (2015). Copyright © The Guilford Press.

Emotion Regulation: Wise Mind Values and Priorities List

What is important to me?: Examples

Use the blanks to fill in your priority ranking for each item. Add your own examples at the bottom.

☐ _____ **Achieve things** (examples: get good grades, work hard, etc.)

☐ _____ **Have fun** (examples: enjoy what I do, go out and have a good time)

☐ _____ **Focus on family** (examples: see family often, keep family relationships strong, do things for family)

☐ _____ **Contribute** (examples: help people in need, make sacrifices for others, improve society)

☐ _____ **Be part of a group** (examples: have close friends, have people to do things, be part of a sports team, feel a sense of belonging)

☐ _____ **Build character** (examples: be honest, stand up for my beliefs, keep my word, be responsible, keep growing as a human being)

☐ _____ **Be responsible** (examples: earn money, take care of myself more and more, become more independent, be reliable)

☐ _____ **Be a leader** (examples: be seen by others as successful, be in charge of something [like a club or team], be respected by others, be popular and accepted)

☐ _____ **Be healthy** (examples: be physically fit, exercise, eat well, develop physical strength, practice yoga)

☐ _____ **Learn** (e.g., seek knowledge and information, read, study)

☐ _____ **Strive for moderation** (e.g., avoid excesses, achieve balance)

☐ _____ **Others:** _____

☐ _____ _____

☐ _____ _____

☐ _____ _____

☐ _____ _____

Adapted with permission from Rathus and Miller (2015). Copyright © The Guilford Press.

Emotion Regulation: Practice with Accumulating
Positive Experiences (Short- and Long-Term)

Name: _____

Due Date: _____

In the Short term:

1. Engage in at least one activity from your list each day. Please write down each activity on the list below. Add more rows if you need them.
2. Rate your mood *before* you start the activity and then *after*. Use the rating scale below.
3. Remember to try to *stay mindful* of activity and unmindful of worries.

```
 -5            -2.5            0           +2.5          +5
 |---+---+---+---+---+---+---+---+---+---+---|
I feel very upset  I feel somewhat upset   I feel OK   I feel pretty good   I feel great
```

Date:							
	Monday	Tuesday	Wednesday	Thursday	Friday	Saturday	Sunday
Activity							
Before/After	/	/	/	/	/	/	/
Activity							
Before/After	/	/	/	/	/	/	/

4. Were you mindfully participating in each activity? If yes, describe the effect on your emotional state. If no, what happened?

_____

_____

In the Long Term:

1. List one of your values and a goal that it is associated with. _____

_____

2. What is the first step in achieving your goal? _____

_____

3. Take the first step. Describe how taking the first step made you feel. _____

_____

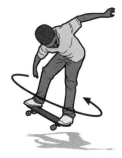

Emotion Regulation:
Building Mastery and Coping Ahead

Build Mastery

1. Plan on doing at least one thing each day to feel competent and in control of your life.

    Example: _____

2. Plan for success, not failure.
    • Do something difficult, BUT possible.

3. Gradually increase the difficulty over time.
    • If the first task is too difficult, do something a little easier next time.

Cope Ahead of Time with Emotional Situations
Rehearse a plan ahead of time so you are prepared.

1. **Describe** a situation that is likely to create negative emotions.
    • Be specific in describing the situation. Check the facts! What's the threat?
    • Name the emotions you are most likely to experience in the situation.

2. **Decide** what coping or problem-solving skills you want to use in the situation.
    • Be specific. Write it out: _____

3. **Imagine the situation** in your mind as vividly as possible.
    • Imagine yourself *in* the situation *now*.

4. **Rehearse in your mind coping effectively**.
    • Rehearse in your mind exactly what you could do to cope effectively.
    • Rehearse your actions, your thoughts, what you say, and how to say it.
    • Troubleshoot: Rehearse coping with problems that might arise.

Adapted with permission from Rathus and Miller (2015). Copyright © The Guilford Press.

Emotion Regulation:
PLEASE Skills

How to **reduce** vulnerability to emotion mind

Treat **P**hysica**L** illness: Take care of your body. See a doctor when necessary.
                              Take medications as prescribed.

Balance **E**ating: Don't eat too much or too little. Stay away from foods that
                              may make you overly emotional.

Avoid mood-altering drugs: Stay off nonprescribed drugs, like alcohol, marijuana, or
                              other street drugs. Limit your use of caffeine.

Balance **S**leep: Try to get the amount of sleep that helps you feel good.
                              Stay on a regular schedule in order to develop good sleep
                              habits.

Get **E**xercise: Do some sort of exercise every day, including walking.
                              Start small and build up to it!

Emotion Regulation: Food and Your Mood

Step 1: Observe how certain foods affect your mood (both negatively and positively).*

Negative examples:

- Soda and sugary snacks might make you feel tired and irritable.
- Heavy, fatty foods (e.g., French fries, potato chips, fried chicken, greasy foods) might make you feel sluggish.
- Caffeine might make you feel jittery and anxious and interfere with your sleep.

Positive examples:

- Complex carbohydrates and fiber (e.g., sweet potatoes, whole-wheat pasta, oatmeal, whole-grain cereals, salads) give you slow and steady energy.
- Proteins (e.g., lean meats and poultry, beans, nuts, fish, and eggs) also provide your body with steady energy that helps you stay active and strong both physically and mentally.
- Dairy foods (e.g., low-fat milk, cheeses, yogurts) have protein and calcium, which help with energy and bone strength.
- Fruits and vegetables provide you energy, boost your health, and give you a sweet or crunchy treat without zapping your energy or making you feel guilty.

*Once you know what foods make up a balanced diet, you can determine what changes might be needed.

Step 2: Notice whether you are eating too much or too little.

Step 3: Start thinking about changes.

How can you begin to increase the amounts of healthy foods you eat? Keep track of your food choices on your food diary every day, so you see your progress!

Step 4: Start small.

Don't try to make dramatic changes to your diet all at once. You might feel overwhelmed and might set yourself up to fail. Start slowly, and gradually change your habits. For example:

- Cut down on processed foods and add more fresh foods.
- Add more fruits and vegetables to meals, and have them for snacks.
- Add lettuce, tomato, cucumber, and onion to sandwiches.
- Add fruit to cereal.

Step 5: Notice the effects of eating well on your mood.

Adapted with permission from Rathus and Miller (2015). Copyright © The Guilford Press.

Emotion Regulation: 12 Tips for Better Sleep Hygiene

Maintaining a balanced sleep pattern will decrease your emotional vulnerability.

1. **Stick to a schedule,** and don't sleep late on weekends. If you sleep late on Saturday and Sunday morning, you will disrupt your sleep pattern. Instead, go to bed and get up at about the same time every day.

2. **Establish a bedtime routine.** This might include shutting off screens, changing into comfy PJs, sipping herbal tea, lowering bright lights, reducing noise, and reading.

3. **Don't eat or drink a lot before bed.** Eat a light dinner about 2 hours before sleeping. If you drink too many liquids before heading to bed, you'll wake up repeatedly for trips to the bathroom. Watch out for spicy foods, which may cause heartburn and interfere with your sleep.

4. **Avoid caffeine and nicotine.** Both are stimulants and can keep you awake. Caffeine should be avoided for 8 hours before your desired bedtime.

5. **Exercise.** If you're trying to sleep better, the best time to exercise is in the afternoon. A program of regular physical activity enhances the quality of your sleep.

6. **Keep your room cool.** Turn the temperature in the room down, as this mimics the natural drop in your body's temperature during sleep. Use an air conditioner or a fan to keep the room cool. If you get cold, add more layers. If you are hot, take some layers away.

7. **Sleep primarily at night.** Daytime naps steal hours from your nighttime sleep. Limit daytime sleep to less than 1 hour, no later than 3 P.M.

8. **Keep it dark and quiet, and NO SCREENS.** Use shades or blinds, and turn off lights. Silence helps you sleep better. Turn off the radio and TV. Use earplugs. Use a fan, a white-noise machine, or some other source of constant, soothing background noise to mask sounds you can't control. No laptops, iPads, phones, or screens for at least 1 hour before bedtime.

9. **Use your bed only for sleep.** Make your bed so it is comfortable and appealing. Use it only for sleep—not studying or watching TV. Go to bed when you feel tired, and turn out the lights. If you don't fall asleep in 30 minutes, get up and do something else relaxing, such as reading books or magazines—NO SCREENS! Go back to bed when you are tired. Don't stress out! This will make it harder to fall asleep.

10. **Soak and sack out.** Taking a hot shower or bath before bed helps relax tense muscles.

11. **Don't rely on sleeping pills.** If they are prescribed to you, use them only under a doctor's close supervision. Make sure the pills won't interact with other medications!

12. **Don't catastrophize.** Tell yourself, "It's OK. I'll fall asleep eventually."

Adapted with permission from Rathus and Miller (2015). Copyright © The Guilford Press.

Emotion Regulation: Practicing with Build Mastery, Cope Ahead, and PLEASE Skills

Name: _____

Due Date: _____

How to increase positive emotions and reduce your vulnerability to emotion mind

Build mastery:

List two ways that you built mastery this week.

1. _____

2. _____

Cope ahead of time with emotional situations:

Describe your plan to effectively manage a future emotional situation. Include skills you will use.

_____

_____

_____

Check off two PLEASE skills to practice during the week:

_____ Treat PhysicaL illness

_____ Balance Eating

_____ Avoid mood-altering drugs

_____ Balance Sleep

_____ Get Exercise

Describe specifically what you did to practice your PLEASE skills:

_____

_____

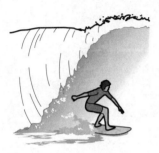

Emotion Regulation: The Wave Skill— Mindfulness of Current Emotions

EXPERIENCE YOUR EMOTIONS

- When you have an emotion, observe it.
- Step back and just notice it.
- Get unstuck.
- Experience it as a WAVE, coming and going.
- Don't try to GET RID of it or PUSH it away.
- And don't try to HOLD ON to it.

PRACTICE MINDFULNESS OF EMOTIONAL BODY SENSATIONS

- Notice WHERE in your body you are feeling emotional sensations.
- Experience the SENSATIONS as fully as you can.

REMEMBER: YOU ARE NOT YOUR EMOTIONS

- You don't need to ACT on a feeling.
- Remember times when you have felt differently.

DON'T JUDGE YOUR EMOTIONS

- Radically accept an emotion as part of you.
- Invite it home for dinner; name the emotion.
- Practice *willingness* to experience the emotion.

Emotion Regulation: Review of Skills for Components of the Emotion Model

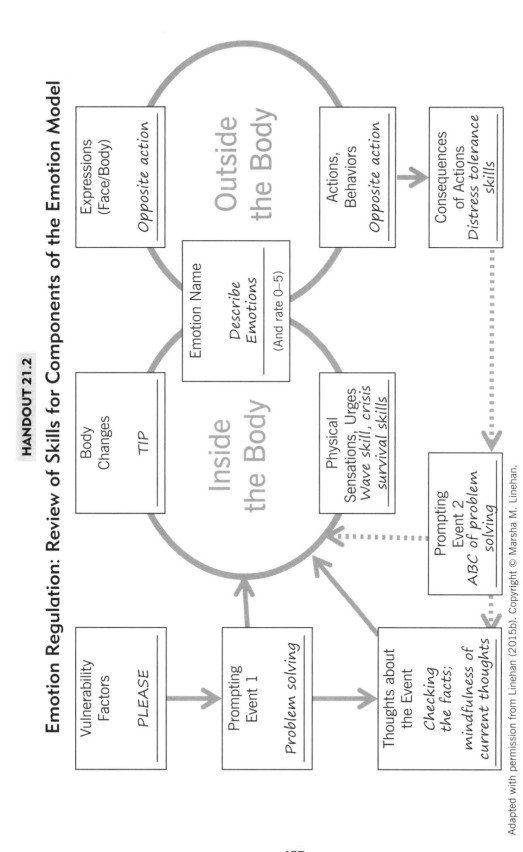

Emotion Regulation:
Practicing the Wave Skill

Name: _____

Due Date: _____

Emotion Name: _____ **Intensity (0–5) Before:** ____ **After:** ____

Describe a situation that prompts emotion. _____

_____

_____

_____

When emotional intensity is extreme, use your **crisis survival skills first**. With any emotion, high or low, practice radical acceptance with **MINDFULNESS OF CURRENT EMOTIONS.**

Check off any of the following that you did:

☐ Stepped back and observed the emotions.

☐ Experienced the emotions as WAVES, coming and going.

☐ Noticed where in my body I was feeling the emotional sensations.

☐ Paid attention to the physical sensations of the emotions as much as I could.

☐ Just noticed the urge to act that went with an emotion.

☐ Got myself to avoid acting on my emotion.

☐ Reminded myself of times when I have felt different.

☐ Let go of judgments about my emotion.

☐ Practiced radically accepting my emotion.

(continued)

☐ Tried to love my emotion by "naming it and inviting it home for dinner."

☐ Practiced willingness to have unwelcome emotions.

Other: _____

Comments and description of experiences: _____

_____

_____

_____

_____

_____

_____

_____

_____

_____

_____

_____

_____

_____

_____

_____

_____

_____

_____

_____

_____

_____

_____

_____

_____

_____

Mindfulness: Getting into Wise Mind

Name: _____

Due Date: _____

Emotion Mind

One example of emotion mind this week was (please describe your emotions, thoughts, behaviors): _____

_____

_____

Reasonable Mind

One example of reasonable mind this week was (please describe your emotions, thoughts, behaviors): _____

_____

_____

Wise Mind

One example of wise mind this week was (please describe your emotions, thoughts, behaviors): _____

_____

_____

Mindfulness: Observing, Describing, Participating Checklist

Name: _____

Due Date: _____

Check off three mindfulness skills that you use during the week. If you choose to practice more than three skills, you are certainly encouraged to do so.

Practice observing: Check off an exercise each time you do one.

_____ 1. Notice what you see: watch without following what you see; observe something you pick up.

_____ 2. Observe sounds: sounds around you, the pitch and sound of someone's voice, music.

_____ 3. Notice smells around you: aroma of food, soap, air.

_____ 4. Observe the taste of what you eat and the act of eating.

_____ 5. Observe your body sensations: the sensation of walking, your body touching something.

_____ 6. Notice thoughts coming in and out of your mind; imagine your mind as a conveyor belt.

_____ 7. Observe your breath: notice the movement of your stomach, sensations of air coming in and out of your nose.

Practice describing: Check off an exercise each time you do one.

_____ 8. Describe what you see outside your body.

_____ 9. Describe thoughts, feelings, and body sensations inside yourself.

_____ 10. Describe your breathing.

Practice participating: Check off an exercise each time you do one.

_____ 11. Dance to music.

_____ 12. Sing along with music you are listening to.

_____ 13. Sing in the shower.

_____ 14. Sing and dance while watching TV.

_____ 15. Jump out of bed and dance or sing before getting dressed.

_____ 16. Go to a church that sings and join in the singing.

_____ 17. Play karaoke with friends or at a karaoke club.

_____ 18. Go running, riding, skating, walking; focus only on your activity; become one with it.

_____ 19. Play a sport and throw yourself into playing.

Mindfulness: Nonjudgmentalness, One-Mindfulness, Effectiveness Checklist

Name: _____

Due Date: _____

Check off three mindfulness skills that you use during the week. If you choose to practice more than three skills, you are certainly encouraged to do so.

Practice nonjudgmentalness: Check off an exercise each time you do one.

_____ 1. Say in your mind, "A judgmental thought arose in my mind."

_____ 2. Count judgmental thoughts.

_____ 3. Stay very concrete and describe your day nonjudgmentally.

_____ 4. Change judgmental expressions, posture, or voice tone.

_____ 5. Imagine the person you are most angry with. Imagine understanding that person.

_____ 6. Write out a nonjudgmental description of an event that prompted an emotion.

Practice one-mindfulness: Check off an exercise each time you do one.

_____ 7. Be fully aware while cleaning the house.

_____ 8. Be fully aware while washing the dishes.

_____ 9. Be fully aware while taking a slow-motion bath.

_____ 10. Be fully aware while making tea or coffee.

Practice effectiveness: Check off an exercise each time you do one.

_____ 11. Give up being right.

_____ 12. Drop willfulness.

_____ 13. Do what works.

Adapted with permission from Linehan (2015b). Copyright © Marsha M. Linehan.

Interpersonal Effectiveness:
Overview of Building Interpersonal Effectiveness

Clarifying Priorities
How important is:

1. Getting what you want/obtaining your goal?

2. Keeping the relationship?

3. Maintaining your self-respect?

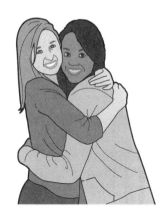

Objectives Effectiveness: DEAR MAN
When it is important to:

1. Be effective in asking clearly for what you want and saying no.

Relationship Effectiveness: GIVE
When it is important to:

1. Act in such a way that you maintain positive relationships, *and*

2. That others feel good about themselves and about you.

Self-Respect Effectiveness: FAST
When it is important to:

1. Act in such a way that you keep your self-respect.

Factors to Consider
When it is important to:

1. Decide how firm or intense you want to be in asking for something or saying no.

Adapted with permission from Linehan (2015b). Copyright © Marsha M. Linehan.

Interpersonal Effectiveness: What Is Your Goal?

Keeping and maintaining healthy relationships (GIVE skills)

Question: How do I want the other person to feel about me?

Example: If I care about the person or if the person has authority over me, act in a way that keeps the person respecting and liking me.

Getting somebody to do what you want (DEAR MAN skills)

Question: What do I want? What do I need? How do I get it? How do I effectively say no?

Example: How do I ask for something, resolve a problem, or have people listen to me? Act in a way that will increase the chances of getting what you want.

Keeping your self-respect (FAST skills)

Question: How do I want to feel about myself after the interaction?

Example: What are my values and personal beliefs? Act in a way that makes me feel positive about myself.

Practice Exercise:

Think about these as priorities to help you decide which skill(s) to use.

Describe an interaction (what I want to say, to whom, why, where): _____

_____

_____

_____

_____

Rank them in order of importance to you (1–3, with 1 being most important).

Keep relationship: _____

Get what you want: _____

Keep your self-respect: _____

Adapted with permission from Rathus and Miller (2015). Copyright © The Guilford Press.

Interpersonal Effectiveness:
What Stops You from Achieving Your Goals?

1. **Lack of skill**

   You actually **don't know** what to say or how to act.

2. **Worry thoughts**

   You have the skill, but your **worry thoughts** interfere with doing or saying what you want.

   - Worries about bad consequences:
     "They won't like me," "He will break up with me."

   - Worries about whether you deserve to get what you want:
     "I am such a bad person, I don't deserve this."

   - Worries about being ineffective and calling yourself names:
     "I won't do it right;" "I'm such a loser."

3. **Emotions**

   You have the skill, but your **emotions** (anger, frustration, fear, guilt, sadness) make you unable to do or say what you want. Emotions, instead of skill, control what you say and do.

4. **Not being able to decide**

   You have the skill, but you **can't decide** what you really want. Or you can't figure out how to balance your priorities:

   - Asking for too much versus not asking for anything.
   - Saying no to everything versus giving in to everything.

5. **Environment**

   You have the skill, but the **environment** gets in the way:

   - Other people are too powerful (sometimes despite your best efforts).
   - Other people may have some reason for not liking you if you get what you want.
   - Other people won't give you what you need unless you sacrifice your self-respect.

Interpersonal Effectiveness:
Clarifying Priorities in Interpersonal Situations

Name: _____

Due Date: _____

Use this sheet to figure out your goals and priorities in any situation that creates a problem for you, such as ones where:

1. Your rights or wishes are not being respected.
2. You want someone to do or change something or give you something.
3. You want or need to say no or resist pressure to do something.
4. You want to get your position or point of view taken seriously.
5. There is conflict with another person.
6. You want to improve your relationship with someone.

Observe and describe in writing, as close in time to the situation as possible. Write on the back of the page if you need more room.

Prompting event for my problem: Who did what to whom? What led up to what? Why is this a problem? Remember to *check the facts*!

My **wants and desires** in this situation:

Objectives: What **specific results** do I want?

What do I want this person to do, stop, or accept?

Relationship: How do I want the **other person** to feel and think about me **because of how I handle the interaction** (whether or not I get what I what from the other person)?

Self-Respect: How do I want to feel or think about **myself because of how I handle the interaction** (whether or not I get what I what from the other person)?

My **priorities** in this situation: Rate priorities 1 (most important), 2 (second most important), or 3 (least important).

_____ **Objectives**   _____ **Relationship**   _____ **Self-Respect**

Interpersonal Effectiveness:
Getting Someone to Do What You Want

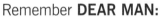

Remember **DEAR MAN:**

Describe	(be) **M**indful
Express	**A**ppear confident
Assert	**N**egotiate
Reinforce	

Describe: Describe the situation. Stick to the facts. For example, you might say, "My paper says I got a C– on the test."

Express: Express your feelings by using "I" statements ("I feel . . . ," "I would like . . . ," "I think . . ."). Do not assume that the other person knows how you feel. Stay away from "you should." For example, you might say, "I am frustrated because I studied for 4 days. I think some of my answers are correct."

Assert: Ask for what you want or say "no" clearly. Remember that the other person cannot read your mind. For example, you might ask, "Would you please go through the problems with me so I can understand why my answers were not correct?"

Reinforce: Reward (reinforce) the person ahead of time by explaining the positive effects of getting what you want. Also, reward him or her afterward. For example, you might say, "I would be better able to understand the material and be able to participate more in class."

(be) **M**indful: Keep your focus on what you want, avoiding distractions. Come back to your assertion over and over, like a "broken record." Ignore attacks; keep making your point. For example, you might say, "I have been working hard in your class, and this test score doesn't show my true abilities."

Appear confident: Make (and maintain) eye contact. Use a confident tone of voice—do not whisper, mumble, or give up and say "whatever."

Negotiate: Be willing to **give to get**. Ask for the other person's input. Offer alternative solutions to the problem. Know when to "agree to disagree" and walk away. For example, you might say, "I understand you are really busy, and I really need to go over my exam with you. What do you suggest we do so I can get some feedback on my exam?"

Adapted with permission from Rathus and Miller (2015). Copyright © The Guilford Press.

———————————

Practice Cards for Learning the DEAR MAN Skills

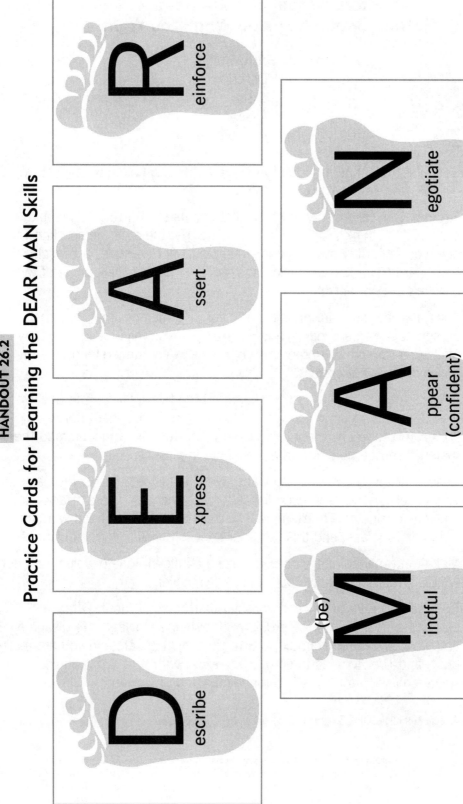

D escribe

E xpress

A ssert

R einforce

(be) M indful

A ppear (confident)

N egotiate

Interpersonal Effectiveness: Practicing DEAR MAN Skills

Name: _____

Due Date: _____

Choose one situation during the week in which you used your DEAR MAN skills, and describe below.

What happened? (Who did what? What led up to what? What was the problem?)

_____

_____

What did you want from the other person?

_____

_____

DEAR MAN skills used (write down **exactly** how you used each one):

Describe (the situation—just the facts): _____

_____

Express (feelings): _____

Assert: _____

Reward: _____

(be) **M**indful: _____

Appear confident: _____

Negotiate: _____

What was the result of using your DEAR MAN skills? _____

_____

_____

_____

_____

Interpersonal Effectiveness:
Building and Maintaining Positive Relationships

Remember **GIVE:**

(be) **G**entle
(act) **I**nterested
Validate
(use an) **E**asy manner

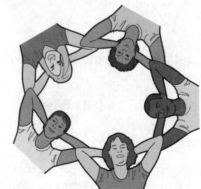

(be) **G**entle:	Be nice and respectful!
	Don't attack, use threats, or make judgments.
	Be aware of your tone of voice.
(act) **I**nterested:	Listen and act interested in what the other person is saying.
	Don't interrupt or talk over the other person.
	Don't make faces.
	Maintain good eye contact.
Validate:	Show that you understand the other person's feelings or opinions. Be nonjudgmental out loud.
	"I can understand how you feel, . . . and . . ."
	"I realize this is hard . . ."
	"I see you are busy, and . . ."
	"That must have felt . . ."
(use an) **E**asy manner:	Smile.
	Use humor.
	Use nonthreatening body language.
	Leave your attitude at the door.

Adapted with permission from Rathus and Miller (2015). Copyright © The Guilford Press.

Interpersonal Effectiveness: Practicing GIVE Skills

Name: _____

Due Date: _____

Choose two situations during the week in which you used your GIVE skills, and describe below.

Remember **GIVE:**

> (be) **G**entle
>
> (act) **I**nterested
>
> **V**alidate
>
> (use an) **E**asy manner

Situation 1:

With whom are you trying to keep a good relationship? _____

What was the situation in which you chose to use your GIVE skills? _____

_____

_____

What was the outcome? _____

_____

How did you feel after using your skills? _____

Situation 2:

With whom are you trying to keep a good relationship? _____

What was the situation in which you chose to use your GIVE skills? _____

_____

_____

What was the outcome? _____

_____

How did you feel after using your skills? _____

Interpersonal Effectiveness: Maintaining Your Self-Respect

Remember **FAST:**

    (be) **F**air

    (no) **A**pologies

        Stick to values

    (be) **T**ruthful

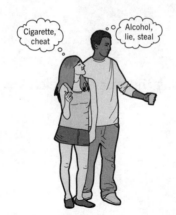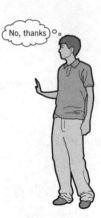

(be) Fair: Be fair to *yourself* and to the *other* person.

(no) Apologies: Don't *over*apologize for your behavior, for making a request, or for being you. (If you wronged someone, don't underapologize.)

Stick to values: Stick to your own values and opinions.

                    Don't sell out to get what you want, to fit in or to avoid saying no.

                    (Refer to the list of values and priorities in Handout 19.5 of the Emotion Regulation module.)

(be) Truthful: Don't lie.

                    Don't act helpless when you are not.

                    Don't make up excuses or exaggerate.

Interpersonal Effectiveness: Practicing FAST Skills

Name: _____

Due Date: _____

Choose two situations during the week in which you used your FAST skills, and describe below.

Remember **FAST**:

> (be) **F**air
> (no) **A**pologies
> **S**tick to values
> (be) **T**ruthful

Situation 1:

In what way are you trying to maintain your self-respect? _____

_____

_____

_____

What was the situation in which you chose to use your FAST skills, and how did you use them? _____

_____

_____

What was the outcome? _____

_____

_____

How did you feel after you used your skills? _____

_____

_____

(continued)

Situation 2:

In what way are you trying to maintain your self-respect? _____

_____

_____

_____

What was the situation in which you chose to use your FAST skills, and how did you use them? _____

_____

_____

What was the outcome? _____

_____

_____

How did you feel after you used your skills? _____

_____

_____

Interpersonal Effectiveness: Evaluating Your Options

Before asking for something or saying no to a request, you have to decide how intensely you want to hold your ground.

Options range from **very low** intensity (you are very flexible and accept the situation) to **very high** intensity (try every skill you know to change the situation and get what you want).

OPTIONS
Low intensity (let go, give in)

Asking	Intensity Level	Saying no
Don't ask; don't hint.	1	Do what the other person wants without being asked.
Hint indirectly; take no.	2	Don't complain; do it cheerfully.
Hint openly; take no.	3	Do it even if you're not cheerful about it.
Ask tentatively; take no.	4	Do it, but show that you'd rather not.
Ask gracefully, but take no.	5	Say you'd rather not, but do it gracefully.
Ask confidently; take no.	6	Say no confidently, but reconsider.
Ask confidently; resist no.	7	Say no confidently; resist saying yes.
Ask firmly; resist no.	8	Say no firmly; resist saying yes.
Ask firmly; insist; negotiate; keep trying.	9	Say no firmly; resist; negotiate; keep trying.
Ask and don't take no for an answer.	10	Don't do it.

High intensity (stay firm)

Adapted with permission from Linehan (2015b). Copyright © Marsha M. Linehan.

Interpersonal Effectivenes: Factors to Consider

When deciding how firm or intense you want to be in asking or saying no, think about:

1. The other person's or your own **capability.**
2. Your **priorities**.
3. The effect of your actions on your **self-respect.**
4. Your or the other person's moral and legal **rights** in the situation.
5. Your **authority** over the person (or the person's over you).
6. The type of **relationship** you have with the person.
7. The effect of your action on **long- vs. short-term goals.**
8. The degree of **give and take** in your relationship.
9. Whether you have done your **homework** to prepare.
10. The **timing** of your request or refusal.

1. Capability:
- Is the person able to give me what I want? If YES, raise the intensity of ASKING.
- Do I have what the person wants? If NO, raise the intensity of NO.

2. Priorities:
- Are your GOALS very important? Increase intensity.
- Is your RELATIONSHIP shaky? Consider reducing intensity.
- Is your SELF-RESPECT on the line? Intensity should fit your values.

3. Self-respect:
- Do I usually do things for myself? Am I careful to avoid acting helpless when I am not? If YES, raise the intensity of ASKING.
- Will saying no make me feel bad about myself, even when I am thinking about it wisely? If NO, raise the intensity of NO.

4. Rights:
- Is the person required by law or moral code to give me what I want? If YES, raise the intensity of ASKING.
- Am I required to give the person what he or she is asking for? Would saying no violate the other person's rights? If NO, raise the intensity of NO.

(continued)

From *DBT Skills in Schools: Skills Training for Emotional Problem Solving for Adolescents (DBT STEPS-A)* by James J. Mazza, Elizabeth T. Dexter-Mazza, Alec L. Miller, Jill H. Rathus, and Heather E. Murphy. Copyright © 2016 The Guilford Press. Permission to photocopy this material is granted to purchasers of this book for personal use or use with individual students (see copyright page for details). Purchasers can download additional copies of this material (see the box at the end of the table of contents).

5. Authority:
- Am I responsible for directing the person or telling the person what to do? If YES, raise the intensity of ASKING.
- Does the person have authority over me (e.g., my boss, my teacher, my parent)? And is what the person is asking within his or her authority? If NO, raise the intensity of NO.

6. Relationship:
- Is what I want appropriate to the current relationship? If YES, raise the intensity of ASKING.
- Is what the person is asking for appropriate to our current relationship? If NO, raise the intensity of NO.

7. Long-term vs. short-term goals:
- Will not asking for what I want keep the peace now but create problems in the long run? If YES, raise the intensity of ASKING.
- Is giving in to keep the peace right now more important than the long-term welfare of the relationship? Will I eventually regret or resent saying no? If NO, raise the intensity of NO.

8. Give and take:
- What have I done for the person? Am I giving at least as much as I ask for? Am I willing to give if the person says yes? If YES, raise the intensity of ASKING.
- Do I owe person a favor? Does he or she do a lot for me? If NO, raise the intensity of NO.

9. Homework:
- Have I done my homework? Do I know all the facts I need to know to support my request? Am I clear about what I want? If YES, raise the intensity of ASKING.
- Is the other person's request clear? Do I know what I am agreeing to? If NO, raise the intensity of NO.

10. Timing:
- Is this a good time to ask? Is the person "in the mood" for listening and paying attention to me? Am I catching the person when he or she is likely to say yes to my request? If YES, raise the intensity of ASKING.
- Is this a bad time to say no? Should I hold off answering for a while? If NO, raise the intensity of NO.

Other factors: _____

_____

_____

_____

Interpersonal Effectiveness: Figuring Out How Strongly to Ask or Say No

To figure out how strongly to ask for something or how strongly to say no, read the instructions below. Circle the dimes you put in the bank, and then add them up. Then go back over the list and see if some items are much more important than others. Check wise mind before acting if some items are much more important than others.

Decide how strongly to ask for something Put a dime in the bank for each of the questions that get a yes answer. The more money you have, the stronger you ask. If you have a dollar, then ask very strongly. If you don't have any money in the bank, then don't ask; don't even hint.		**Decide how strongly to say no.** Put a dime in the bank for each of the questions that get a no answer. The more money you have, the stronger you say no. If you have a dollar, then say no very strongly. If you don't have any money in the bank, then do it without even being asked.	
10¢	Is this person able to give or do what I want?	**Capability**	Can I give the person what is wanted?	10¢
10¢	Is getting my objective more important than my relationship with this person?	**Priorities**	Is my relationship more important than saying no?	10¢
10¢	Will asking help me feel competent and self-respecting?	**Self-respect**	Will saying no make me feel bad about myself?	10¢
10¢	Is the person required by law or moral code to do or give me what I want?	**Rights**	Am I required (for example, by law) to give or do what is wanted, or does saying no violate this person's rights?	10¢
10¢	Am I responsible for telling the person what to do?	**Authority**	Is the other person responsible for telling me what to do?	10¢
10¢	Is what I want appropriate for this relationship? (Is it right to ask for what I want?)	**Relationship**	Is what the person is requesting of me appropriate to my relationship with this person?	10¢
10¢	Is asking important to a long-term goal?	**Goals**	In the long term, will I regret saying no?	10¢

(continued)

Adapted with permission from Rathus and Miller (2015). Copyright © The Guilford Press.

Interpersonal Effectiveness: Figuring Out How Strongly to Ask or Say No *(page 2 of 2)*

		Asking		Saying no	
10¢	Give and take	Do I give as much as I get with this person?	Do I owe this person a favor? (Does the person do a lot for me?)		10¢
10¢	Homework	Do I know what I want and have the facts I need to support my request?	Do I know what I am saying no to? (Is the other person clear about what is being asked for?)		10¢
10¢	Timing	Is this a good time to ask? (Is the person in the right mood?)	Should I wait a while before saying no?		10¢
$		**Total value of asking** (Adjusted ± ____ for wise mind)	**Total value of saying no** (Adjusted ± ____ for wise mind)		$

Asking	Total value	Saying no
Don't ask; don't hint.	10¢	Do it without being asked.
Hint indirectly; take no.	20¢	Don't complain; do it cheerfully.
Hint openly; take no.	30¢	Do it, even if you're not cheerful about it.
Ask tentatively; take no.	40¢	Do it, but show that you'd rather not.
Ask gracefully, but take no.	50¢	Say you'd rather not, but do it gracefully.
Ask confidently; take no.	60¢	Say no firmly, but reconsider.
Ask confidently; resist no.	70¢	Say no confidently; resist saying yes.
Ask firmly; resist no.	80¢	Say no firmly; resist saying yes.
Ask firmly; insist; negotiate; keep trying.	90¢	Say no firmly; resist; negotiate; keep trying.
Ask and don't take no for an answer.	$1.00	Don't do it.

Interpersonal Effectiveness:
Using Interpersonal Effectiveness Skills at the Same Time

Name: _____

Due Date: _____

Choose a situation during the week that required more than one interpersonal effectiveness skill.

Describe the situation: _____

_____

_____

What were my priorities? (Check all that apply)

____ Build/maintain relationship.

____ Get what I want, say no, or be taken seriously.

____ Build/maintain self-respect.

What I said or did: (check and describe)

____ (be) **G**entle	____ **D**escribe	____ (be) **F**air
____ (act) **I**nterested	____ **E**xpress	____ (no) **A**pologies
____ **V**alidate	____ **A**ssert	____ **S**tick to values
____ (use an) **E**asy manner	____ **R**einforce	____ (be) **T**ruthful
	____ (be) **M**indful	
	____ **A**ppear confident	
	____ **N**egotiate	

_____

_____

_____

_____

_____

Adapted with permission from Rathus and Miller (2015). Copyright © The Guilford Press.

_____

References

American Psychiatric Association. (2013). *Diagnostic and statistical manual of mental disorders* (5th ed.). Arlington, VA: Author.

Atienza, F. L., Balaguer, I., & Garcia-Merita, M. L. (1998). Video modeling and imagining training on performance of tennis services of 9- to 12-year-old children. *Perceptual and Motor Skills, 87,* 519–529.

Burns, B. J., Costello, E. J., Angold, A., Tweed, D., Stangl, D., Farmer, E. M. Z., et al. (1995). Children's mental health service use across service sectors. *Health Affairs, 14,* 147–159.

Catron, T., & Weiss, B. (1994). The Vanderbilt school-based counseling program: An interagency, primary-care model of mental health services. *Journal of Emotional Behavioral Disorders, 2,* 247–253.

Collaborative for Academic, Social, and Emotional Learning (CASEL). (2013). *2013 CASEL guide: Effective social and emotional learning programs—Preschool and elementary school edition.* Chicago: Author. Retrieved from *www.casel.org/guide/preschool-and-elementary-edition-casel-guide.*

Collaborative for Academic, Social, and Emotional Learning (CASEL). (2015). *2015 CASEL guide: Effective, social and emotional learning programs—Middle and high school edition.* Chicago: Author. Retrieved from *www.casel.org/guide/middle-and-high-school-edition-casel-guide.*

Cook, C. R. (2015, Spring). *Universal screening and selective mental health services within a multi-tiered system of support: Building capacity to implement the first two tiers.* Paper presented as part of the Washington State Association of School Psychologists Lecture Series.

Cook, C. R., Burns, M., Browning-Wright, D., & Gresham, F. M. (2010). *Transforming school psychology in the RTI era: A guide for administrators and school psychologists.* Palm Beach Gardens, FL: LRP.

Cook, C. R., Frye, M., Slemrod, T., Lyon, A. R., Renshaw, T. L., & Zhang, Y. (2015). An integrated approach to universal prevention: Independent and combined effects of PBIS and SEL on youths' mental health. *School Psychology Quarterly, 30,* 166–183.

Cook, C. R., Gresham, F. M., Kern, L., Barreras, R. B., & Crews, S. D. (2008). Social skills training for secondary EBD students: A review and analysis of the meta-analytic literature. *Journal of Emotional and Behavioral Disorders, 16,* 131–144.

Dimeff, L. A., & Koerner, K. (Eds.). (2007). *Dialectical behavior therapy in clinical practice: Applications across disorders and settings.* New York: Guilford Press.

Dimeff, L. A., Woodcock, E. A., Harned, M. S., & Beadnell, B. (2011). Can dialectical behavior therapy be learned in highly structured learning environment?: Results from a randomized controlled dissemination trial. *Behavior Therapy, 42,* 263–275.

Durlak, J. A., Weissberg, R. P., Dymnicki, A. B., Taylor, R. D., & Schellinger, K. B. (2011). The impact of enhancing students' social and emotional learning: A meta-analysis of school-based universal interventions. *Child Development, 82,* 405–432.

Gould, M. S., Greenberg, T., Velting, D. M., & Schaffer, D. (2003). Youth suicide risk and preventive interventions: A review of the past 10 years. *Journal of the American Academy of Child and Adolescent Psychiatry, 42,* 386–405.

Gould, M. S., Marrocco, F. A., Kleinman, M., Thomas, J. G., Mostkoff, K., Cote, J., et al. (2005). Evaluating iatrogenic risk of youth suicide screening programs: A randomized controlled trial. *Journal of the American Medical Association, 293,* 1635–1643.

Harned, M. S., Rizvi, S. L., & Linehan, M. M. (2010). Impact of co-occurring posttraumatic-stress disorder on suicidal women with borderline personality disorder. *American Journal of Psychiatry, 167,* 1210–1217.

Hashim, R., Vadnais, M., & Miller, A. L. (2013). Improving adherence in adolescent chronic kidney disease: A DBT feasibility trial. *Clinical Practice in Pediatric Psychology, 1,* 369–379.

Haskell, I., Daly, B. P., Hildenbrand, A., Nicholls, E., Mazza, J. J., & Dexter-Mazza, E. T. (2014, September). *Skills training for emotional problem solving for adolescents (STEPS-A): Implementation and program evaluation.* Paper presented at the annual conference on Advancing Mental Health, Pittsburgh, PA.

Hoagwood, K., & Erwin, H. (1997). Effectiveness of school-based mental health services for children: A 10-year research review. *Journal of Child and Family Studies, 6,* 435–451.

Jeannerod, M., & Frak, V. (1999). Mental imaging of motor activity in humans. *Current Opinion in Neurobiology, 9,* 735–739.

Johnston, L. D., O'Malley, P. M., Bachman, J. G., & Schulenberg, J. E. (2007). *Monitoring the Future: National results on adolescent drug use. Overview of key findings, 2006.* Bethesda, MD: National Institute on Drug Abuse.

Kabat-Zinn, J. (1994). *Wherever you go, there you are: Mindfulness meditation in everyday living.* New York: Hyperion.

Kabat-Zinn, J., Massion, A. O., Kristeller, J., Peterson, L. G., Fletcher, K. E., Pbert, L., et al. (1992). Effectiveness of a meditation based stress reduction program in the treatment of anxiety disorders. *American Journal of Psychiatry, 149,* 936–943.

Kataoka, S. H., Zhang, L., & Wells, K. B. (2002). Unmet need for mental health care among U.S. children: Variation by ethnicity and insurance status. *American Journal of Psychiatry, 159,* 1548–1555.

Kaviani, H. J., Javaheri, F., & Hatami, N. (2011). Mindfulness-based cognitive therapy (MBCT) reduces depression and anxiety induced by real stressful setting in non-clinical population. *International Journal of Psychology and Psychological Therapy, 11,* 285–296.

Kazdin, A. E., & Mascitelli, S. (1982). Covert and overt rehearsal and homework practice in developing assertiveness. *Journal of Consulting and Clinical Psychology, 50,* 250–258.

Kilgus, S. P., Reinke, W. R., & Jimerson, S. R. (2015). Understanding mental health intervention and assessment within a multi-tiered framework: Contemporary science, practice and policy. *School Psychology Quarterly, 30,* 159–165.

Linehan, M. M. (1993). *Skills training manual for treating borderline personality disorder.* New York: Guilford Press.

Linehan, M. M. (2015a). *DBT skills training manual* (2nd ed.). New York: Guilford Press.

Linehan, M. M. (2015b). *DBT skills training handouts and worksheets* (2nd ed.). New York: Guilford Press.

Mazza, J. J., & Hanson, J. B. (2014a, February). *Dialectical behavior therapy (DBT) in public schools.* Paper presented at the annual conference of the National Association of School Psychologists, Washington, DC.

Mazza, J. J., & Hanson, J. B. (2014b, October). *Multi-tiered approach to dialectical behavior therapy (DBT) in schools.* Paper presented at the annual conference of the Washington State Association of School Psychologists, Skamina, WA.

Mazza, J. J., & Reynolds, W. M. (2008). School-wide approaches to intervention with depression and suicide. In B. Doll, & J. A. Cummings (Eds.) *Transforming school mental health services: Population-based approaches to promoting the competency and wellness of children* (pp. 213–241). Bethesda, MD: National Association of School Psychologists (co-published with Corwin Press).

McMain, S. (2013, November). *The effectiveness of brief dialectical behavior therapy skills training for suicidal behavior in borderline personality disorder: Findings from a randomized control trial.* Paper presented at the annual conference of the International Society for the Improvement and Teaching of Dialectical Behavior Therapy, Nashville, TN.

Mehlum, L., Tormoen, A. J., Ramberg, M., Haga, E., diep, L. M., Laberg, S., et al. (2014). Dialectical behavior therapy for adolescents with repeated suicidal and self-harming behavior: A randomized trial. *Journal of the American Academy of Child and Adolescent Psychiatry, 53,* 1082–1091.

Miller, A. L., Mazza, J. J., Dexter-Mazza, E. T., Steinberg, S., & Courtney-Seidler, E. (2014, November). *DBT in schools: The do's and don'ts.* Paper presented at the annual conference of the International Society for the Improvement and Teaching of Dialectical Behavior Therapy, Philadelphia.

Miller, A. L., Rathus, J. H., Leigh, E., Landsman, M., & Linehan, M. M. (1997). Dialectical behavior therapy adapted for suicidal adolescents. *Journal of Practicing Psychiatry and Behavioral Health, 3,* 78–86.

Miller, A. L., Rathus, J. H., & Linehan, M. M. (2007). *Dialectical behavior therapy with suicidal adolescents.* New York: Guilford Press.

Miller, D. N. (2011). *Child and adolescent suicidal behavior: School-based prevention, assessment, and intervention.* New York: Guilford Press.

Monahan, K. C., VanDerhei, S., Bechtold, J., & Cauffman, E. (2014). From the school yard to the squad car: School discipline, truancy, and arrest. *Journal of Youth and Adolescence, 43,* 1110–1122.

Moreland, R. L., Levine, J. M., & Wingert, M. L. (1996). Creating the ideal group: Composition effects at work. *Understanding Group Behavior, 2,* 11–35.

Neacsiu, A. D., Rizvi, S. L., Vitaliano, P. P., Lynch, T. R., & Linehan, M. M. (2010). The Dialectical Behavior Therapy Ways of Coping Checklist: Development and psychometric properties. *Journal of Clinical Psychology, 66,* 1–20.

Rathus, J. H., & Miller, A. L. (2002). Dialectical behavior therapy adapted for suicidal adolescents. *Suicide and Life-Threatening Behavior, 32,* 146–157.

Rathus, J. H., & Miller, A. L. (2015). *DBT skills manual for adolescents.* New York: Guilford Press.

Rubinstein, R. S., Meyer, D. E., & Evans, J. E. (2001). Executive control of cognitive processes in task switching. *Journal of Experimental Psychology: Human Perception and Performance, 27,* 763–797.

Sayrs, J. H. R., & Linehan, M. M. (in press). *Developing therapeutic treatment teams: The DBT model.* New York: Guilford Press.

Vøllestad, J. N., Nielsen, M. B., & Høstmark, G. (2012). Mindfulness- and acceptance-based interventions for anxiety disorders: A systematic review and meta-analysis. *British Journal of Clinical Psychology, 51,* 239–260.

Wagner, B. M. (1997). Family risk factors for child and adolescent suicidal behavior. *Psychological Bulletin, 121,* 246–298.

Wegner, D. (1989). *White bears and other unwanted thoughts: Suppression, obsession, and the psychology of mental control.* New York: Viking.

Weissberg, R. P., & Cascarino, J. (2013). Academic learning + social-emotional learning = national priority. *Phi Delta Kappan, 95,* 8–13.

Index

Note: *f or t* following a page number indicates a figure or a table; handouts and homework forms are in italics.